T0073617

ADDITIONAL PRAISE FOR
FIGHTING FOR RECOVERY

"The subtitle condenses the promise of this book: a bracing account by both committed activist and seasoned social historian, *Fighting for Recovery* is a textual double for the story it tells. Underscore *struggle*: messy, divisive, unresolved, leaving wreckage in its wake. The roster includes players of various stripes (clinicians, families, bureaucrats, service users/refusers, researchers, even venture capitalists), pitting power politics against street theatre, professional defensiveness against first-person testimony, and even (on rare occasion) discussing relevant research. You may have wondered why 'psychiatry has been slow to adopt recovery programs.' That verdict (coming after more than three hundred pages of painstakingly documented history) will be less mysterious—but not one iota less sad—to any reader of what came before it. The epilogue, a brave coda in its own right, brings the story up to date with shout-outs to promising changes in policing and prisons . . . and a weary, final call for action."

—KIM J. HOPPER,
author of *Reckoning with Homelessness*

"I am in awe of this generation-spanning, much-needed history about efforts to improve our tragically inadequate mental health system. Born out of love for a brother, executed with storytelling flair, and featuring a parade of impassioned individuals, *Fighting for Recovery* introduced me to waves of brilliant reforms—and reminded me of the villains who thwarted them. But part of what makes Phyllis Vine's book such a find is the effect it had on my morale. While at times it made me cry out in frustration, by the end I took away an empowering message: You are not alone. You are in fellowship with many who envisioned something better—and many who still do. Armed with that sense of solidarity and this illuminating history, I feel newly resolved to keep fighting."

—RACHEL SIMON,
author of *Riding the Bus with My Sister*

"Hardly ever does a single text so capably conjoin the personal with both policy and practice in mental health care. Through the lens of her own family's experience with mental illness, Phyllis Vine illuminates key problems and achievements in mental health care over the past half century, while simultaneously giving the reader a detailed view of the development and evolution of the consumer movement and peer support. The results of her efforts are must-reading for anyone who wants to understand how the mental health field has developed and where it must go in the future."

—RON MANDERSCHEID,
former president/CEO, National Association of
County Behavioral Health and Developmental Disability
Directors and the National Association for Rural Mental Health

"*Fighting for Recovery* is a groundbreaking history of the mental health recovery movement in America. It covers both the family advocacy movement and, more importantly, the consumer/ex-patient/survivor movement, from its beginnings with the Mental Patients Liberation advocacy work of the early 1970s through today's peer-support and advocacy organizations, which now provide services in most of the country. I highly recommended it to anyone interested in the mental health recovery movement in America."

—MIKE FINKLE,
founder and former executive director,
On Our Own of Maryland

FIGHTING
FOR
RECOVERY

FIGHTING

FOR

RECOVERY

An ACTIVISTS' HISTORY *of*
MENTAL HEALTH REFORM

Phyllis Vine

BEACON PRESS, BOSTON

BEACON PRESS
Boston, Massachusetts
www.beacon.org

Beacon Press books
are published under the auspices of
the Unitarian Universalist Association of Congregations.

25 24 23 22   8 7 6 5 4 3 2 1

This book is printed on acid-free paper that meets the uncoated paper
ANSI/NISO specifications for permanence as revised in 1992.

Text design and composition by Kim Arney

Library of Congress Control Number: 2022013002
Hardcover ISBN: 978-08070-7961-4
Ebook ISBN: 978-08070-7974-4

For
Matthew

CONTENTS

DRAMATIS PERSONAE

Priscilla Allen, a former patient from California who served on the President's Commission of Mental Health.

Bill Anthony (1944–2020), a psychologist who founded Boston University's Center for Psychiatric Rehabilitation, and a pioneering leader on behalf of rehabilitation and recovery.

Bernard "Bernie" Arons, served administrative positions at St. Elizabeths Hospital and was director of the Center for Mental Health Services in the Clinton administration.

John Beard, executive director of Fountain House, New York City, the flagship of the clubhouse model providing affiliation for patients discharged from Rockland State Hospital in the 1950s.

Arthur "Art" Bolton, a California social worker leading reform of court commitments, ending in Lanterman-Petris-Short (LPS), and head of the lieutenant governor's campaign for an integrated service system.

Bertram "Bert" Brown (1931–2020), a psychiatrist and a protégé of Robert Felix who cowrote the federal regulations for JFK's Community Mental Health Act. He directed the National Institute of Mental Health from 1970 to 1977 and emphasized the social context of health environments.

Neal Brown, an NIMH administrator who continued support for consumers and peer initiatives when he assumed leadership of the Community Support Program in 1980s.

Su Budd, a Kansas-based ex-patient.

William "Will" Carpenter, a research psychiatrist starting at NIMH before moving to the University of Maryland, who worked on the John Hinckley Jr. defense team and later became editor of the *Schizophrenia Bulletin*.

Bernard "Barney" Carroll (1940–2018), an Australia-born psychiatrist who chaired the FDA's evaluation committee hearing about clozapine. He was credited with a laboratory test for a hormone associated with melancholia, a type of depression. From 1983 to 1991 he chaired the psychiatry department at Duke University.

Judi Chamberlin (1944–2010), a first-generation activist, leader, speaker, organizer, and author of *On Our Own*, who is credited with the rally cry "Nothing About Us Without Us."

Paolo del Vecchio, a Philadelphia-based activist who became the first consumer working at the Center for Mental Health Services and rose to become director at Substance Abuse and Mental Health Services.

Anne (McCuan) Drissel, the lead author organizing Towards a National Plan, explaining the component parts of the Mental Health Systems Act.

Robert Felix (1904–1990), author of the National Mental Health Act in 1946, director of the National Institute of Mental Health (NIMH), and the architect of President John F. Kennedy's community mental health centers.

David Ferleger, a Pennsylvania lawyer representing the rights of institutionalized people with disabilities.

Laurie Flynn, the executive director of the National Alliance on Mental Illness from 1984 to 2000.

Larry Fricks, a Georgia-based activist who networked with peers and developed a peer service model receiving Medicaid reimbursement.

Howie the Harp (1953–1995), the founder of the Mental Patients' Liberation Front, an advocate for self-help and peer services, and promoter of social justice.

Howard Goldman, a research psychiatrist, editor of *Psychiatric Services,* and a consultant on state and federal matters.

Frederick Goodwin (1936–2020), a research psychiatrist with a specialty in mood disorders who rose quickly through the ranks at the NIMH but ended his tenure in controversy.

Courtenay Harding, a psychologist whose study of a cohort of patients who were discharged from a Vermont state hospital laid the groundwork for recognizing recovery for people with a diagnosis of schizophrenia.

Agnes Hatfield, a family organizer in Maryland and NAMI leader.

Tony Hoffman (1923–2000), a parent who organized other parents in San Mateo, California, in the 1970s, and eventually led a delegation to the first meeting of NAMI in 1979.

Sam Keith, a psychiatrist who came to the NIMH as a Yellow Beret, and remained for two decades becoming head of the Center for Schizophrenia Research and editor of *Schizophrenia Bulletin*.

Frank Lanterman (1901–1981), a powerful California assemblyman from Orange County with a lifelong commitment to serving people with a mental illness and those with disabilities. He worked to limit court-appointed commitments in the 1960s, and was the "L" in LPS.

Jay Mahler (1947–2021), a first-generation California activist and member of the team working for California's law AB3777 authorizing integrated services.

Ron Manderscheid, a research sociologist in public service at the NIMH, later SAMHSA.

Lucy Ozarin (1914–2017), coauthor of the regulations for JFK's Community Mental Health Act, and assistant director for mental health services at NIMH initiating the Community Support Program.

Herbert Pardes, an academic psychiatrist who continued his leadership after stepping down from NIMH, where he was director from 1978 to 1984.

Darby Penney (1952–2021), a first-generation activist in New York who became the Department of Mental Health's first director of recipient affairs, and a national leader working for social justice and human rights.

Joseph Rogers, a Philadelphia activist who headed the National Mental Health Consumers' Self-Help Clearinghouse and was employed by the Mental Health Association of Southeastern Pennsylvania.

Harvey Rosenthal, consumer activist and executive director of the New York Association of Psychiatric Services.

Max Schneier (1917–2002), a founding member of NAMI, an activist exposing abuses in New York's Willowbrook State School for the Mentally Retarded, and a housing pioneer for independent living called "halfway" houses.

John Strauss, a research psychiatrist at NIMH early in his career, later at Yale University working with Courtenay Harding, and an early proponent of recovery.

John Talbott, a leader of psychiatry who worked to ameliorate the catastrophic effects of deinstitutionalization as editor of the journal *Hospital and Community* (later *Psychiatric Services*) and became president of the American Psychiatric Association.

Mary Ann Test, a research psychologist at Mendota State Hospital in Madison, Wisconsin, and coauthor and proponent of assertive community treatment (ACT).

Boswell "Bos" Todd spearheaded a housing program in Lexington, Kentucky, and was a founder of the National Association for Research on Schizophrenia and Depression (NARSAD).

E. Fuller Torrey, a psychiatrist who worked at NIMH, with NAMI, and founded the Treatment Advocacy Center (TAC) promulgating controversial opinions about outpatient commitment to prevent violence in untreated people.

Judith Turner (Crowson) was brought into the NIMH to head the Community Support Program and helped community groups, former patients, and families develop services.

Laura Van Tosh, a West Coast activist and an independent consultant for state and federal policy initiatives.

Dan Weisburd (1933–2019), a California parent activist who campaigned for integrated services, which led to the creation of the Village in Long Beach.

Sally Zinman, a leader of the ex-patient movement who organized the California Network of Mental Health Clients.

ACRONYMS
AND ABBREVIATIONS

ACT	assertive community treatment
ADAMHA	Alcohol, Drug Abuse, and Mental Health Administration
APA	American Psychiatric Association
ARP	American Rescue Plan
CAMI	California Alliance on Mental Illness
CMHC	community mental health center
CMHS	Center for Mental Health Services
CSP	Community Support Program
DOJ	Department of Justice
ECT	electroconvulsive therapy
GAO	Government Accountability Office
GMHCN	Georgia Mental Health Consumer Network
LPS	Lanterman-Petris-Short
MHA	Mental Health Association
MPLP	Mental Patients' Liberation Party
NAMHC	National Advisory Mental Health Council
NAMI	National Alliance on Mental Illness (originally National Alliance for the Mentally Ill)
NAMP	National Alliance of Mental Patients
NARPA	National Association for Rights Protection and Advocacy
NARSAD	National Association for Research on Schizophrenia and Depression
NASMHPD	National Association of State Mental Health Program Directors
NIH	National Institutes of Health

NIMH	National Institute of Mental Health
PAIMI	Protection and Advocacy for Individuals with Mental Illness
PCMH	President's Commission on Mental Health (during the administration of President Jimmy Carter)
SAMHSA	Substance Abuse and Mental Health Services Administration
SMRI	Stanley Medical Research Institute
SSDI	Social Security Disability Insurance
TAC	Treatment Advocacy Center
TD	tardive dyskinesia
VA	Veterans Administration
WRAP	Wellness Recovery Action Plan

A NOTE ON LANGUAGE

M ANY OF THE TERMS used by contemporaries changed over the course of this story. Some have fallen out of use because they are inaccurate or misleading, or they have been redefined due to scientific discovery and are no longer used today. I have used the language that was current at the time of any given chapter, even if today it offends, as examples of how words, ideas, and understandings change over time.

BJ'S STORY

O N A MARCH EVENING IN 1977, I walked my younger brother BJ into the emergency room of St. Luke's Hospital on Manhattan's Upper West Side. Snow was falling and people were brushing white powder from their coats as they barged through the fogged-up double doors of the glass vestibule. Like us, they gave their names to a nurse sitting behind a Plexiglas barrier.

The nurse glanced quickly at BJ. "Another one," she shouted, looking behind her to nobody in particular. BJ was shifting his weight from one foot to the other, with a frothy half smile and vacant eyes, and reaching his hands deep into the pockets of greasy pants that had once belonged to a much larger person. BJ was in his late twenties and resembled people I had seen sitting under awnings holding cardboard signs scribbled with the word *HOMELESS*.

The nurse motioned for us to take seats on the orange plastic chairs under flickering fluorescent lights. Condensation trickled down the windows, and the overheated emergency room was thick with the smell of damp woolen scarves and mittens. I masqueraded calm, pretending not to be startled each time my brother jerked wild glances at someone coming in the door. I didn't respond, but I couldn't ignore the guttural sounds, or the occasional *No* as if he were ejecting a foreign object that was only sound. Pushing panic away, I stared at the linoleum floor watching snow puddle beneath our feet. Fortunately, we didn't wait long.

Until the day before, I had thought BJ was in Los Angeles, where we'd grown up. Somehow he'd managed to get to New York City, clearly unwell. The doctors called his delusions, paranoia, and hallucinations "textbook." That's when I first heard the word "schizophrenia." They said it was a "wastebasket" diagnosis before they loaded him up with drugs that made him sleep. Turning to me, they explained that our mother had caused this. "Of course," they said. They even had a term for her: schizophrenogenic. It didn't seem "of course" to me, but what did I know? I had grown up thinking doctors were semi-gods, so I answered their questions about her as best I could. She'd had lupus and had died a couple of years before.

"Father?"

"Bad heart." He'd died ten years earlier.

"Could it have been their early deaths?" I asked. "Or did this have something to do with our mother's chronic illness?"

They had no idea. Probably not, they said.

"What will help him get better?" I asked.

"Nothing." They were emphatic. He'll be this way for the rest of his life.

"For the rest of his life?"

"Look around at the people you see on the streets," the young doctor said matter-of-factly.

It might have been routine to them, but to me it felt like shrapnel. Naive, or perhaps still a novice, I had faith in medicine and expected BJ to get better. But before that could happen, he made a quick getaway. Staying two days, no more, he left against medical advice. Damn, I thought, hearing this as I stepped off an elevator carrying magazines and snacks. Now what?

Thus began the future—his, mine, ours.

I took BJ to the hospital with an innocence time would cure. I had no idea that psychiatry was ill equipped to treat him, that its scientific tools were few, or that his prognosis was based on a vague understanding. Schizophrenia was defined as "disturbances of thinking, mood and behavior" that led to a "misinterpretation of reality and sometimes to delusions and hallucinations, which frequently appear psychologically self-protective."[1] That description of schizophrenia came from the American Psychiatric Association's second edition of the *Diagnostic and Statistical Manual*

(*DSM-II*), which was published in 1968. When I later read this, I thought it very unhelpful.

There would be four revisions of the diagnostic manual in BJ's lifetime. The first revision, the *DSM-III*, became a turning point for modern psychiatry. It aimed to move the field away from its reliance on Freudian theories and adopt terms more resonant of a medical specialty. After 1980, the *DSM-III* would frame symptoms as a "manifestation of a pathological condition," not developmental conflict or neurosis. Groups of symptoms, called "syndromes," were something less than a disease such as leukemia or polio. Those had known causes. But no pathogens were associated with the mental illnesses. Offering diagnostic guidance, the *DSM-III* carried the patina of science but lacked clues from biology. There were no laboratory analyses of fluids such as blood or urine, no imaging tools such as X-rays. There was no microscope to detect bacteria. Diagnosis would henceforth derive from an agreement about observable behaviors and the statistical reliability of people rating symptoms. This is how they would reorganize psychiatry.

When BJ received his diagnosis, I had no idea that the theoretical framework informing his doctors dated from the nineteenth century. Working in psychiatric hospitals in Germany, a psychiatrist named Emil Kraepelin studied hospitalized patients with active delusions, paranoia, and hallucinations. He named the disorder *dementia praecox*, Latin for premature dementia. This condition was apparent in younger people, and because the patients he studied were hospitalized, it led to a tautology: people diagnosed with *dementia praecox* must end up in the hospital, perhaps for a lifetime. In his schema, recovery was not possible. Long after Swiss psychiatrist Eugen Bleuler renamed *dementia praecox* "schizophrenia," in the first decade of the twentieth century, pessimism about prognosis continued to dictate expectations.

By the time psychosis led to BJ's hospitalizations, canon presumed he would not recover. Despite psychiatry's new embrace of science and its efforts to medicalize diagnosis, the *DSM-III* perpetuated that mischaracterization. It meant that some patients would be hospitalized indefinitely. Although a diagnosis of schizophrenia, or manic depression (later renamed bipolar disorder), contributed to this fate, other diagnoses were added, layering one on the other as if each were discrete, and adding more reason to be pessimistic. In BJ's lifetime, each revision of the diagnostic manual modified its description of schizophrenia with additional qualities, but the prognosis never included recovery.

The impressionistic process of arriving at a diagnosis did not mean that psychiatry paid little attention to basic science. It was the opposite. Kraepelin was himself a scientist employing observational techniques to organize and group patterns of patients' symptoms. Bleuler too used an observational method then considered scientific. In Western Europe and Australia starting in the 1950s, research labs were steeped in the study of chemicals and electrical impulses reaching nerves. In America, at the National Institute of Mental Health (NIMH) in Bethesda, Maryland, research was also underway on the fourth floor of the Clinical Center where laboratories pulsed with basic discoveries about synapses, enzymes, metabolism, and pharmacological agents.

It wasn't until a decade after BJ's diagnosis, in the mid-1980s, that scientists confirmed the brain's centrality for behavior, a pivot as important as any in the history of medicine. After years of studying anatomy and physiology, mediated by philosophy and theology, there would be incontrovertible evidence that the brain, a walnut-shaped organ weighing two to three pounds, with folds and wrinkles and parts called lobes and hemispheres, could be linked specifically to hearing or vision or hunger, emotions or pain. This was far greater than an abstraction about the mind or the soul. It meant the brain would no longer be considered a recipient of activity, including the cleansed fluids from the heart, liver, or kidneys. It was more than a metaphorical switchboard coordinating and connecting. There was proof that it was an engine for feelings, memory, emotions, action, behavior, and so much more.

Scientists at NIMH had paved the way for these discoveries under the leadership of Dr. Robert H. Felix, a psychiatrist who drafted the National Mental Health Act of 1946, signed by President Harry S. Truman that year. NIMH would join the nation's health research institutes pursuing knowledge about allergies, infectious diseases, and the heart. Felix became its first director, and two imperatives guided him before mandatory retirement forced his departure in 1967, at the age of sixty-five. The first came from an offhand remark his father, a circuit-riding doctor in rural Kansas, made after a house call: "Everything in medicine has a cause, even if you don't know it."[2] That set Felix's unimpeachable ambition to unlock the secrets of human biology to better humanity and alleviate suffering.

Felix's other guiding principle, which took shape during internship training in Colorado in the 1930s, stemmed from the conviction that psychiatric hospitals had become a blight. They locked patients away. They weren't helping people have better lives. When he later studied public health at Johns Hopkins University, he conceived of an alternative to hospitals. Care in local communities, not remote and uncaring institutions, was what was needed.

Felix directed NIMH with these twin goals for research and services, to which he added a third, educating professionals—nurses, social workers, and psychologists as well as psychiatrists—for a workforce that would bind them. He called it the three-legged stool.

In addition to the accomplishments of Nobel Prize–winning scientists at NIMH, one of Felix's proudest moments came when President John F. Kennedy appeared before a joint session of Congress to propose community services to treat mental illness and (what was then called) mental retardation. Joint sessions to Congress were infrequent, and JFK's on February 5, 1963, outlined "a bold new approach." He described "a problem unpleasant to mention, easy to postpone, and despairing of a solution." But the federal government didn't have to tolerate problems because states hadn't solved them. State mental hospitals amounted to little more than custodial care, and JFK proposed bypassing them to work directly with local communities to build mental health centers that would house community clinic services. Sixteen hundred centers are all that were needed.

Felix's fingerprints were all over JFK's Community Mental Health Act. He had been coaching Mike Feldman, a Kennedy aide, and had already discussed these ideas with cabinet secretaries, members of Congress, and the leadership of the US Public Health Service, where he was chief of the Mental Hygiene Division. Kennedy's message unfurled facts to make people wince: more than half of the 279 state hospitals housed more than three thousand patients; three-quarters of the hospitals had opened before World War I; and people with schizophrenia, who could be discharged within six months, remained hospitalized for an average of eleven years.[3] This would be one of JFK's last accomplishments before he was assassinated three weeks later, on November 22, and it would become part of the legacy friends and family cherished and protected.

The federal government's robust interest in mental health intended to bypass state budgetary authority to subsidize local construction of facilities.

Each would have five core services, and four of them weren't found in state hospitals: outpatient services, day treatment, emergency services, and consultation and education services. The centers could contract for the fifth, inpatient services in local general hospitals.

Felix had been writing and lecturing about community services for nearly two decades. As head of NIMH, as a past president of the American Psychiatric Association, and as a leader in the Mental Health Section of the American Public Health Association, his opinion mattered to lawmakers. During the Senate subcommittee hearings on health in March 1963, he predicted the next generation "would see the day when the State mental hospitals as we know them today would no longer exist."[4] With utmost confidence he wrote in the *American Journal of Orthopsychiatry*, "The shape of the future is ours to mold. The time has come for action." So convinced was he, he predicted that by 1984 hospitals would exist only as museums to show "what the care and treatment of our mentally ill once was."[5]

None of Felix's vision, or subsequent congressional measures expanding services, benefited BJ. Fewer than half of the sixteen hundred mental health centers JFK anticipated had been constructed for people like him, those who left hospitals not once, not twice, but many times in many cities. He roamed from New York to New Jersey, Chicago, Baltimore, Philadelphia, Denver, and Vancouver, British Columbia, before he returned to Los Angeles. I don't think he ever met staff in a clinic under the authority of a community mental health center.

Eventually I began to understand that the course of his illness consisted of multiple short hospitalizations, interspersed with arrests for vagrancy. When he left a hospital, a social worker might have arranged for him to go to a sheltered place, and depending on where he was living it could have been called a board and care home, a halfway house, or a group home. In New York City people diagnosed with mental illness often found their way to an SRO—a single resident occupancy. Not-for-profit agencies operated some, unscrupulous profiteers feeding off federal poverty programs operated others. Usually BJ was kicked out of community housing options because he wouldn't comply with their rules about medication, or curfew hours, or smoking. He left as quickly as he arrived, and without a forwarding address.

For years BJ disappeared, reappeared, called to demand money or announce he had disowned me. He bellowed grievances I eventually stopped hearing. The list was endless. Sometimes phone calls came every ten minutes, and my only relief was to smother the phone's shrill rings under a pile of pillows and blankets, or leave my apartment for a couple of hours.

And then he changed. BJ's energy depleted, his bluster passed, and the rants dissipated when he was about fifty. Relatives took him to lunch. He called me to ask about my family, not to demand money. He asked about my children, whose genetic quilt I had worried about from the day they were born, and about my husband, whom he had never met. He sent me birthday cards, cards for Hanukkah, Passover, and all the other Jewish holidays. By the end of his life, at the age of sixty-seven, he was living in a studio apartment in a cohousing program for senior citizens in Los Angeles. He was proud of where he lived in a well-kept, low-slung building with big windows, ample sunlight, and a lush verdant courtyard thick with tall plants. The familiar neighborhood was close to our childhood home. And his neighbors knew and valued him. He was getting services. I appreciate the intrepid work of an aunt who located the Edelman West Side Mental Health Agency, associated with UCLA, which included a visiting psychiatrist, nurse, and social worker. He was never happier. Or better cared for. Or safer.

I saw all this when I visited two or three times a year. I stayed long enough to assure myself that he was managing. On these trips, we shopped. Mostly we went to Staples to buy paper and pens so he could draw, and batteries for his transistor radio. Or to Ralphs, the local supermarket, where we would shore up his pantry. We walked around the La Brea Tar Pits. It was now a fenced site for tourists, but as kids we played there, pretending to be dinosaurs while sidestepping seeping goo. His favorite part of my visits was going out for lunch and dinner. Binging on restaurants was wonderful for a couple days, while we were both on our best behavior. Anything longer was taxing, and I would take leave before the inevitable fight erupted. We were well scripted.

Occasionally he called to tell me about something that caught his attention, that reminded him of time he spent in Israel, or his student days at the London School of Economics. Did I remember those years? he asked.

Did I still have the gift, a cameo pin, he had given me the year he lived in Italy? I was then reminded of his unstinting generosity, his sparkling eyes, his mischievous grin, and the whimsy of his youth. I hurt for what could have been while I grieved for us both.

Planning for recovery hadn't existed for psychiatry, with its near-exclusive use of medication to abate symptoms when BJ got sick. I had no idea that the field was in its nadir, or that recovery was considered as preposterous as melting glaciers or driverless cars. Or that psychiatry was wrestling with the dilemmas of untreated people for whom it was responsible yet lacked adequate tools or resources or even interest. John Talbott, author of *Death of the Asylum* and a psychiatrist emerging as one of the field's leaders, asked why "psychiatry continues to be frustrated by the elusiveness and intractability of this severely vulnerable and impaired population."[6]

Fifteen years after Felix prophesied the death knell of hospitals, Talbott pondered why they persisted. Clearly, he said, they were "designed to avoid treating patients." There was little interest in improving them. "We have a huge mental hospital system—with buildings, employees, and patients. . . . It is not working, and something needs to be done." On his long list of needed repairs were new attitudes, responsibilities, and accountabilities. He included "a public constituency for the severely and chronically mentally ill." Doubtful that families and patients could deliver this powerfully needed constituency, he confessed to having no ideas about how it would develop.[7]

Former patients and families would show him, and they would set the path for that constituency. Their experiences shaped suspicion of authorities who intended to help and guide them yet denied them voice. They would organize, protest, and challenge the system. They would do it themselves.

BJ never aligned with the emerging coterie of former patients who wanted to resume a life hospitalization had paused. Drugs, the standard treatment, had been used as a weapon to beat back their symptoms. When BJ was hospitalized, the drugs he received were in the same chemical family as chlorpromazine, which was discovered in the 1950s. At the time, it was considered a miracle helping hospitalized patients who would otherwise bang their heads against the walls and leave concrete bloodstained, thereby becoming candidates for the monstrous lobotomies. Chlorpromazine checked that. After it was understood that this drug had major tranquilizing qualities, it became the primary tool on the wards. Soon, drugs in the same chemical family of phenothiazines—Haldol, Mellaril, Loxitane, and Prolixin—promised to attack schizophrenia. All of the sudden, psychiatry had what the rest of medicine used, pills, or in some instances, injections or even liquid medications.

Around the time BJ was hospitalized in the 1970s, drugs were advertised widely in professional journals, including the American Psychiatric Association's house organ, *Psychiatric News*. Squibb, the maker of Prolixin, boasted that an injection could "save time, it could save money, and it can even save people" who were on "maintenance therapy." Lithium was added to the armamentarium treating depression, and the makers of the antidepressant Elavil promised to "penetrate the symptom barrier," enabling psychotherapy to "take direction." Another tranquilizing antidepressant, Etrafon, claimed to beat back symptoms of constipation, sweating, early morning wakening, weight loss, anorexia, apprehension, and eleven additional items, according to its advertising.[8]

Could treatments really be as clear-cut as these ads implied? What of their brutal side effects? Or of patients finding them noxious as well as toxic, patients who, on discharge, refused to take them, or sought control of their treatments outside of a hospital's confines? Challenging pharma's drugs became a process of reclaiming authority over patients' own lives, actually engaging in discussions about what they would need to do to achieve their goals. If BJ had been asked about his goals, he would not have put drugs on the short list; drugs were agents leading to twitchy muscles that compromised his self-respect. He would have said his goals included permanent shelter keeping him off the streets, out of the emergency room. He would have wanted choice about his bedtime and meals, and a quiet space. When he started working with a psychiatrist who was more of a coach guiding him than a traffic cop monitoring the stop-and-go of his symptoms, he started to engage differently with me, the world, and himself.

Originally, the word "recovery," both as a process and a result, applied only to people struggling with addictions. But it has come to include people whose lives have been interrupted while they learned to manage a major mental illness. It can include medication, psychotherapy, peer support, exercises in mindfulness, and accepting help from psychiatrists, psychologists, or social workers. Or none of the above. When symptoms of schizophrenia upended BJ's life there was no consensus, as there is none today, that help could be tailored to a person's unique situation and speed their reengagement. For some people, recovery meant they could resume life pretty much where it had been paused, in the midst of an education, a career, or a family plan; most would learn how to chart a course managing their symptoms as they set out to achieve their goals; some would struggle more, take longer, and have to modify their goals and aspirations.

The following pages explore these changes from multiple points of view. Some came by way of psychiatrists and psychologists, others by way of bench research scientists, still others by way of politicians. But it was coalitions of former patients who put recovery on the agenda. That their movement grew in tandem with similar campaigns for social justice is no accident. Inspired by contemporaries fighting to upend racism, sexism, and militarism, they saw their work on the same continuum. Initially, it was to halt the exercise of authority based on force. Former patients opposed social profiling—"the mentally ill" or "a schizophrenic"—long before social profiling referred to discrimination, or to social or ethnic qualities. Later they would advance understanding about engaging people in a healing process, one with an opportunity to recover.

Pulitzer Prize–winning author Siddhartha Mukherjee explains why he wrote about cancer survivors in *The Emperor of All Maladies*. It wasn't only because they had beat the odds "miraculously." Mukherjee knew that oncologists had to become inured to losing patients. "But when medicine inures you to the idea of life, to survival," he said, "then it has failed utterly."[9] In a similar vein, the history of recovery for psychiatry is the story of becoming unshackled to expectations of chronicity or bare maintenance.

In many ways, recovery always existed for people diagnosed with a mental illness, but it stayed in the shadows. Robert Felix once said, "There are shadows only when the sun shines,"[10] and his buoyant optimism seemed realistic by the 1990s, when recovery could no longer be credibly ignored. Call it a tipping point, in the style of Malcolm Gladwell, or a paradigm shift, according to the teachings of Thomas Kuhn. Credit belongs to people who told their stories while they lobbied, campaigned, and denounced those who would ignore that recovery could not only be achieved but should be central to guiding policy and program. As Surgeon General David Satcher would proclaim in 1999, treatments for serious mental illness worked. Recovery was real.

———————

Had recovery been one of BJ's options, he would have enjoyed a different quality of life. On the streets, he was half starved, fearful, untrusting, and suspicious. His was a fight to survive while managing a heart condition, as well as the loss of caring friends and a welcoming synagogue. He gained the stigma of menial jobs, working off the books, and living in fear that his government would tax his Social Security Disability benefits, as it once did when he reported a modest birthday present with pride-filled innocence. This punitive policy has since changed, but it was another of the insults undermining his dignity, something else he learned to manage.

BJ would have been a good fit for today's person-centered, self-determining care for those with mental illness. He knew what he wanted and was quick to express it. Living on his own, and with family help, first in a small apartment taking him off the streets, later in a cohousing apartment bearing the influence of programs in Australia, he was happy. His world grew with an iPad, a birthday present bringing him music and movies and the explosion of color with the touch of a finger. In his later years, he cherished the bustle of Beverly Boulevard. He lived three long blocks from a drugstore, and two from the iconic Farmers Market. His routine included a weekly trip with a neighbor to Trader Joe's. He loved shopping at Goodwill, which, in his neighborhood, carried high-end merchandise—the dapper shirts and leather jackets that his heart desired and his frugal budget could manage. He went regularly to Du-par's Pancake House, where they called him Mr. Vine.

———————

A paradigm about recovery was evolving in the decades BJ hustled to survive. Once it was apparent that a combination of services could lead to recovery, different challenges confronted tens of thousands still in the grip of a flagging medical model based exclusively on decisions coming from doctors in white coats. Activists, who called themselves consumers, survivors, or ex-patients, articulated ideals of health and wellness with recommendations for action. Rehabilitation, like that available to men and women who lost limbs or had to repair their lives following a stroke, carried the challenge of emphasizing "what's strong, not what's wrong." No longer would sheer maintenance and a lingering assumption of hopelessness and chronicity suffice.

The stepping-stones to this paradigmatic shift fill the following pages. It is a story depending on the intermixture of politics, science, and citizen activists. Former patients mounted campaigns to shape reform, as did distraught parents, daring professionals, unorthodox administrators, unconventional politicians, and tireless public servants. They were bold and stubborn, and often in conflict. The essential question reverberated: who controls the mental health agenda?

———————————

People who championed recovery intrigued me. By the time I started writing this book, I had given up a practiced career teaching college-level history. An earlier book, *Families in Pain*, focused on the family experience I knew so well. I had come across ex-patient protests, but I wanted to know more, where they had come from and where they wanted to go. I didn't initially link protests to recovery until I dug deeper, and until I understood it as I do now. Already I knew the difference between hearing that a family member would forever be disabled by a psychotic episode and arriving at recovery's door by way of hope. I saw it in my own family. I knew the difference between stereotypes and newspaper headlines, and actual people whose recovery had inspired others. Those role models hadn't existed for BJ, or any of his generation. They certainly hadn't existed for families like mine. How different would it have been for either of us had we known about the possibilities that opened in the fight to recover?

The question of how the concept of recovery replaced the "wastebasket" diagnosis during BJ's lifetime, 1949–2015, brings me here. *Fighting for Recovery* is organized in three parts. Part 1 introduces circumstances leading activists to challenge received wisdom about the intractability of serious mental illness. In the 1960s and 1970s, distinct groups of citizen activists and government players incited reform in parallel spheres. Part 2 explores how their fight for remedies in the 1980s allowed them to bridge, expand, and collaborate when they were not competing. Part 3 shows how a coalition led by ex-patient activists birthed a constituency for recovery and imagined a reformation.

Recovery may have revolutionized ideas about how best to assist people with mental illness with transformed services, but the idea is only the beginning. And there's been pushback because not all have agreed with recommendations about solutions. What they agreed about is how the current mental health system is in shambles. Of the 10.4 million adults with serious mental illness in 2016, only 65 percent received mental health services. That figure has held steady for ten years.[11] As many as two-thirds of those experiencing a psychotic disturbance waited six months or longer for treatment services.[12] People in a psychiatric crisis can spend days waiting in an emergency room. So common is this that there's even a term for it: "boarding." Suicide, the tenth leading cause of death overall, is the leading cause of death for people between the ages of ten and thirty-four.[13] These are not recovery-oriented practices. Not even close. However inadequate the mental health system was before COVID-19, a pandemic has worsened them and laid them bare.

On the eve of sweeping political activism in the 1960s, historian Warren Susman wrote, "An intelligent reading of the past might make possible man's intelligent direction over the future course of history."[14] Susman's injunction was synchronous with historians who tired of viewing the past as quaint artifact. The next generation of scholarship also proposed that it was not sufficient to acknowledge how the past had shaped culture: what was needed was to mine the past for clues to a dynamic future. In *A People's History of the United States*, Howard Zinn writes that history can "emphasize new possibilities by disclosing those hidden episodes of the past when . . . people showed their ability to resist, to join together, occasionally to win."[15] And this generation's most prolific public historian, Jill Lepore, writes, "To study the past is to unlock the prison of the present."[16]

That theme resounds for ex-patients who heaved to challenge doctrines once codified by psychiatry and enshrined in law. What Zinn called "hidden episodes" have been hiding in plain sight. They include moments when former patients insisted that doors open to them, not as supplicants but as participants. This remains an ongoing fight. Hidden episodes include campaigns to end injustice as a way of life. Ex-patient activists began testing the feasibility of change before launching a redesign. Others channeled an assault on the paradigm that threatened authority empowering professionals. Science and social science have given us new tools. It is time to use them. It is worth repeating what Tipper Gore said more than twenty years ago when the surgeon general released a landmark study anointing recovery: "It is time for America to act."[17]

PART 1

SETTING THE STAGE

CHAPTER 1

TEAR 'EM DOWN

T HIS STORY BEGINS on a July day in 1964 when the California heat pushed past ninety degrees, and Art Bolton, a thirty-eight-year-old social worker, drove thirty-five miles from his home in Sacramento to the town of Auburn, at the foothills of the Tahoe National Forest. Bolton was on assignment from "Big Daddy" Jesse Unruh, speaker of the California State Assembly, to learn what he could about state psychiatric hospitals. A hundred years earlier, people had rushed to Auburn to dig for the glory of gold. Now it was a faded town with faded lives in the service of Dewitt State Hospital.

To reduce overcrowding and improve California's public hospitals, Governor Earl Warren had acquired Dewitt from the federal government two decades earlier. Warren said he wanted to take "California out of the asylum age and put it in the hospital age where emphasis is on prevention, treatment, and cure in place of mere custody." As a former district attorney, he knew the police escorted people to hospitals, and now he wondered about judges sentencing someone to treatment against their wishes. He had been struck by *Life* magazine's photographic essay after World War II featuring deplorable hospital conditions. With this in mind, Warren, who had been governor since 1943, toured California's public hospitals. The misery he saw gave him nightmares. Patients resembled Holocaust survivors. Makeshift buildings were susceptible to earthquakes or fire. Medieval and barbarous, he thought, and he vowed to change this. He announced a new division would oversee what was then called "mental hygiene." Next, he ordered the demolition of forty-seven buildings. To address overcrowding, he added beds in the remaining facilities. Under his leadership, by 1952 California started building new hospitals.[1]

Two years later, Warren left California to become the chief justice of the US Supreme Court, and reform stalled. One scandal at Modesto State Hospital revealed how staff routinely tortured patients. They would twist arms hard enough to break shoulders with spiral fractures. Perceived misdeeds led to beatings with toilet plungers; reprobate staff painted Epsom salts on a woman's vagina. Lawsuits, damning publicity, and recommendations about fixing psychiatric hospitals were available to the next governor, Goodwin J. Knight. Still, little had changed by the time Bolton, a sandy-haired chain-smoking father of five, started his journey that July morning.

Bolton knew that the late president John F. Kennedy had called for revamping mental health services, setting the stage for his assignment. The Kennedy family's remorse about his sister Rosemary's exile to Wisconsin after a lobotomy undoubtedly contributed to JFK's dislike of the "social quarantine" of people "out of sight and forgotten."[2] He criticized the "desultory interest in confining patients in an institution to wither away." In some ways, America needed to catch up to Great Britain's "open hospital" ideas about less confining and more flexible services.

Under Robert Felix's leadership at the National Institute of Mental Health, there had been steady support for community services throughout his two decades at the helm. Federal grants pumped energy into local communities, and they were showing results with innovative designs. One came in the 1950s, in Bronx, New York, supporting doctors' design of the nation's first day hospital to replace twenty-four-hour locked wards for inpatients. NIMH also invested in Vermont's use of community housing and rehabilitation for discharged patients. Felix appreciated George Fairweather's ambition in California to develop housing for veterans who were rebuilding skills to live independently. Scattered in local communities, they reflected local circumstances, unique needs, and an autonomy unlike the national planning for health systems underway in Europe.

Assembly Speaker Unruh wasn't particularly interested in mental health reform.[3] But he wanted to remain within the Kennedy circle of influence. He had managed JFK's successful California campaign, and he had stayed close to Robert Kennedy. But even that wouldn't would have mattered had he, the state's most seasoned politician, not been touched by the grief of desperate parents whose children suffered from institutional care. His compassion must have been genuine, his biographer writes, saying he could "not have found a more daunting or politically unrewarding challenge."[4] He had assigned Bolton responsibility for reforming kids' services, and he built regional satellite programs, satisfied families, and thereby earned a trip to the White House and JFK's praise. Pleased, Unruh now wanted Bolton to succeed for thirty-four thousand adults in California's public psychiatric hospitals, which, in 1964, cost the state $99 million. Reforming state hospitals could burnish California's image; it could cement Jesse Unruh's leadership. And it might improve the lives of thousands.

Bolton believed in hands-on research, and driving himself to Dewitt State Hospital was how he worked. When he had assessed the state's programs for disabled children, he surveyed parents of the three thousand kids on a waiting list for public services. "What is it that you want?" he asked them. He would adopt similar strategies for assessing the adult system. It too teetered while it had grown larger, cost more, and accomplished less.

For the next two years, as director of the Assembly Office of Research, Bolton spoke to patients, interviewed their families, reviewed hospital policies, and observed operations. Everything he saw convinced him that reform was impossible. In a stunning display of speaking truth to power, he returned to the assembly speaker with an answer. Unruh was called Big Daddy—and it wasn't just for his love of power, or because he was the second most important politician in California. Jesse Unruh, who weighed 280 pounds, was known for intemperate outbursts. Still, Art Bolton, of average size and cautious deportment, told Big Daddy that the hospitals were beyond repair. They could not be fixed or improved or reformed. They were incompatible with humanity. They should be closed. "Tear 'em down," he said. "Tear 'em down."[5]

It took Bolton two years to reach this epiphany, but he had been thinking about hospitals steadily since visiting Dewitt State. Dewitt was among California's newer facilities, acquired after World War II as a transfer station for patients hospitalized elsewhere. Located on 216 acres, with Quonset huts lined up like the teeth of a comb, and a central corridor joining forty-five wards,[6] it still looked more like its original military base than an asylum for troubled people. By the time Bolton visited, it housed three thousand more patients than it should have. Like most of California's remote psychiatric hospitals, it was invisible to all but the most purposeful set of eyes.

DeWitt's seven hundred employees powered Auburn's economy. There were secretaries, housekeepers, telephone operators, guards, pharmacists, maintenance crews, kitchen crews, groundskeepers, nurses, a few social workers, and one or two psychiatrists. Staff sandwiched their duties between meeting patient needs and satisfying superintendents who controlled their domain like fiefdoms with few rules, no accountability, and raw power.

Bolton did not accept this assignment naively. Previously he had seen crowding and restraints, aging facilities and short staffs, and he knew the sickly smell of feces painting the halls. He had seen children restrained and shackled in cages. He knew of bedsores and hunger and near-starvation diets. Could there be anything worse? Yes. He would learn degradation was measured differently for the adults at Modesto State Hospital, where they were required to mop the floors while naked. Although the practice was decades old, at a hospital in Stockton forced sterilization still attached to its image. DeWitt's dire conditions, worthy of tabloids, now fed his curiosity. Only recently a patient had died there, and the culprit was said to be an alcoholic technician whose principal advocate was allegedly an alcoholic doctor. People could, and actually did, get lost in these hospitals, which held up to five thousand patients. The actress Helen Chandler spent five years recovering from alcoholism at DeWitt, and Martin Ramirez, whose pen and pencil drawings would later be acclaimed as folk art, spent half of his thirty-two hospitalized years at DeWitt. Fighting with neighbors over a property line got one couple trapped behind the hospital's one-way gate. Before family could get them out, they had received unwanted electroshock treatments (known as electroconvulsive therapy, or ECT).[7]

At first he thought it odd that his request to tour the grounds without staff was denied. When he tried to open a locked door, staff tried to dissuade him. Nothing to see in there, the escort said. Nonsense, Bolton thought while opening the door to a cavernous dormitory, 235 feet long and 30 feet wide. Cots were jammed together, filled with idle, urine-soaked patients. "Some of them were just old people that nobody wanted," he thought. "Just elderly people who often died shortly after being admitted to the state institution." Others had a history of alcoholism. Most were poor. Some, he guessed, actually suffered from a mental illness.[8] Leather belts and cuffs strapped one elderly man to his bed. He didn't seem to be agitated, out of control, or in need of restraints. He was "lying there, looking miserable, old, and feeble," and Bolton wondered if there could be a "psychologically therapeutic value of being stripped naked and tied to a bed." What kind of behavior warranted still using physical restraints when the Department of Mental Hygiene had outlawed them six months earlier?[9]

Walking down another hall, he asked his escort, "What's behind those doors?"

"Oh, you don't want to bother. That's a laundry."

"Really, I'd like to go see the laundry," he said, opening the door to an unbearably hot room. "Dante's inferno," he said to himself. In the middle stood an attendant on an elevated observation deck watching men and women work. A hot iron landing on moist cloth hissed, sending clouds of steam floating upward. Bolton strolled up and down the aisles, pausing here and there to look more closely at one of the forty patients operating the industrial pressers.

"How long have you been doing this?" he asked one man working on sheets.

Despite Bolton's well-honed cynicism, he was surprised to hear this man say five years.

This was called industrial therapy. "Everything was labeled therapy," Bolton told me. "If they didn't call it industrial therapy, they said it was milieu therapy." At the time he believed there was no therapy. He considered it slave labor.[10]

Other California facilities were just as shocking. One time, at Sonoma State Hospital, Bolton was sitting with three people from the professional staff—a nurse, a physician, and a psychologist—when a patient had an epileptic fit. Spasms, tight muscles, rapid eye movements, drooling—it was unmistakable. Barely twenty feet away, staff sat impassively. The patient fell to the floor. Other patients came to his aid. Bolton asked, shouldn't they be helping? No, nothing to worry about, said one of them. "We see this all the time."[11]

The size of Sonoma State Hospital, five thousand patients, led Bolton to doubt it could truly help people with serious mental illness. "You can imagine what kind of thinking went into that," he said sarcastically during an interview for a PBS documentary. "Imagine," he said, "we're gonna take five thousand people who have difficult problems, and put them all in one place, and good things will come of that." He laughed at the very thought. "What a crazy idea to begin with but, you know, when these institutions were created . . . they were created mainly with the idea of finding a place to get these people out of our community. They're a nuisance, they're difficult, they create problems, we don't want 'em and we don't wanna spend money on 'em."[12]

Courts committed 84 percent of California's inpatients. Why? What had people with a mental illness done that was so wrong as to have broken the law? What was so terrible that district attorneys and judges had to get involved? For the next two years, all of 1965 and most of 1966, Bolton's seven-person staff determined to find out. They sent questionnaires to fifteen hundred people—patients, representatives of public and private hospitals, and the courts in forty counties. They visited doctors, psychologists, and hospital staff.[13] Public hearings followed.

Bolton came to believe that the courts' intractable role in sentencing people to hospitals was driving California's catastrophic mental health system. It might have originated with a phone call to the police after a family conflict or an incident involving an elderly person who drank too much or someone's problem with dementia.[14] Many people were agitated, but most were not dangerous. Three-quarters needed emergency services for a short-term emotional disturbance.[15] That led to a police escort to a hospital for up to seventy-two hours. For many, it was the first step toward what would become a civil commitment.

Once someone was admitted, it fell to staff to determine if that person seemed "normal." They used a checklist for actions which Bolton ascribed to a middle-class bias about behavior, starting with the criterion of *self-control*: "The normal person can control his impulses." Another concerned the *planned life*: "The normal person 'plans ahead.'" And *good relations*: "The normal person gets along well with his spouse."[16] People of means usually got themselves discharged; the rest got pajamas, limited phone calls, and censored letters.

A medical exam took place in a hospital. Assemblyman Jerome Waldie, who had also worked with Bolton investigating children's services, observed one of these exams at the San Francisco General Hospital. This is what he saw: doctors sat knee to knee across from patients. There was no privacy. Other patients surrounded them, listening to the interview. Respondents with vague answers were thought to lack "insight or judgment." They were labeled "mental defects." Lack of insight and judgment were among schizophrenia's signature symptoms in the 1960s, and it was all too easy to conclude that the person needed to remain beyond the evaluation phase.[17]

A doctor's evaluation was mandatory. In rural areas, a general practitioner met the need. In Los Angeles County, which contained three of the state's nine hospitals, one psychiatrist evaluated as many as ten people a day. Court-ordered hearings followed to decide if the restrained person should be legally committed; two public defenders could represent as many as 120 people a week.[18] But they did so weakly. This was the process sending fourteen thousand people to a public psychiatric hospital in California in 1965.

Bolton asked, was this needed?

Legal statutes foreclosed judicial independence and constrained sentencing choices. According to Section 5550 of the Welfare and Institutions Code, a medical examiner could recommend involuntary commitment if a person was "in need of supervision, treatment, care or restraint." Rarely did judges challenge a doctor's recommendation. Ventura County Superior Court judge William Reppy said it would mean he would be telling a doctor, "You think this man is mentally ill but I don't." San Francisco's Judge Joseph Karesh told Assemblyman Waldie at a subcommittee hearing in December 1965 that he didn't ask questions. "Since they were there," he said, "they were presumed to be mentally ill." Karesh later acknowledged feeling ashamed about his role in the process. It also bothered Judge John Racanelli. He described a circuslike atmosphere in his Santa Clara County courtroom where patients, dressed in hospital-issued pajamas, sat lined up on wooden benches. After a couple of hours, those who were not bored became agitated. Racanelli felt constrained by the doctors' orders. Still, he felt obliged to ask people who came before him if they wanted to say anything. Only once did someone answer yes. And what did he say? "Fuck you."[19]

California was not unique. A similar line of pajama-clad patients waited in the corridors of New York's courtrooms. As with California,

New York didn't guarantee patients' rights, and there was no minimum constitutional protection.[20] To expedite the woeful process, Illinois built a courtroom for patients on the premises of a hospital.[21]

Bolton was aghast that courts treated sick people as if they were criminal lawbreakers, which furthered an impression about people with a mental illness being dangerous. Given the vague, imprecise, and idiosyncratic diagnostic process, he was dumbfounded. He had come to believe that "the term 'mental illness' does not describe any particular condition; it does not reveal the cause of an individual's difficulty, nor does it suggest any specific course of remedial action." It was, he said, "a catchall concept." Like beauty, madness "may exist in the eye of the beholder."[22]

Although imprecision was a problem, Bolton was a social worker, not a psychiatrist. His lever for change came from working for the legislature, which had the power to pass laws. The most disturbing of all his findings was how quickly someone's life could be upended by an involuntary commitment to a state hospital. Trained observers used a stopwatch to measure the time it took to complete a commitment hearing for fifty-eight patients appearing before a county lunacy commission. The hearings averaged 4.7 minutes.[23] If there were a headline, a sound bite, a photo caption, it was knowing how quickly someone could be "committed indefinitely to a state institution in California."[24] That became his handle for reform.

———————

Bolton would have had similar misgivings had he toured hospitals in Pennsylvania, Oregon, Alabama, or Illinois, where seven thousand men filled the state hospital.[25] Constitutional protections didn't apply to institutionalized patients in any of these places. But his task was understanding what to do in California, and his findings raised two questions: how should lawmakers protect the rights of people before they ended up arbitrarily confined to hospitals, and how should the state provide mental health services for those who needed them? Answers filled two hundred pages for a report, *The Dilemma of Mental Health Commitments in California*, which he delivered to the Assembly's Subcommittee on Mental Health Services in November 1966. He expected this report to inform the bicameral legislature, which would then pass a reform law before adjourning the next summer. Already he was drafting a bill and anticipating that a new system would take root within a year.

Bolton intended to choke a commitment process he deemed vague. This he would change and *The Dilemma* threaded long-standing problems. Staffing patterns hadn't changed since Earl Warren was governor in 1952 and poor management with overcrowding was the norm. He would individualize service needs with a plan, not the "lumping and dumping" practices he considered "legally, medically, and socially unsound." He would impose standards for people he considered "mentally disordered," not "mentally ill." This would mean that courts would have to cease sending a thousand people a month to California's public hospitals.

———————

"The central feature of the proposed new system," Bolton wrote, was an emergency service unit (ESU) to replace the commitment court.[26] It would become a local referral agent, "close to home," and available to people who sought help voluntarily as well as those who had been accompanied by family, friends, doctors, or the police. Staffed with psychologists, social workers, or psychiatrists, it could also contract with universities, hospitals, and private or public clinics to conduct evaluations, including in "the citizen's own home."

The Dilemma broadened the conversation by asking new questions. Would an evaluation prevent a suicide? Was it a medical emergency? Might an unspecified social service avert a crisis? What service existed locally? Voluntarily? And if the recommendation was a hospital or a doctor, as confining as that might be, the person should have freedom of choice during the selection process to decide which doctor or hospital.

The process was more complicated than the services clinics, called Short-Doyle, already offered. Counties managed the decade-old clinics, and each local program differed. The ESU of Bolton's imagination required consistency, and because of its importance, he recommended that the state fund this new system. Bolton further assumed that it would be rare to encounter someone so "gravely disabled" that they were incapable of feeding, clothing, sheltering, or communicating—criteria for involuntary detention—or that they were so overtly destructive that they should be forced into a hospital.

A typical ESU evaluation could hold someone for up to seventy-two hours. If more time were needed because of a crisis, the evaluator could recommend an additional fourteen involuntary days at a hospital. Still, the ESU endorsed patient choice. Patients "shall be free to reject treatment, and . . . to terminate treatment at any time." This essentially ended forced lobotomy, which had pretty much been sidelined by the 1960s. Choice could curtail other involuntary treatments, notably ECT, loathed by hospitalized patients and civil libertarians alike.

Psychiatrists would later question the assumptions guiding Bolton's recommendations. They disagreed about ending involuntary ECT. It was both common and controversial, and doctors feared ending it would tie hands when it came to prescribing treatments. Psychiatrists also questioned the wisdom of limiting an involuntary admission to fourteen days. Bolton introduced basic patient rights for people held longer: they could wear their own clothes, have visitors and uncensored phone calls, and send and receive uncensored letters.[27] If, at the end of this time, someone remained gravely disabled, only then should court proceedings begin.

Intending to divert people from the hospital, he proposed the ESU arrange for financial or legal counseling, recreation programs, employment services, housing agencies, senior citizen centers, child welfare services, and civic or ethnic service organizations—all of which could be enlisted to assist "a mentally disordered person to remain in the community." Social workers could provide these services before people went into a hospital, not only when they left. To establish a measure of accountability, *The Dilemma* proposed a citizens' advisory council with oversight authority.

Bolton didn't want in his report to be leaked. He wanted a bombshell to grab public interest while lawmakers considered the bill he put before them. His strategy worked. When the press got a copy of *The Dilemma* in November 1966, there was a "small explosion." The *San Francisco Examiner* shouted, "Thousands Locked Up Erroneously." The *Los Angeles Times* accused the existing system of being "legally, medically weak." Words like "archaic," "defective," and "drastic overhaul" peppered headlines. Bolton had hoped his work would create a thunderbolt, and it did when reporters wrote that current practices allowed for the indefinite commitment of someone to a state hospital in less time, 4.7 minutes, than it takes to boil an egg.[28]

Practices such as these also troubled Judge David Bazelon, chief judge of the influential US Court of Appeals for the District of Columbia. The case of a man named Charles Rouse, who wanted to be discharged from St. Elizabeths Hospital, the federal hospital in Washington, DC, piqued his interest. The Washington, DC, district court had considered Rouse's request based on claims that he had received only custodial care, not treatment, in four years of confinement. In February 1967 the court said custodial care was okay, that it counted as treatment. The American Psychiatric Association found this unacceptable, as did Bazelon.

Judge Bazelon's inclination toward social justice was evident as early as 1954 in *Durham v. United States*, a case charging Monte Durham with breaking and entering a house. Durham also had an extensive history of hospitalizations for an "unsound mind." In a decision that would provoke debate about the overlap of law and medicine, as well as revise the insanity defense for years to come, Bazelon's decision swapped punishment in a jail for rehabilitation in a hospital. The key factor addressed an assailant's mental status at the time of the alleged crime.

Rouse's mental status became just such a factor in his appeal. He had originally been charged with carrying a Colt .45 and six hundred rounds of ammunition in Washington, DC. He was eighteen years old, and a conviction would normally be a misdemeanor. As he was judged to be symptomatic at the time of his arrest, his disposition, "not guilty by reason of insanity," sent him to St. Elizabeths Hospital for treatment. Four years later, claiming he had not received treatment, he asked the courts to discharge him.

Ruling on another case involving insanity excited Bazelon. He prevailed on a young attorney, Charles Halpern, to handle Rouse's appeal. The case would ask whether it was constitutional to send someone to a hospital yet withhold the remedy, which was treatment. Without treatment, "the hospital is "transform[ed] into a penitentiary where one could be held indefinitely for no convicted offense," Bazelon said.[29] Halpern eventually got Rouse released, but not because he proved he was not mentally ill and shouldn't be at St. Elizabeths; nor did Halpern persuade the appeals court that what was considered milieu therapy of a ward was really a sham. Rouse's release turned on a flaw in the original trial. Still, this case was unprecedented, Halpern writes, asking courts "to protect the rights of mental patients confined in public mental hospitals against their will." Also unprecedented was asking if hospitals met their treatment obligations.[30] For the first time, it seemed jurists had opened the doors of a hospital to look inside.

The Mental Health Law Project, which Halpern later founded, subsequently brought many landmark cases. The facts spoke for themselves, and one of the staff attorneys described it this way: "When we do institutionalize people for any duration beyond crisis intervention, we should not engage in euphemisms that we are helping them. The evidence is almost entirely to the contrary."[31]

In the Rouse decision Judge Bazelon asked whether everybody who commits a crime is mentally ill. If that were the case, Bazelon said, "our whole system of criminal law would have to break down."[32] Bolton knew of the Rouse decision, of course. His own work posed the opposite question: was everybody with a mental illness a criminal?

As director of the Office of Assembly Research, a nonpartisan position, Bolton had to balance competing political interests with the skill of a high-wire acrobat while writing the Mental Health Act of 1967 to revamp California's hospital-based system. During this period, Eugene Bardach was working on a doctorate in political science at UC Berkeley. He shadowed Bolton, watched him navigate the channels of power, compromise, and cajole while he denounced the misery and misfortune of decisions made after a brief sham hearing. The process revealed Bolton's qualities—shrewd, insightful, intelligent, even cunning—that earned his staff's respect.[33]

Bardach marveled that Bolton could overlook pronounced philosophical differences among power brokers, knowing he had to turn them into allies. While tasked with reforming children's services, he had developed a working relationship with legislators, notably Republican Frank Lanterman and Democrat Nicholas Petris. Now they would team to reform the state's adult hospitals.

The two lawmakers were polar opposites. Lanterman represented the affluent, white-gloved Orange County where constituents lived in Spanish-style villas with curated art collections. Living in the county that was home to the anti-communist, far-right John Birch Society, many of his constituents mistrusted government and believed that psychiatry was part of an international Jewish communist conspiracy.[34] A portly bachelor with a receding hairline, Lanterman lived in the La Cañada family home where he'd grown up, and from which he was elected in 1953. The day's major political issue was water shortages. Lanterman wielded considerable power as a fiscal conservative and senior member of the Ways and Means Committee. He saw himself as a guardian of the civil liberties of elderly patients with dementia who had been inappropriately committed. Bardach writes that mental health policy was regarded as his territory and that "no significant changes in that area could be made without his consent or, alternatively, without having him exact a price."[35]

Petris also represented his birthplace, in his case Oakland, in northern California. The son of Greek immigrants, elegant and fit, he served a constituency that included the Berkeley campus of the University of California, Oakland's immigrant families from Europe and Latin America, and African Americans who had come north during the Great Migration. He championed labor protections and wanted to expand opportunities for education and protection of tenants. Many of his priorities carried public health benefits, such as his campaigns against car pollution.

Lanterman and Petris were more than figureheads appending their names to bills. They spoke regularly to Bolton or one of his staff members while they drafted the Mental Health Reform Act of 1967. Lanterman could be depended on to harness Republicans in the assembly. Petris had since moved over to the Senate, thereby losing the influence he had previously wielded, but Speaker Unruh could deliver Democratic votes. While the major thrust ended indefinite involuntary court-ordered commitments, the package elbowed existing unions, psychiatrists, the state's Department of Mental Hygiene, Short-Doyle clinic directors, and their patrons.

California's mental health services were controlled by counties through the ten-year-old Short-Doyle system, named after the legislators who designed the program. At first, it was a backstop to the soaring numbers of hospitalized patients in 1958. Most patients were middle class, predominantly white, needing outpatient counseling services for a "neurosis," nothing as severe as schizophrenia. These clients didn't need shelter, food, or clothing, as did the poorer patients whom Short-Doyle didn't treat, sending them instead to psychiatric hospitals.

The press showered enthusiasm when *The Dilemma* was released in November 1966, and again with the bill's introduction five months later. Supporters expected to save millions because people would be served and wrongs could be righted.[36] "'Civil Rights' Bill on Mental Health Sets Goals," wrote the *Los Angeles Times* when *The Dilemma* appeared. Judge Karesh called it the "Magna Carta of the Mentally Ill." Dr. Stanley Yolles, who that year succeeded Robert Felix as NIMH director, told Bolton he hoped it would become a national model.[37] But all this was on the chopping block after the election of a governor whose disdain for mental health services had been part of his campaign to unseat the incumbent governor, Edmund G. "Pat" Brown.

Ronald Reagan's 1966 victory changed the California landscape. As governor, he intended to make good on his campaign promises to cut budgets. He lowered business taxes, hiked student fees, and cut $20 million and 3,700 jobs from the Department of Mental Hygiene. He claimed the department was overstaffed and bragged about saving costs in a system that was ranked twenty-fifth—exactly in the middle—of national quality assessments. The biggest cuts targeted hospitals, which he called "hotel operations," a place "where the slothful went for a rest."[38] Cuts also targeted day treatment centers, geriatric screening centers, and the handful of aftercare clinics in the Bay Area. Broken toilet seats would not be replaced, said Health and Welfare Secretary Spencer Williams. He called wooden seats a weapon in the wrong hands. Besides, patients didn't need seats, he later boasted.[39]

Confusion sent reporters into hospitals to see for themselves. Roughly two-thirds of the editorial pages of California papers criticized Reagan's policies: a "false economy," charged the *Los Angeles Times*, and "callous regression," said the *Sacramento Bee*.[40] It turned ugly when the governor accused hospital employees of sabotaging patient safety and boycotting discussions. Psychiatrists fought back, saying it was the governor who had snubbed them.[41] Before his visit to Camarillo State Hospital in Ventura Country, patients got new clothes, making them appear well cared for. To upgrade the shabby grounds of an aging Spanish-style hospital, staff painted dead grass green. The local press had a field day.[42]

Reagan risked feuding with Frank Lanterman, who told the governor to back down. Not wanting to wrestle with the most powerful member of the Ways and Means Committee, Reagan soon voiced support, a presumed turn-around, but it was a publicity stunt, more guile than genuine, and inaction ruled.

———————

Praise for principles guiding Bolton's work often coupled with doubts about specific recommendations. Ending involuntary commitment laws threatened to overwhelm the county-run clinics by discharging scores of people needing a different kind of help. At the same time, state financing of local services, which Bolton recommended, seemed anathema to politicians fearing a creeping authority careening toward socialism. And counties such as Modesto, with two state hospitals, or Auburn, with DeWitt's staff, feared the economic debacle that closing hospitals would bring.

Complicating everything was Alan Short, who chaired the committee on government efficiency that had to vote to release the bill for a Senate vote. Senators finding fault with the Mental Health Act of 1967 were in no hurry to follow in the assembly's footsteps to pass Bolton's bill, which Lanterman submitted under the new name Lanterman-Petris-Short (LPS). The Senate's procrastinations perplexed Lanterman, who wanted to avoid a fight. Reject the "antiquated," "barbaric," "reprehensible" system, he begged Republicans. Do it now, before the first week of August when they were scheduled to adjourn for the customary two years.

Bolton felt a quandary tighten. Grotesque images of surrender—naked old men strapped to their beds, the flailing limbs of an epileptic seizure, stench-filled dormitories, helpless patients abandoned to their minders— had haunted him since his trip to DeWitt three years earlier. To conciliate, and to allay Short's fears about threats to the clinics, Bolton had to gut programs he wanted. There would be no emergency services to curtail hospitals, no aftercare for people needing help once they left, no robust citizen oversight, no central vision to unify more than fifty county operations. Now, in August 1967, deadlines loomed as the bicameral legislature prepared to recess.

Bolton faced this, his personal dilemma, asking himself how much reform was enough. Could he live with himself if his only accomplishment was ending involuntary commitment? As long as hospitals remained the centerpiece of the mental health system, Bolton believed they would dictate essential choices. People would ask how they should be changed, not whether they were the best way to help people with mental illness. He struggled for the rest of Saturday night and into the morning hours, sitting at his kitchen table to construct out of whole cloth a budget to accompany the bill that would be voted on the next and last day of the legislative session. The bill didn't have the guts or the heart or the brains that had informed *The Dilemma*. But there would also be no courts involuntarily committing people to institutions from which they might not return whole.

At the legislature's last day for that session, Sunday, August 6, 1967, the Senate passed LPS. Implementation was planned for 1969, but delays postponed this until 1972. In the meantime, Lanterman drafted several amendments to fill service gaps. One of the most notable consequences, which became apparent two years later, was a reduction by one-third in the number of hospitalized patients. Soon it became apparent that the doors had opened to unimaginable chaos. Failure to plan hung from the shoulders of political power brokers, and critics charged LPS with swelling the streets; they called patients "criminals and dangerous."[43] Some might have said the failure belonged to power brokers who rejected *The Dilemma*'s plans for an emergency service, aftercare, and a coordinated policy establishing coherence. Fragmentation—the opposite of Art Bolton's intention, of Lanterman's mission, and of Unruh's ambition—overwhelmed the organized planning *The Dilemma* would have delivered. Not in Illinois, New Jersey, or Minnesota, or in any of the thirty states revising their commitment laws in the wake of LPS, would adequate planning take place for patients whom they dumped. Bedlam was laid bare. There would be chaos on the streets and in the statehouse; one-way bus tickets to nowhere, so-called Greyhound therapy; and a new trend would be called deinstitutionalization.

In California, where political opportunities and lofty ideals merged, winds shifted radically after 1967 when LPS was passed. Within a year, Bobby Kennedy would be assassinated, and Unruh would lose his national influence. He suffered a commensurate upset in the state when he lost his speakership in 1968. Two years later, he was defeated in his campaign for governor when California reelected Ronald Reagan.

After a short time, Bolton left government service. He and his wife, Ruth, opened a guest lodge for people touring the Redwoods. With his degree in hand, Gene Bardach visited and found them content welcoming their guests. Soon, however, Bolton was drawn back into a good fight, helping other states accomplish what California had left incomplete. He opened a consulting group and worked with other states attempting to get it right. Twenty years later, he would have another chance when he was recruited back into action for California.

CHAPTER 2

"NOTHING ABOUT US WITHOUT US"

N OT FOR A MINUTE DID JUDI CHAMBERLIN believe that she was giving up her civil rights when she signed herself into a private psychiatric hospital in 1966. She was twenty-one years old and had experienced a miscarriage three months before. She was crying all the time and unable to get her bearings despite having seen a psychiatrist. At her first appointment, he prescribed Stelazine and Thorazine, two heavy-hitting antipsychotic drugs. They didn't ease her turmoil. She couldn't snap out of it, as her husband and parents urged, or as her doctor preferred. Seeing little improvement, her psychiatrist recommended a hospital.[1]

Thus began a journey that would take Chamberlin to five hospitals in six months, starting with a posh private institution that had a floor for psychiatric patients, New York City's Mount Sinai Hospital, and ending at a long-term state facility for indefinite involuntary patient care and basic research, Rockland State Psychiatric Institute.

Although Chamberlin had initially checked herself into Mount Sinai, grave doubts about her decision gripped her almost immediately. She wanted to talk to people, but her roommates were remote. So was her doctor, a white-coated psychiatric resident who was less available than her private psychiatrist. He prescribed different medications, which caused agitation and insomnia. With hopes for emotional relief crumbling, and with the support of her parents and husband, she left two and a half weeks later. Still, there was nothing to quell her nearly inconsolable sadness, which received an official diagnosis of depression.

She felt no better at home. Most days she stayed in bed and argued with her husband. In desperation, she went to Bellevue, part of New York City's public system, even though she'd heard it described as "a place that will take anybody," which didn't bode well. At admission, staff took her glasses, and terrifically nearsighted, she could barely see more than a few feet. Someone had to guide her "to a bed in a corridor" and told her to "lie down and go to sleep." To go to the bathroom, she groped her way through the hall, only to be returned by staff. Again she regretted her decision. All this she would later describe in her autobiography *On Our Own*.

There were two more elective hospitalizations before Chamberlin was admitted to an inpatient hospital at Rockland State Psychiatric Institute, a last stop for people diagnosed with stubborn illness. Taken involuntarily in an old school bus marked "ambulance," she was delivered to the female reception area where she undressed for a rectal examination. Authorities searched her body for identifying marks. She received a shapeless cotton dress with the initials RSH stamped across the back. She walked through dark hallways to quarters with barred windows. Terror and fear filled her. To console herself, she sat on a wooden bench, drew up her knees, put her head down, and started to cry.[2]

"Do not do that," another patient cautioned. "They will think you are depressed."[3]

Chamberlin's previous hospitalizations had left a mark, and except that this was a sixty-day involuntary commitment, it seemed little different. Doctors were glacially remote, locked doors led to other locked doors, and halls opened onto drab, colorless rooms with steel bars fitted over the windows. The drugs made her drowsy. When she tried to nap, the staff claimed she was uncooperative. By then, doubting she would ever recover, doctors had added chronic schizophrenia and catatonic schizophrenia to her diagnosis. It seemed "a death sentence," she said, and she begged them to let her "go someplace where I can get treatment." Staff discouraged her hopes of ever living outside of a hospital, attempting to convince her that Rockland would be the best place for her long-term custodial care.

Everything fed an image of the diminished person she feared she was becoming, and her fears turned into anger and resentment. Television filled the hours she spent locked in a dayroom. She hated the lack of privacy, the open toilet stalls, the public gang showers three times a week. She'd been forced to give up her watch and her clothes. Her mouth tasted like cotton balls and there wasn't even a water fountain. Isolation was robbing her of her self-esteem.

Chamberlin realized that survival required thinking strategically. Authority was wielded arbitrarily and the rules were dehumanizing, so she determined to hide her misery and challenge nothing. She had heard that "bad patients" ended up in seclusion rooms or got put onto the "worst wards." She decided to soldier through without complaining about taking pills or group therapy sessions where the therapist did all the talking. Dances and movies broke the monotony, so she went. The occasional afternoon outings with her parents seemed magical, but the mandatory fingerprinting before leaving was demeaning. Yet she couldn't object. "I became a good patient outwardly," she said, "while inside I nurtured a secret rebellion that was no less real for being hidden. . . . I gritted my teeth and told staff what they wanted to hear."[4] When the option for a more open ward came about, she dulled her response to show little emotion. That meant she was in control. "It sounds very nice," she said quietly. When she finally got to the open ward, she thought it was a misnomer. She still needed permission to use the doors.

Chamberlin had never thought of herself as particularly strong, but now she became convinced of her worthlessness. After two months, when her involuntary commitment was up, the staff suggested she stay longer. She didn't consider it a credible recommendation. After leaving Rockland, Chamberlin sought help from a psychologist who seemed horrified by her account of the ordeal.[5]

On a spring day in 1971, Chamberlin picked up a copy of New York City's counterculture weekly newspaper, the *Village Voice*. An article describing Howie Geld, founder of the Mental Patients' Liberation Party (MPLP), caught her eye. The *Voice* called MPLP a "radical lobby for the rights of the mentally incarcerated" and predicted that "sane chauvinism" would be the next cultural battleground, taking a place alongside gender equality, civil rights, and peace. If the MPLP had its way, insane pride would follow. The story announced a meeting Geld planned for June for "our brothers and sisters imprisoned in mental institutions." With a vision for self-help, and barely nineteen years old, he intended to provide alternatives to hospitals.

Geld's drive came from spending three years at Creedmoor Psychiatric Center on Long Island in the late 1960s. After hearing doctors make plans to keep him for another year of treatment, Geld jumped out of a window and escaped. It was 1968, and he was sixteen. A New York State Senate investigation would soon reveal vile and violent conditions, including overcrowding with seven thousand patients.

He spent a couple of years on the West Coast, and with his sister's help he founded the Insane Liberation Front. But he couldn't stay away from New York City. Barely nineteen in 1971, he returned and lived on the streets of the Lower East Side. "Before I went into the hospital," he later said, "I had a home. When I got out, I didn't. It's as simple as that." Street living indelibly marked his understanding of poor people and how class affected choice.[6]

Soon he would be called Howie the Harp, a moniker acknowledging his harmonica, which he learned to play from a night attendant at Creedmoor. His song, "I'm Crazy and I'm Proud," spoke to breaking out of the mold and accepting who he was, and he emphasized the refrain, "Cause I'm Crazeeee and I'm Proud." With wild golden hair and an untamed beard, he posed for pictures wide-eyed, staring into the camera, almost to mimic madness. Coming to New York City's Lower East Side, he opened the MPLP in a storefront on streets thick with smells and sounds, marijuana and music, poetry and protest, poor people, homeless people, and aging immigrants who lived next door to counterculture flower children. He was a mission-driven activist, and his mission promoted self-help.[7] "You can only be helped by a person who has the same problems you do, someone who shares in the insane experience," he said. "You can't be helped by someone merely because he studied your problem in a textbook."[8] He described himself as a rebel without a cause before his hospitalization. Three years in the hospital gave him a cause. Now, the story in the *Village Voice* was a giant opportunity to reach others. It certainly got Judi Chamberlin's attention.

On a Sunday afternoon in mid-June 1971, Chamberlin made her way to the Washington Square Methodist Church in Greenwich Village, where a couple dozen people were planning a demonstration at the Off-Broadway opening of *One Flew Over the Cuckoo's Nest*. The play, like Ken Kesey's book, depicts a tug-of-war, with staff using electroshock to control defiant patients. Chamberlin was motivated. What patients endured wasn't just on the stage, she said. "This was real."

Meanwhile, in San Francisco, Leonard Roy Frank found it inconceivable that, as a graduate of Pennsylvania's Wharton School of Business and a veteran of the US Army, he could be forced into a psychiatric hospital. Frank had come to Northern California in the early sixties by way of New York and Florida. He had been fired from one job, quit another, burned through his savings, sold his belongings, grown a beard, let his hair flow to shoulder length, and become a vegetarian. He spent a lot of time in the library. What he called a process for reviewing his life when he was living in San Francisco and unemployed for two years, his parents deemed withdrawn and bizarre behavior. They thought he was hiding from them and worried themselves sick before his father flew from New York to have Leonard committed.

Hospital doctors noted that, on admission, Frank, thirty years old, had a black beard and lived "like a beatnik."[9] He claimed secret work and wouldn't answer questions. Clinical notes described a "pre-psychotic personality"—"withdrawn, schizoid, autistic." Staff called him delusional, mostly involving food, with a tendency for religious preoccupations. Other than that, he was well groomed, neatly dressed, taller than most, and pencil thin at 144 pounds. His mother was described as overprotective and hysterical, his father as a successful businessman. And they were frantic. Nobody doubted that he should be in a hospital except for Frank himself, who refused all forms of treatment. That alone was enough to convince everybody that he needed to be there. He was diagnosed as Schizophrenic Reaction, Paranoid Type, Chronic Severe, and his doctors wanted him to "have the benefit of an adequate course of treatment to see if this illness can be helped." The course of treatment included electroshock and insulin coma therapies.

After two months, attendants noted he was amenable to reason even though he was "as paranoid as ever." A month later, they would write that he was "more spontaneous." He gained weight. But his full beard still bothered his doctor. And "his religious preoccupations remain rather steadfast." Doctors approved his request to attend Jewish services on Saturdays. Still, they were guarded: "plenty of room for pessimism, to put it mildly." They recommended more treatments to induce an insulin coma and more ECT.

Frank loathed the treatments. Over eight and a half months, at three different hospitals, he received thirty-five ECT treatments and thirty-five insulin-induced comas, none with his permission. They led to memory loss, including memories from his childhood. He suffered knowing that he had forgotten a lot, but what he never forgot were the battles in the hospital over his beard and long hair.

Frank's medical records refer to his hair twelve times. The initial assessment described a "beard, [and] piercing eyes." His progress report noted a "big black bushy beard," making him look "sloppy." Another note mentioned "long black curly hair and a full-face black beard." Spittle stuck to his beard during the insulin coma treatments, and staff claimed it was difficult to attach electrodes for ECT. Doctors wanted him to shave. No, said Frank. The hospital recruited his rabbi. No luck. Administrators worried about a lawsuit charging assault and battery if they shaved his beard without permission, so they petitioned the local district attorney for permission and the courts approved. Now they could make a plan: doctors would subdue him with a five-day schedule of ECT. The treatments would keep him confused and pliable, unable to resist them when they shaved his beard during an insulin coma treatment. After the deed had been done, they told his father that this "caused him no great amount of distress." Consistent with prevailing theories about the psychodynamics of personality, one of his doctors boasted that the intervention would "provoke anxiety and make some change in his body image."

Frank was furious. The medical staff feared suicide. Their chart notes revealed fears he would elope, a euphemism for "escape" or "run away." Thinking that the doctors were collaborating with his parents to restore their authority enraged him.

Frank left the hospital in June 1963. Although his diagnosis was unchanged, doctors marked his condition "improved" and recommended medication over "an extended period of time which may run into years." Relapse was a possibility, they said, recommending what they called supportive therapy with frequent contact—emphatically not psychoanalysis. Frank, who would become one of the most eloquent critics of forced ECT, never fully regained the memories he'd lost, despite his doctors' promises. These were among the reasons he dedicated his life to writing, organizing, and framing his personal experience as a window unto a larger evil. He would later tell the American Society of Law and Medicine that psychiatry was "masquerading as medicine and science" when he railed against forced treatment. His doctors' confidence that ECT would modify his beliefs about his diet, appearance, or beard convinced him that psychiatrists oppressed patients. He called it mind control, a tool of the state used to exact conformity, criticisms that carried the force of an unremitting rage at a humiliating and damaging hospital experience.

Of the four hundred thousand people confined to psychiatric institutions in the early 1970s, about one-third (32 percent) were diagnosed with schizophrenia, nearly one-quarter (22 percent) with alcoholism, and about one-tenth (11 percent) with depression.[10] People diagnosed with a mental illness filled one bed out of every three in community hospitals. Many left these hospitals angry, thinking that they had been robbed of agency, that their voices had been silenced, that they had been denied choice in their treatments.

Nobody expected patients to ignite a protest movement. Yet protest ripened while inpatients compared notes during group sessions, or on the wards, or on the unpaid teams doing the maintenance work in state hospitals in California, New York, Vermont, Pennsylvania, Connecticut, Ohio, and Florida. Leonard Roy Frank, Judi Chamberlin, and Howie the Harp were among those calling themselves survivors, psychiatric prisoners who had been oppressed.

In the fall of 1971, two female patients who had met at Agnews State Hospital in Northern California organized a conference for therapists: "Encountering Psychosis, or Everything You Always Wanted to Know About Madness but Were Afraid to Ask."[11] Within months they formed the Psychosis Validation Coalition "to affirm both to psychiatric patients and to the community, that the experience of psychosis is a valid one." Toward that aim, they published an eight-page newsletter, *Madness Network News*, which they distributed to patients, former patients, and sympathetic hospital workers. In the coming decade, *Madness Network News* would become the voice of protest and an affirmation of community, studded with humor, satire, news, and the politics of the mental patients' liberation movement.[12]

Counterculture newspapers flourished wherever activists lived during the signature days of 1960s protests. *Madness Network News*, whose motto was "All the fits that's news to print," took root in the Bay Area, already home to the *San Francisco Oracle*, *Good Times*, and the *Berkeley Barb*. Surviving on shoestring budgets and volunteers, these counterculture papers—with their bold cartoons and dizzying psychedelic art—celebrated guerrilla theater, alternative lifestyles, and the overthrow of the ruling class.

Leonard Roy Frank volunteered for *Madness Network News*. Nearly every issue included something he had written: a book review, an editorial, an interview with one of psychiatry's critics. It became an opportunity to feature people such as Thomas Szasz, author of *The Myth of Mental Illness*, a psychiatrist Frank called a Freedom Fighter. Szasz was an iconoclast, both celebrated and denigrated for challenging psychiatry's premise that nonconforming behavior was an illness. He abhorred using force to send people to hospitals; he decried involuntary treatments.

In 1972, Frank invited Szasz to speak at a meeting in San Francisco of the American Association for the Abolition of Involuntary Mental Hospitalization, where he told three hundred people that mental patients were "essentially prisoners."[13] Frank loved that. Szasz called psychiatry "quackery" with "cures for which there are no diseases." Another applause line! But it was Szasz's conclusion—"Psychiatry, as we know it, can't be reformed: it must be abolished"—that carried the moment.

The next year, Frank invited another psychiatrist, Peter Breggin, whose opposition to antipsychotic medication sounded subversive. One hundred people came to San Francisco's First Congregational Church for Breggin's talk about "Psychosurgery, Psychiatry, and Nazi Germany."[14]

To rally readers, document his claims, and build a movement protesting ECT, Frank printed his hospital records in *Madness Network News*.[15] In what would become a regular column, he listed Bay Area facilities performing shock treatments. Two years later, he added sixteen names to a list of "shock doctors." Every issue added new names from Kansas or Minnesota or Massachusetts. Within five years, by 1979, the names of 350 psychiatrists appeared in *Madness Network News.*[16]

At the same time, a renewed interest in ECT was percolating in the medical community. The mechanism behind ECT was unclear. Research from Europe, based on both empirical observations and anecdotal evidence, suggested that it worked, especially for people with depression who had not responded to conventional drugs.[17] But nobody then, or even now, could explain why this was so.[18] Explanations for its success diverged widely. Psychoanalytically trained clinicians offered fanciful notions about self-preservation in the face of psychopathology or the restoration of sanity coming from the release of inner tensions. Others postulated that the sudden jolts destroyed diseased nerve cells. There was suspicion that it might damage brain tissue, but this stood alongside a hypothesis about the dubious benefits of amnesia.[19]

Portable boxes no bigger than a suitcase packaged the electroconvulsive device, making it suitable for offices or even house calls. The electricity carried a jolt between 70 and 150 volts—about the power of a 100-watt light bulb—enough to induce a seizure mimicking an epileptic fit. In the higher ranges, it could cause breathing problems, while severe muscle contractions pulled and pushed at the same time. Yet, for many, it worked when nothing else had.

Patients forced to have ECT considered it detestable. They called it zapping, brain fry, and a human rights violation. Staff didn't always provide tongue depressors or mouth guards, and they usually failed to administer muscle relaxants. In addition to broken bones and chipped teeth, patients sustained memory loss.[20] Insurance paid for ECT in private hospitals, and they ordered more episodes. How much was just right, and how much was too much, was unclear. In 1973, the Massachusetts Department of Health capped ECT to thirty-five sessions for adults and outlawed it for children under the age of sixteen.[21] Former patients thought this didn't go far enough and considered ECT torture.

Involuntary ECT inspired political action in San Francisco where, in 1974, demonstrations started on the doorsteps of the Langley Porter Neuropsychiatric Institute at the University of California. Demonstrators moved to other hospitals and attended public hearings of the San

Francisco Health Advisory Board at the behest of the Network Against Psychiatric Assault, organized by Frank. He brought a platoon of survivors to witness and record the hearings. Former patients spoke, and a guerrilla theater group, Proud Paranoids, performed.[22] A couple of psychiatrists went on record opposing ECT. It was "overused by most practitioners," said one. It just so happened that a team from Washington's Mental Health Law Project, which filed lawsuits for class-action cases, was consulting with California lawyers about constitutional protections for people with mental health conditions. Naturally Frank interviewed one of them for *Madness Network News*.[23]

In the fall of 1974, a liberal California assemblyman, John Vasconcellos of Santa Clara, introduced a bill restricting involuntary ECT. To the surprise of many, it passed. Alarmed psychiatrists went into a tailspin. They feared for their prestige, their image, and, potentially, their medical independence. Were $10,000 fines and a possible loss of license government overreach? What was next? Vasectomy? Tonsillectomy?[24] The pressure mounted for an entire year until the legislature rescinded the law.[25] By February 5, 1975, California's controversy reached a national audience on the pages of the American Psychiatric Association's newsletter, *Psychiatric News*.

Psychiatrists were keenly aware of lawsuits and grumblings from former patients.[26] Polemics and zeal infused discussions about ECT and respect for a patient's voice. But the American Psychiatric Association could not remain mute while clashing professional opinions spilled into public view. Where did patient well-being fit in this dilemma? Between 1974 and 1976, the association surveyed a sample of its twenty thousand members, asking about ECT's effectiveness, benefits, and long-term consequences, including adverse effects.[27] This was more than a public relations exercise, and the survey results were unambiguous. Roughly two-thirds of the sample reported favorable opinions about the benefits of ECT; nearly three-quarters thought it was "the safest, least expensive, and most effective form of treatment." Fully 87 percent doubted that medications made ECT obsolete. At the same time there was broad support for more explicit guidelines surrounding its use. Based on its survey, the American Psychiatric Association concluded that ECT was more beneficial than not.[28]

The APA's decision, however, did not satisfy Leonard Frank. He continued his campaign challenging ECT's efficacy and the injustice of involuntary treatments.

Activists saw force of any kind as a power play. That was as true of drugs as it was of ECT. Forcing patients to take drugs involuntarily diminished and infantilized them, and created a battleground over choice and dignity.[29] In psychiatric hospitals, when staff detected that patients had "cheeked"— hadn't swallowed—their Thorazine, nurses could force-feed them. Liquid burning down your throat seemed another form of torture. Defiant patients were also hit with "snowing," getting a shot with three or four times more than the prescribed dose, or "sheeting," constraining patients by tying them up like mummies.[30]

Heavy doses of drugs led to uncontrollable twitches, with muscles jerking and pulling at the same time. It created a loathsome feeling that one's body was in combat with itself. Phenothiazines—a class of heavy tranquilizers—stiffened muscles. A contemporary documentary, *Hurry Tomorrow*, filmed on the ward of a Los Angeles hospital, portrayed how a grown man was felled by one shot of medicine in the butt. A psychiatrist writing for *Madness Network News*, under the pseudonym Dr. Caligari, explained the side effects of commonly prescribed psychiatric drugs—Thorazine, Haldol, Mellaril, Stelazine, Elavil—and how they led to varying degrees of insomnia, weakness, dizziness, vertigo, headaches, excessive perspiration, agitation, mania, low blood pressure, difficulty urinating, and blurred vision. Other side effects included anxiety, dry mouth, restlessness, a rolling or protruding tongue, smacking, chewing, or pouting. Jerky muscular movements, called tardive dyskinesia, or TD, could be irreversible.

While side effects appeared in early clinical experiments, psychiatrists considered them less urgent than hammering symptoms. Delusions and hallucinations were the most conspicuous, but others included so-called symptoms of defiance or disagreeableness like Leonard Frank's. Proof that the drug worked could be seen in TD's shuffle or stiffness, akin to people with Parkinson's disease. Activist ex-patients hated them. Was there any better evidence of oppression than being subjected to a dangerous drug ostensibly "for their own good"?[31]

The most pernicious of all unwanted interventions was psychosurgery, a practice that included excising brain tissue, targeting ultrasound at specific areas, or implanting electrodes.[32] Most psychiatrists considered psychosurgery fringe, but some doctors—and they got a disproportionate share of the attention—said it was acceptable for treating "maladaptive" behavior such as political protest, urban riots, and violent assaults including rape.

After Detroit burnt itself into a heap during a summer of racial strife in 1967, three doctors in Boston claimed rioters had pathological irregularities and abnormal brains. They asserted that a "brain dysfunction related to a focal lesion plays a significant role in the violent and assaultive behavior of thoroughly studied patients."[33] Their letter to the editor, which appeared in the *Journal of the American Medical Association*, presaged a growing controversy about operating on the brains of prison inmates. In the fall of 1971, California's head of the Department of Corrections, Raymond Procunier, sought Federal Safe Streets Acts funds through the California Council of Criminal Justice to implement brain surgery to alter the personality of violent prisoners. The request was denied at the end of the year, but it opened a news peg for a rash of stories starting in 1972.[34] The *Los Angeles Times* headlined a story, "A Convict's Brain: Is It Really His Own?" The *Christian Science Monitor* pointed to a "deepening moral crisis." The *Washington Post* described operations on convicts in California. Some called it the "Clockwork Orange Approach," alluding to the Stanley Kubrick film that dramatized the use of aversion therapy to punish prisoners into compliance. Soon came reports about sixteen psychosurgeries at VA hospitals, leading Senator Edward "Ted" Kennedy to call for hearings. Writing for the *New York Times*, Jane Brody said that a Michigan court had denied a patient's request for psychosurgery in exchange for release of his involuntary confinement. Brody reported that about five hundred psychosurgeries were conducted annually.

Psychosurgery had once seemed a bad joke touching on civil rights violations, medical ethics, and Eighth Amendment constitutional protections. But now psychosurgery no longer seemed conjecture or remote. In California, controversy circled UCLA's proposal for a Center for the Study and Reduction of Violence at the Neuropsychiatric Institute. *Madness Network News* pointed out how the center would focus on the "major known correlates of violence[, which] are sex (male), age (youthful), ethnicity (black), and urbanicity." It raised the specter of "social oppression, racism and neglect."[35] For an odd bedfellows twist, political dissidents in the Black Panther Party aligned temporarily with psychiatry's opponents in the Church of Scientology to oppose the center.[36] Governor Reagan, who had initially taken pride in the funding partnership with the federal government for this first-of-a-kind center, let it go.

Psychiatrist Peter Breggin attempted a wake-up call about the dangers of brain surgery in a public lecture in Washington, DC. He failed to propel outrage and asked Congressman Cornelius Gallagher (D-NJ) to insert his remarks into the *Congressional Record*, which Gallagher did in the spring of 1972, shortly before he was indicted for tax evasion and perjury.[37]

When the American Psychiatric Institute devoted a morning session of its 1973 meeting in Los Angeles to discussing brain surgery for behavior disorders, about fifty people protested outside the Century City hotel.[38] Could it ever be justifiable to operate on a person's brain to change someone's behavior? The question was rooted in the presumption that mental illness was an organic disease that could be treated, despite how little was truly known about the brain at the time. Lobotomy, a heinous procedure in which an ice pick was inserted behind a person's eye socket to sever the frontal lobe, had already been discredited, and its horrifying image lingered.[39] What about amygdalotomy to destroy tissue in the part of the brain influencing social behavior and emotions?[40] Or cingulotomy to tame anger and aggression by creating lesions on the cingulate cortex in those diagnosed with an obsessive-compulsive disorder? Was any alteration of brain tissue using a scalpel, electricity, or radiation merely a laundered lobotomy?[41] These procedures affected real lives, often irreversibly and traumatically. In 1973, Oregon required an independent board to review a clinician's petition for psychosurgery.[42]

What alarmed Leonard Frank, and other former patients, was using psychosurgery as an instrument to control behavior. To them it was illicit and political. Their suspicions were confirmed when Senate hearings revealed that the CIA was implicated in a quarter century of secret drug experiments.[43] On the heels of a federal commission's refusal to repudiate psychosurgery for research purposes, *Madness* staff writer Tanya Temkin wrote a blistering critique, assailing political expediency and repression. No safeguards, she said—whether institutional reviews, benevolent concern, or surgical refinements—disguised such visible threats to patients' rights.[44]

Su and Dennis Budd met when each was an inpatient at Yale New Haven Hospital in the 1960s, and their respective experiences turned them into activists. Dennis's awakening began his first night on a twelve-person ward when another patient kept yelling, "I'm gonna kill 'em. I'm gonna kill 'em. I'm gonna kill 'em." To manage him, staff ordered ECT. On that and subsequent nights Dennis saw a new personality emerge in that man. He had no memory. Su thought he seemed down for weeks. She asked herself, "Is he really better off than he was before?"[45]

Su and Dennis married, over the objections of the floor's nurses. They eventually moved to Kansas so Su could keep her job running the immunoassay lab for her boss, a pediatric endocrinologist. Shortly after settling in Kansas, they heard about a group called Freedom in Mental Health. A protest was afoot challenging the hospitalization of a white student who was involuntarily committed because she was dating a Black student at Kansas University. The following year, they attended a conference in Detroit organized by a psychologist at Northfield State Hospital to discuss human rights and psychiatric oppression. There they met Howie the Harp, who had helped plan the event.

Driving east for the Christmas holidays, Su and Dennis stopped in New York City to catch up with Howie, who was organizing former patients for a self-help coalition. On that visit they discussed having another conference on human rights and psychiatric oppression. They aimed for Topeka, Kansas, which called itself "The Psychiatric Capital of the World" and was home to the world-renowned psychiatric training center and hospital, the Menninger Clinic. This would become the Second Annual North American Conference on Human Rights and Psychiatric Oppression. Aiming for ex-patients who self-disclosed and were seeking mutual support and affiliation, Dennis wrote the flyer, inviting people who believed, as they did, that "psychiatry must no longer have the power to force incarceration and 'treatment' on unwilling victims." They wanted to engage people who agreed with the proposition that "the psychiatric power to oppress in the name of mental health threatens the civil liberties of every citizen."[46]

Organizers expected about a hundred people (professionals, students, and former patients) for the Labor Day weekend, which turned out to be beset by sudden fog, rain, and wind. Howie arrived first; Judi Chamberlin and her soon-to-be-husband, Ted Chabasinski, followed. Leonard Frank came from San Francisco. Already in Kansas, the Budds had but a short commute from Lawrence to Topeka.

Organizers chose the Forest Park Campground of the United Methodist Church to host the conference. Detroit's meeting had taken place at a swank hotel with red-velvet wallpaper and white tablecloths, and it had hurt both their pocketbooks and their message.[47] Participants believed that every gesture—where people met, what they wore, what they called themselves—mattered. Howie was a roll-up-your-sleeves kind of guy, and his ethical imperatives demanded that nobody sit at the head of a table or wear a jacket. He frowned on the university students whom the Budds had recruited to volunteer. It should be *us* doing this, not *them*, he insisted. Judi agreed. She wanted former patients only. She had overlooked, if she had ever known, the fact that students and professionals had started the organization Freedom in Mental Health.

These were not the only tensions. Su and Dennis wanted to democratically decide breakout sessions. Judi thought that empowered the few professionals who were present. They also clashed about which symbols best conveyed the movement. Su wanted a tethered horse fighting to be free; Judi preferred a clenched fist. Through it all Leonard Frank kept to himself until they discussed terminology, at which time he perked up and insisted that they call themselves inmates. Don't accept a brainwashed psychiatric label, he said, or behave like "victims of the shrinks and the whole mental health system."[48]

———————

While plans were underway for Topeka's conference, a newly minted lawyer in Philadelphia, David Ferleger, was filing briefs on behalf of inpatients at Haverford State Hospital whose forced labor violated the Thirteenth Amendment's prohibition of involuntary servitude. Waiting for the court's decision in this case, he went to Kansas.

Civil rights activism and social justice filled his soul. As the son of Polish Holocaust survivors, he knew that people with disabilities were among the first victims of Nazi eugenics campaigns. He was an undergraduate at the University of Pennsylvania during the heyday of student protest and felt at home at demonstrations and protests. Once, for an entire week, he waged a solo protest sitting in the president's office to call attention to the secret germ warfare research on campus. An elective he took during his last year of law school in 1972, "Asylums and Jails," was co-taught by a forensic psychiatrist and a law professor who introduced him to Haverford State Hospital. For that class, he observed patients on locked wards and analyzed the relevant legal issues pertaining to their treatments and their rights.

Haverford State Hospital was a relatively new facility located in a Philadelphia suburb. Reasonably clean and well staffed, including with many psychiatrists, it had six hundred beds, private rooms, a bowling alley, a gymnasium, a soda fountain, and a library. The six-story brick building with a circular drive resembled a hotel and was offhandedly called the Haverford Hilton.

Practices inside the contemporary building were less modern. Haverford patients were locked out of their rooms during the day, a theoretical holdover promoting engagement to discourage inertia. They were assigned a work routine up to five hours a day, which expected them to landscape, repair furniture or outdoor benches, sew rags, deliver messages, sell food in the snack bar, launder, operate elevators, staff the mail room, cook, and wash dishes, cars, and floors. They also did chores for which employees would have been paid. Ferleger estimated that in this way patients saved the state between $33 million and $44 million. Civil rights were curtailed. Fresh air or telephone calls were privileges. Staff censored incoming and outgoing mail, used mechanical punishments, and were quick, Ferleger would say, to put a "needle in the ass" of patients who refused oral medication. Ferleger wrote, "Patients' concern about what is being done to them and under what authority is very real." He turned this project into a law review article, "Loosing the Chains: In-Hospital Civil Liberties of Mental Patients," which was an unprecedented analysis of patients' rights inside hospitals.[49]

When he graduated, he opened an office in Center City Philadelphia for his newly founded Mental Patients Civil Liberties Project. Two grants, a total of $10,000, supported him. With a door from a lumber yard, which he placed over two sawhorses, he had a desk. With a borrowed electric typewriter, he had office equipment. And with a passion for overturning the hardships patients endured, especially the loss of liberties, he negotiated an agreement with Pennsylvania to become an in-house ombudsman at Haverford.

Haverford's superintendent appreciated Ferleger's desire to help individual patients who had legal issues, mostly around commitment hearings. Supervising a team of twenty law students and a couple of interns from Temple University, he became a safety valve for the hospital, fielding patient complaints and monitoring relationships. Housing the team in an office between the morgue and the loading dock, between the dead and the garbage, was telling.[50] The hospital considered them irrelevant, something that shielded them while they gathered facts to document unconstitutional work practices. In 1973, Ferleger filed *Downs v. Department of Public Welfare*, a class-action lawsuit charging peonage, a violation of the Thirteenth Amendment's ban on involuntary servitude. After Ferleger started filing lawsuits, the state canceled the arrangement and the hospital locked them out. *Downs* was heard by Judge Clifford Scott Green, an African American judge known for promoting civil rights, in US District Court for the Eastern Pennsylvania District.

Green's decision, which he handed down in December, ruled that the work had been coercive and not therapeutic. "The source of coercion," Green wrote, "is said to be the boredom of institutional life and the belief of patients that it will be advantageous to them to appear to cooperate with the institution." Coercive action on the part of the institution included harassment, intimidation, and malice, and patients' rights had been deprived and their activities restricted when work "assignments are not performed." Saying that the Department of Public Welfare and Haverford State Hospital had violated the Eighth, Thirteenth, and Fourteenth Amendments, Green dismissed Pennsylvania's claim that the court lacked jurisdiction to hear the case.[51] When Green handed down his decision, the state, unable to pay the 6,346 patients, discharged all but roughly six hundred people.[52]

Madness Network News grew in tandem with conferences like Topeka's. Featured stories described events and parsed elements of legitimacy, a recurring concern. Should their work, including their conferences, be open to any self-proclaimed friend, or should participation be limited to people who had been hospitalized? Or only to people who had been forcibly hospitalized? Or just to those who had spent a night in the hospital?

Disagreements about authenticity threatened a movement seeking voice and the suitability of their motto, "Nothing About Us Without Us."

In 1976, former patients again met, this time in Boston, and as they had previously, they added a demonstration to their agenda. For the national bicentennial, between sixty and a hundred people marched to the Boston State Hospital, where the year before a class action lawsuit known as *Rogers v. Okin* had tested whether a competent person could make decisions about their treatment in situations short of an emergency.[53] Marching to the hospital, demonstrators carried signs rebuking psychiatry: "Therapy Is Social Control," "I Am the Expert of My Own Head," "Lobotomize Shrinks," "End Shock Treatments." It was a hot summer day, and marchers sat down in the middle of the street in front of the hospital. They read from a long list of demands: end censored communication; provide more information about drugs and shock treatments; end seclusion, restraint, physical punishment, involuntary commitment, and behavior modification. As in Topeka, they could see patients standing at the windows, gesturing and appealing for help.[54]

The fifth annual conference in 1977 took place at Griffith Park Boys Camp in Los Angeles. Participation was now limited to "ex-inmates and activists in the anti-psychiatry movement."[55] The signature demonstration marched to UCLA's Neuropsychiatric Institute, a potent symbol of the psychosurgery controversy. That year, none of the internal conflicts about who could participate, or who should represent what point of view, derailed them. Su Budd rejoiced, calling it the "rightness of our cause."[56]

———

Judi Chamberlin left Rockland Psychiatric Institute in 1967, and three years later she gave birth to a daughter. Continued marital strife and a move to Boston eventually led to a divorce with a bitterly contested custody battle in 1972 over whether she was "too mentally ill to be a fit mother."[57] Massachusetts law required a doctor's approval for former patients to see their medical or psychiatric records. The judge had them, as did her husband's lawyer, but she was denied. She was livid. The veil of professional protection became another barrier undermining autonomy for people with a psychiatric history, and she launched a test case through the newly formed

Mental Patients Legal Front (MPLF), seeking to establish the ability of former psychiatric patients to obtain their records.[58]

Again, Chamberlin was not alone. Activist Janet Gotkin, who had sought her medical records so she could write about her voluntary hospitalizations in New York, cited the First, Fourth, and Fourteenth Amendments in her failed attempts.[59] College students had access to their school records, and medical patients could see their health records. People who had received psychiatric services were disenfranchised and treated as children.

Vivacious and petite, Chamberlin packed a quick wit and a sharp tongue. She had become a respected, if contentious, spokesperson, a de facto leader in the presumably leaderless collective of former patients. She expected to weigh in on issues of the day and was furious when Massachusetts bypassed her. "We are the people locked up in DMH facilities euphemistically called hospitals," she shouted at a meeting about charging patients for their costs in state hospitals. Rather than bill poor patients for their treatment, she said, they should seek alternative placements. Sitting down, she jotted herself a note: "I testify—get lots of applause."[60]

By 1977 Chamberlin sensed she had a broader audience. Meticulous records, carbon copies of lengthy outgoing letters, and handwritten notes filled her drawers. "They don't want to pay me," she scribbled while talking to Walter Menninger, who had invited her to appear on a panel. "Really gave him a piece of my mind," she wrote. "[I] really laid a guilt trip on him. Lots of embarrassed laughter on his part."[61]

After Sally Zinman freed herself from forced treatment, she was living in Loxahatchee, Florida, helping people leave an inpatient psychiatric hospital, and she discovered *Madness Network News*. It had become the liberation movement's organizing tool, and this particular issue, Fall 1977, referenced testimony from four people—Judi Chamberlin, Tanya Temkin, Ozzie Bozarth, and Bob Harris—at First Lady Rosalynn Carter's hearings about mental health reform. Zinman was delighted to learn that other people were also advocating for patients and helping them leave hospitals. She studied every word of each person's testimony.

Each of their accounts resonated. Zinman knew the credibility of Chamberlin's assertion that services were forced on mental patients, and that they were "qualitatively different from [other] medical treatments." Tanya Temkin's discussion of coercion, and how drug therapy benefited the staff and not the patients, rang true. She could relate to Ozzie Bozarth's comparison of human rights violations in Russia with what was happening right here in America. And she recognized Bob Harris's lament about housing shortages and flophouses resegregating former patients where he lived in Philadelphia. Zinman found this thrilling and terrifying at the same time: thrilling because she realized she shared a vision with people she had never met, terrifying because *Madness Network News* would be considered quite radical where she lived near Palm Beach. She quickly tore out the pages before anybody could see how revolutionary it was.[62]

Earlier that year, Zinman had seen an ABC documentary, *Madness and Medicine*. Narrator Howard K. Smith opened the hour-long special by calling mental illnesses "the most baffling of human afflictions" and "its victims the most abused." One scene portrayed a patient rocking back and forth; another zoomed through the window of a seclusion room where leather straps restrained a man. Standing in front of a wall of bookshelves, Smith said: "Our ignorance far exceeds our knowledge." Before us, he said, was the "nagging question": "What are we trying to treat? What is mental illness?"

The documentary's sympathetic portrayal of patients captivated Zinman. Members of the Mental Patients Liberation Front discussed isolation, forced treatments, diets of bread and water, or being torn from one's parents. Should these be considered therapeutic? What about discounting patient complaints as a sign of one's illness? "What does that do to your head?" former patient Ted Chabasinski asked rhetorically.

Zinman burned to meet them. After a few phone calls she learned that there was a meeting in September—ex-patients were now holding annual conferences—this one in Los Angeles, at Griffith Park. That was where she needed to be, and she got herself and her two-year-old daughter out to California.

At Griffith Park, Zinman met Su and Dennis Budd, Leonard Frank, Judi Chamberlin, and Tanya Temkin. They, and the hundred other people at the park, were devoting themselves to helping patients get out of hospitals and build the lives they might have once they were free. All over the campground, people worked on a shared agenda. Self-determination, democracy, and participation propelled them. And now she was part of it. "I was not alone," Zinman wrote. "Everywhere I listened, I heard reverberations of myself."[63]

Judi Chamberlin, Tanya Temkin, and Sally Zinman were invited to speak at the 1978 meeting of the American Psychiatric Association. Over the last half dozen years their activism had publicly challenged orthodoxy, and they had stood outside and picketed hotels and conferences protesting psychiatry. In 1978, they would be inside the conference center where psychiatrists were meeting in Atlanta, Georgia.

Speakers at the national conventions found the demonstrators a sideshow, perhaps a nuisance, but also irrelevant. But nobody could be more relevant than they were to addressing the topic "The Patient's Perspective." NIMH psychologist Louis Kopolow, who had worked with Chamberlin on the National Committee on Patients Rights, organized the panel. She considered Kopolow a "mentalist," a term used in the movement to refer to people who accepted traditional mental health services. But she believed his views were evolving, as was evidenced by this event.[64]

Each of the panelists could speak about "the patient's experience." Only Chamberlin had already done so extensively. For nearly two years, she had traveled the nation challenging "mental healthies," another term for service providers. Days before the APA meeting she appeared at the Edna McConnell Clark Foundation, answering the question "Who Should Speak for Patients' Rights?"

The same psychiatrists they had spent years maligning would fill the audience. Excited about this, she wrote to Temkin, "I think we can really shake them up. . . . The movement's been popping up everywhere (this really scares them), and suddenly, here we are at *their* [emphasis original] convention. We should give them indigestion over their expensive dinners . . . A lovely thought. A hotel full of psychiatrists tossing and turning all night, clutching their stomachs."[65]

Psychiatrists presumed they knew, as benevolent caregivers invested in the art of treating disease, what was best for patients. That was basic to the medical model in which they had been trained. Hearing from their patients about the value of their services would be new. Yet that is how the moderator introduced Chamberlin, Zinman, and Temkin, who would introduce "points of view seldom heard at a meeting such as this—those of the consumers of mental health services."[66] These panelists weren't asking for more medical services or more psychiatric treatments. They weren't focused on helping psychiatrists do a better job. Instead, each explained her opposition to the medical model and involuntary treatments, and outlined priorities of self-determination. These were the essence of political liberation. They clarified why their own understanding of patients' needs differed from that of the professionals in the audience.

From the stage, Temkin could see many people sitting with crossed arms. It occurred to her that the audience might consider them "a freak show." She hoped that was not the case and that they had come to learn something; perhaps they would leave with a better understanding of the former patient's point of view.[67] She couldn't tell. One news account reported, "Psychiatrists Listen to Mental Health Consumers."[68] But neither Chamberlin nor Temkin nor Zinman could be sure how much they had heard—or learned.

To be sure, not all patients became activists in the liberation movement. Not everybody wanted to upend psychiatry or change the mental health system. Not all left hospitals angry. Some had been institutionalized for so many years that they had lost hope and accepted their lot; others had grown old, lost mental capacity, or become demented. Still others believed that they had benefited from the sanctuary to heal and to rest. And many wanted to just put it all behind them, quietly slip back into life's envelope without calling attention to their ordeals. Political activists were different. Intolerant of what they had experienced, they set out to reform it. They were creating alternative services to the hospitals from which they had escaped or fled. They were championing former patients not as victims, not as subjects, but as essential voices in planning and leading a human liberation movement.

CHAPTER 3

BUILDING OPPORTUNITIES FOR COMMUNITY CARE

W HILE JUDI CHAMBERLIN WAS checking out of hospitals in New York, and while Art Bolton was investigating them in California, Mary Ann Test was finishing graduate school at Northwestern University, where she was studying to become a psychologist. And she had doubts about the field she was entering. Rorschach inkblot tests absorbed psychologists interested in personality, emotions, or patterns of thought, and psycho-analytic dogma consumed psychiatrists where she interned at a private hospital in Chicago. How did either of these approaches help people like the patient she'd met at a VA hospital in Heinz, Illinois, who had partially destroyed his face with a self-inflicted gunshot wound?[1]

Test was fiercely independent, a Quaker, and a quiet rebel. Initially, she had hoped political action would bring peace to the world, but she decided to content herself with using psychology to bring peace to individuals. Her single-mindedness and strong will dated from childhood. She had aspired to become a professional baseball player, and her father had built her a pitching mound in the backyard. After school, she would go outside, stand on the mound, and throw to her brother. Had the Little League's governing body not reversed a local decision granting her a uniform, she might have gotten closer to her goal. But these options were closed to girls in the 1950s. By the time she was ready to attend college, she chose Gettysburg, declining the more prestigious Swarthmore because it lacked an intercollegiate sports program. In 1966, in her early twenties,

with one last clinical internship needed to fulfill Northwestern's requirements for a doctorate, an ad for Denver's Fort Logan Mental Health Center caught her eye. Knowing that Fort Logan was considered "the most
progressive mental health center in the country," Test, a tall, slim student
with blunt-cut straight blond hair, hopped into her red Ford Falcon and
headed to Colorado.

Fort Logan was exploring a treatment model that differed from the
conventional hospital-based methods. Paul Polak, the head psychiatrist,
doubted that hospitals were needed, even for a crisis. Unlike the standard
treatments, which kept patients on high doses of heavy tranquilizers for
weeks or months, he tapered them quickly, perhaps after a few days. With
this in mind, he developed a system he called a "foster-family network"
of local community residents who would work with neighbors, friends, or
family in crisis and divert them from hospitals. The network helped even
grossly symptomatic patients and minimized the need for inpatient hospital beds for Denver's nine hundred thousand residents.[2]

When Denver demanded Fort Logan build a conventional brick-and-
mortar hospital for acute or emergency care, it could have ended Polak's experiment. Instead, they settled on a design that could have been
mistaken for a motel—low-slung buildings, large windows, and an open
courtyard. This would be an open hospital, similar to innovations in
Great Britain.[3]

Test loved what she found in Denver. Unlike treatments she'd seen in
previous internships, Fort Logan offered activities anybody would want to
join. Patients and staff played volleyball, picnicked, and hiked in Colorado's mountains. They softened boundaries and muted hierarchy based on
professional training. Mirroring recommendations from Maxwell Jones,
author of *The Therapeutic Community* (1953), Fort Logan's programs aimed
to return patients rapidly to living in the community. When Polak, who
had studied with him, brought Jones to "the Fort," Test was awestruck. She
told me she knew then that this was the kind of place where she wanted to
work when she graduated in 1969.

Test began her career at a time of fertile thinking. For at least fifteen years,
the circle around Robert Felix at NIMH had been weighing how to sup-

port projects building local services.[4] He had worked with a private foundation, Milbank Memorial Fund, to rethink challenges brought on by the pace of change in urban environments. That led the fund to sponsor a research project about the mental health of social groups in New York City, "Midtown Manhattan," in the 1950s.[5] To understand why people called mental health agencies for help, the fund underwrote a project to learn what they asked for.[6]

Projects like these would be essential for a public health campaign to build a mental health workforce, for which Felix sought congressional funding. Scattered yet tangible results began appearing in the 1950s. In Massachusetts, the city of Quincy developed "reaching-out services" to help people in a crisis.[7] Florida created the "mental health worker," a new paraprofessional. Iowa and Missouri considered foster home care services. New York was already operating a day treatment program in the Bronx.[8] By 1959, NIMH counted at least 1,400 of these outpatient clinics.[9]

Felix saw these diverse programs as harbingers of something new.[10] "We were never going to get anywhere if we just continued to take care of the patients in the hospitals. No matter how well we did it," he said. "We had to do something else."[11] Part of that "something else" would be outpatient services in local communities. If they were to work as Felix expected, he needed statistics to prove their worth. Psychiatry would need to evaluate what they were doing by building programs and developing services. None of this mattered when the practice of psychiatry was organized around a typical session treating patients in a fifty-minute psychoanalytic hour.

How to move systems became the topic of the Milbank Memorial Fund's annual conference in 1965. It was the fund's ninth on mental health; Dr. Bertram "Bert" Brown, a Felix protégé, organized the event. Brown had already finished writing regulations for JFK's signature Community Mental Health Act, and he was prepared to consider what was needed for "Evaluating the Effectiveness of Mental Health Services."[12] Brown convened twenty-seven of the world's experts. Four came from England, three from Scotland, and one each from Colombia and Switzerland, joining their American colleagues at the posh Savoy-Plaza Hotel in New York City for three days. This conference represented an opportunity to explore ideas about research and services, and to map a future they hoped would make custodial care obsolete.

Some of the demand for new thinking responded to the fact that hospitals were letting people out. Of those attempting to move patients into the community, the work of psychiatrists Arnold Marx and Arnold Ludwig at Mendota State Hospital in Madison, Wisconsin, stood out. They had been experimenting and had written about their transition program readying long-term patients for discharge. They were looking for a research associate, and Mary Ann Test was looking for a job and arranged for an interview.

A century after Mendota State Hospital had been built on the site of sacred Indian mounds, it had grown into a five-story building with portal windows and a commanding view of its namesake, Lake Mendota. But Marx and Ludwig worked in a single-story dilapidated clapboard structure with a locked patient research ward and walls painted purple, pink, and green. That was Building 2, where Mary Ann Test had come to interview with Marx. Throughout their conversation in his tiny office, he tossed a tennis ball while smoking a cigar. Somehow, she thought to herself, "this is my kind of place."[13] He must have felt the same because he hired her straight out of graduate school to become the associate director of the Chronic Schizophrenia Research Center.

Test joined Building 2's Special Treatment Unit (STU), which Marx and Ludwig had built to break a cycle of keeping people in the hospital so long they became chronic patients. They were careful observers of behavior, anthropologists of a sort, examining how institutions shaped someone's expectations and routines. Ludwig had already coauthored "The Code of Chronicity,"[14] about inpatient ward culture. Within the closed quarters, staff rewarded docile patients and punished aggression, especially in patients using provocative language or overtly sexual behavior. Patients attending group meetings, no matter how useless, were frequently allowed to run an errand or deliver a message. Patients who worked on the grounds, or those who snitched, earned extra time to smoke or have a cup of coffee. Some patients worked a back channel outside the staff's purview where they cultivated companionship and affection, or developed a social economy based on trading money, books, or cigarettes. The so-called chronic patients even developed something called "insanity by convenience" to thwart a system they could not otherwise influence.[15]

Could patients refashion these behaviors, which demonstrated a mastery of their surroundings, to manage outside of a hospital?[16] Could the STU teach them different strategies even if they had already been hospitalized up to thirty-six months? Beyond that they were considered "treatment failures" and there was little hope for them.

It was worth a try. Ludwig and Marx taught work habits to STU patients, taught them how to manage their symptoms, and helped them develop face-to-face interactions.[17] Physical activities and taking medicine became obligatory at the STU, as did participation in team and group activities.[18] It took at least six months for changes to emerge. But when they did, and someone was discharged, the staff threw itself a party to celebrate.[19] The formula for leaving hospitals seemed to be working.

Success on the inpatient unit didn't necessarily lead to success in the community, and even the most well-prepared patients had difficulty sustaining themselves. Many returned with florid psychotic symptoms. And as they did, staff morale deteriorated and disillusionment set in.[20] The one exception were the clients of one particular social worker, Barb Lontz. Test and Leonard Stein, who had replaced Marx, needed to know why the patients discharged to her supervision almost never returned.

Lontz worked differently. When a patient was discharged, she accompanied that person into the community. She helped them search for an apartment. It could be a boardinghouse or the local Y, and once they'd decided, she helped them shop for sheets and then taught them how to make a bed. She partnered with each at the local laundromat where they separated clothes by color, used the coin machines, and measured the detergent. She rode the bus with clients to get their medication at the pharmacy, and she went as many times as she was needed. She sat with anybody attending a sheltered workshop, a protected environment for people with disabilities developing social and job-related skills, and returned as many times as necessary. She gave out her home telephone number for afterhour emergencies. And if patients needed her, she went to them.

Lontz's work was unmatched. That was the good news. But it also underscored that the STU had not succeeded. It wasn't enough to hand a discharged person a list of follow-up addresses with phone numbers for follow-up services. National statistics on community adjustment were uniformly discouraging.[21] As many as 40 percent of the patients from conventional hospital programs returned within six months, half within a year, and three-quarters in three to five years.[22] The best results came from Fort Logan, but even there one person in five had difficulty with community living.[23] A few of the experimental housing programs such as the Fairweather Community Lodges Program in Palo Alto, California,[24] or the psychiatric rehab club programs such as Fountain House in New York, had better results. Fountain House offered a unique job-training program and opportunities for stable housing.[25]

Working with discharged patients in the community, not in a hospital's classroom, led to better outcomes. Test and Stein redesigned Building 2's research. They now asked what helped people after leaving a hospital. They followed sixty patients. One group of thirty received the STU's hospital-based preparation; the other was discharged without preparation but received real-time support in the community.[26] The results showed that teaching patients about managing symptoms, about life, mattered less than continuing to support them in real time.

Test and Stein revised their program again in 1970.[27] Instead of discharging patients with a list of instructions about scheduling appointments, staff needed to understand life on the streets where they would need to mediate common real-world problems: lost keys, lost clients, poor meals, drug use, crummy housing, annoying roommates, vengeful landlords, panhandling, toothaches, the wrong bus, the right bus but the wrong stop, lack of confidence, few incentives, inertia, dependency, a sheltered workshop, fears of failure, forgotten medication, or a family's uncertainty about what to do in a crisis.[28] Some patients got overwhelmed; others became discouraged. Two attempted suicide. Stigma clobbered them in public. No amount of preparation could fully anticipate the challenges. The team, like the patients, had a steep learning curve.

Staff closed Building 2 in 1972 and moved their offices to a refurbished house in the center of Madison. Each day, the eighteen-person treatment team—doctors, social workers, psychologist, nurses, and aides—met to review each client's progress. When a person needed help to manage stress or anxiety, at work or at home, the whole staff knew about it. Round-the-clock services meant anybody on the team could, and often did, step in. Staff measured client outcomes and discovered that in two years, only 10 percent had to be readmitted.[29] This number compared favorably to the more than half (54 percent) of all hospital admissions nationwide that were returning patients.[30] The results convinced Test and Stein they were doing something right. They renamed their project the Program in Assertive Community Treatment, or PACT.

Staff also worked with families to strengthen their coping skills. While their recovering relatives developed new roles, parents would focus on letting go of guilt. Test and Stein frowned on patients living at home. It interfered with independence. Instead, it would be up to the staff to help. One mother remembered the moment PACT told her, "We take over." That put an end to the *what if* questions keeping her awake at night—questions about safety and symptoms, medication and services.[31] It was magical, she said. "My whole world turned around."

Sue Estroff, a medical anthropologist, described PACT's first patients in a book titled *Making It Crazy*.[32] Estroff notes that Madison, in addition to being the state capital, was also home to a university, making for an unusually rich mix of part-time jobs, training and retraining employment programs, and social service benefits offices. Discharged patients shopped locally, met for coffee in the local diner, and lodged in halfway houses, the local YMCA, or apartments near the university's student ghettos.[33] Housing was essential for getting started with independence, but many people remained alone to the point of isolation. Even though they were learning to "manage the details of daily living" and may have been in the community, they were not *of* the community.

Test summarized this phase of her work by saying it was time to focus on achieving mental health rather than treating illness. In 1974, the American Psychiatric Association (APA) awarded its prestigious Gold Award to the Mendota Mental Health Institute for its contributions to "enhance community adjustment, to decrease time spent in institutions, and to prevent the development of the chronic patient role."[34]

After PACT was recognized, Test and Stein traveled like missionaries enlisting kindred spirits and challenging conventional ideas. For Test, it was the fruition of ideas that were planted when she worked at Fort Logan, ideas about how to structure practical support to help someone leave a hospital environment. Just as she was seeing success in Wisconsin, political bickering and a budget crisis in Colorado threatened Fort Logan, making it impossible to sustain its unique authority. In what reads like an obituary, in 1975, the Fort's director, Dr. Ethel M. Bonn, wrote: "If Fort

Logan has accomplished anything at all in its brief existence, it has provided abundant evidence that there is a practical and viable alternative to the classical state hospital."[35] Test's work affirmed that missive.

———————

By the 1970s, it was apparent that the transition to community services had been stalled and leaders at NIMH were itching for change. Federal belt-tightening for NIMH programs had started when President Lyndon Johnson diverted funds to pay for the Vietnam War. Mental health funding also suffered when Richard Nixon impounded congressional allocations, and Gerald Ford subsequently used his veto power vigorously to keep federal spending under control. In a triumphal moment, Congress overrode one of his five vetoes to affirm an expansion of the community mental health centers.[36] Still, a somber mood hugged NIMH after Felix's departure in 1967, and it tightened throughout Stanley Yolles's three years as director. His successor, Bert Brown, opened staff meetings by announcing who had resigned or departed, and who was working in an "acting" capacity.[37]

Lucy Ozarin, another of Felix's protégés, had also become a senior member of the NIMH staff. Unadorned and independent, her spunky style had served her well after graduating from New York Medical College in 1937 and then going on to Harlem Hospital for a two-year residency. The country was still struggling through the Great Depression, and she needed an income only hospitals guaranteed. What would it be: a tuberculosis sanitarium or a psychiatric hospital? People with mental illness were less "catching," she told me, making her decision easy. She went off to Gowanda State Hospital in upstate New York, and after World War II drew the male doctors into service, she became the only psychiatrist for one thousand women patients. Seeing the swollen ankles of the women who sat all day in straitjackets disturbed her. Get them "dancing, prancing, and moving," she told the staff, and requisitioned a record player. When women were allowed to enlist in the service after 1943, she joined the navy and became a lieutenant commander.

Ozarin didn't see herself as a trailblazer even though only two other women psychiatrists became Waves. She saw herself as the Brooklyn-born daughter of poor Jewish immigrants fulfilling her patriotic duty and copying her brother. After the war, she took a job at the Veterans Administration (VA) and discovered that half the men diagnosed with schizophrenia had been hospitalized for between five and ten years. Why? she asked. Discovering the VA's obsolete practices led her to urge changes. Later, she embraced Felix's mission to expand community treatment, and he asked her to work with Bert Brown and turn the vision—and JFK's reform legacy—into practical information guiding implementation of community mental health centers.

Because she had visited 245 centers, she saw the problems alongside the promise. Not enough of them had built clinical staff or retooled services. And politics trimmed NIMH budgets, putting these goals at risk. Budget constraints started when LBJ had to pay for the Vietnam War. Then Nixon wanted to manage inflation and Ford intended to control federal spending.

Although Ozarin was impatient, cautious optimism infused the annual psychiatry meetings in San Francisco in May 1970, where speakers complimented the CMHC initiatives for people addicted to alcohol and street drugs. The school-based initiatives for youngsters and their success keeping people out of hospitals also earned praise. Centers in Philadelphia and San Francisco had built consortia bridging voluntary hospitals with the various service agencies, residential options, rehabilitation programs, and suicide prevention initiatives. Too many CMHCs hadn't provided care for people who were poor and needed access to continuous services. "A center that does not address itself to the mental health needs of the residents of its community is not fulfilling its mission," she said. People with the fewest resources and the least access needed the most help, and she believed middle-class citizens or the local power elite could turn elsewhere for help.

The transition from hospitals to community services seemed to have stalled by 1974. Only 660 centers, barely one-third of the goal, had been built. Despite the number of inpatient beds, which were down to about 220,000 from the all-time high of 550,000 in the 1950s, states still spent up to 80 percent of their mental health budgets on maintenance and staffing the oversized campuses. At the same time, $540 million earmarked for community services sat unused. The failures would soon lead homeless people to gather on street corners, at bridge underpasses, and in tunnels, fields, parks, train stations, bus terminals, and the lobbies of buildings, public and private. Many of the practical questions affecting patients—Where would they live? Where would their meals come from? Who would renew their medical prescriptions?—got submerged in the bureaucracies of the CMHCs.

Ozarin had not anticipated this. Nobody had. Believing she had no time to waste, and staring at mandatory retirement in just five years, she invited a cluster of NIMH staff psychiatrists, sociologists, and psychologists to brainstorm solutions. About twenty people accepted Ozarin's call. There was Frank Ochberg, her boss, a Stanford-trained psychiatrist who headed the institute's Mental Health Services division. There was Sam Keith, a psychiatrist in the schizophrenia bureau. He had come to NIMH fresh out of training at Emory University and was quickly earning a favorable reputation from the families he was meeting. And there was Saul Feldman, a psychologist who, in addition to organizing continuing staff education at NIMH, was in the office overseeing CMHCs. The group needed direction, and by year's end, Ozarin had begun to explore rehabilitation programs to learn how they assisted people leaving hospitals.[38] That's when she met Judy Turner at Federal Rehabilitation Services. She had a quick smile, infectious energy, and a willingness to experiment, all qualities Ozarin found compelling enough to hire her to organize the ad hoc group's work.[39]

Coming on board, Turner was struck that NIMH was working from an oversimplified dichotomy: "If hospitals are bad, then the community is good." The CMHCs had proven success reducing hospital populations: Kentucky's dropped by nearly 50 percent.[40] But they had not succeeded when it came to community living, where discharged patients found life more complicated. She attended the American Psychiatric Association meetings in May 1975, accompanied by Ozarin and Keith, where community-oriented practitioners spent three days discussing the challenges for patients who had been discharged without adequate planning and without a system for community services.[41] That same year, NIMH announced on the pages of *Schizophrenia Bulletin*, a journal it published, that a new group would work on this need, now associated with closing hospitals and called "deinstitutionalization." No federal agency had singular responsibility, but the Work Group on Community Support would identify programs and coordinate and build interagency liaisons. That would be where to start.

NIMH didn't directly fund services, but it did underwrite grants to states and agencies, and she had a list of questions to work from: Where should services be set up? What help did people need when they left a hospital? What was the right balance of services for any single individual? And for how long? Months, years, indefinitely?[42]

To get a better understanding of what already existed, Turner contacted Harry Schnibbe, the founder and executive director of the National Association of State Mental Health Program Directors (NASMHPD). If ever there was an organization ready to lobby for mental health, it was NASMHPD, and Turner was wise to seek him out. But their first meeting was a disaster, according to his deputy Anne McCuan, the in-house expert about how states used Medicaid and Medicare funds.

"Judy arrived with her typical enthusiasm," McCuan recalled. She was going to "put a Fountain House in every city, where people were turning up without homes or families or anything to help them when they left a hospital."[43]

Schnibbe and McCuan thought Turner naive. Nonprofits perpetually struggled to make their budgets, and she was talking about changing the world with bootstrap, grassroots, independent operations. "Oh God, who brought this lady in?" they asked. "She doesn't get it."

But Turner had different ideas. Hers came from a rehabilitation model that presumed people with physical disabilities could get better in communities if they had support and resources. Where were the wheelchairs or crutches for people with mental illness? She asked herself, "Why am I meeting with these people? They don't get it."[44]

When McCuan accepted a job at NIMH the next year, she and Turner renewed their conversation. They met at a local greasy spoon for lunch, bypassing the cafeteria's bastion of male researchers and administrators, and talked about their mutual interests. Little by little—a job promotion for McCuan; hiring a deputy, Bill TenHoor, for Turner; and conversations with the work group—they crafted a strategy helping states develop community services.

By now, as director of NIMH, Bert Brown had expanded social science research. Much of it aligned with one of Felix's original ambitions to address addiction, crime, racism, and the challenges faced by children, especially urban kids. As Brown would later say, NIMH intended to foster an "optimal service system," the best community service program the federal government could sponsor.[45] Meanwhile, his leadership set the stage for Turner's work group to meet with little fanfare, no budget, and an improvised team.

———————

Judy Turner and Mary Ann Test met in January 1976. In the two years since receiving the APA's Gold Award, Test had been on the lecture circuit and widely published in professional journals. Turner was reading everything she could before passing it on to members of her ad hoc group. Both were attempting to check into the Sheraton National Hotel in Alexandria, Virginia, for an NIMH conference, and they learned simultaneously that only one room was available. On the spot they agreed to share it, and they stayed up late into the night talking away about their work, their missions, and their dreams.[46]

This conference was Judy Turner's province, and Test was among the emerging experts NIMH had invited to speak on "current problems in community care." That January weekend, twenty-nine people, lay and professional, discussed what they needed to do to scaffold a system that would sustain services.

Turner insisted that they sharpen their framework and clarify a vocabulary they had begun to use over the last several years. Was an *advocate* an individual or an organization? Did *aftercare* require a community placement, or could it be only medication management? To become a *client*, was it necessary to receive services from an agency? And what about the word *deinstitutionalization*? It was a sweeping term that had made its way into print by the middle of the 1970s, and it was becoming synonymous with an era.[47] To some people, however, *deinstitutionalization* was the wrong word because it conjured up the wrong concept. People who developed community services didn't think of themselves as getting rid of something as much as they envisioned creating opportunities, a new system for care. That is what they were doing when they built networks of community-based services. And that is why Turner and NIMH wanted their project to be known as the Community Support Program.[48]

The CSP recruited innovators—Mary Ann Test, Leonard Stein, Paul Polak, and John Beard, who ran the flagship client-organized support program, Fountain House in New York City—to present at workshops. Initially about a dozen people from local mental health agencies came. No two community programs were alike, but they shared qualities and could become models. Their very names sounded like a litany to hope. In Philadelphia, there was Horizon House; in Savannah, it was Open Door; in South Miami, it was Fellowship House; in Hackensack, it was Friendship House; in Chicago, it was Thresholds; and in Washington, DC, it was the Green Door. Like Fort Logan, like PACT, they were the antithesis of custodial care.

Bernard Ungar directed the Government Accountability Office's (GAO) report about downsizing state hospitals, and he attended CSP workshops. It didn't take Ungar long to realize how the states had failed. It wasn't just California, where local politicians under Paul Short's influence had abandoned people they discharged. In the GAO's draft report to Congress, staff had tracked four hundred discharged patients in five states. The title, "Improvements Needed," said it all. Boldly, it stated: "Care and treatment of the mentally disabled in communities rather than in institutions has been a national goal since 1963." Thirteen years later, that goal was unmet. With details about funding gaps, service gaps, and omissions in "guidance, management, or focus," the GAO ripped into the multiple failures of eleven federal agencies managing 135 programs. The federal government had "not yet developed a comprehensive, systematic, and clearly defined national strategy or plan to achieve the goal."[49] Of course Ozarin and Turner weren't surprised. They had suspected there was "no overall plan and management system." That's what Art Bolton had feared as well.

Among the federal agencies the GAO criticized, the Department of Health, Education, and Welfare (HEW) stood out. Failures included conspicuously shifting services into nursing homes, for which the GAO blamed HEW's Medicaid and Medicare. Discharged psychiatric patients enabled nursing home operators to build a new industry with "a stable, docile, tranquil population." In 1974, Medicaid spent about one-third of its $4.5 billion budget on nursing homes. That transfer undermined ideals of living in the community, nullified the goals of self-determination, and sabotaged expectations of fewer people institutionalized. "Because Federal programs provide the financing," said the GAO report, "States are encouraged to transfer the mentally disabled from institutions to nursing homes and other facilities that often are inappropriate."[50] A new word, *transinstitutional*, entered the conversation to describe the process of shifting people from one to another. Soon prisons would be part of the mix.

The GAO also faulted Housing and Urban Development (HUD) for housing shortages hindering people ready to leave hospitals. In Maryland the commissioner of mental hygiene estimated that more than six thousand people remained hospitalized in 1974 for want of appropriate services. In Texas it was close to twelve hundred people.[51] An NIMH survey of St. Elizabeths Hospital indicated that half of all the patients, about thirteen hundred people, didn't need a hospital. Yet, despite a lawsuit and court-ordered community alternatives, there they were because they had no place to go.[52]

In Brockton, Massachusetts, the earliest CSP staff offered a model of how networking with existing services, including emergency services and social services, could provide housing. They had secured at least one bed for home-based programs in every neighborhood and purchased a house near downtown. The advantage of using a community instead of a hospital was that by going to a private home, clients "don't identify it as a crazy place."[53]

These examples resonated with Unger, and throughout the months he attended CSP conferences, he regularly spoke with Turner and her deputy, TenHoor. Their talks practically guaranteed the GAO report would be informed, comprehensive, and specific.[54] It also turned out to be biting. The final draft reached Congress in 1977, with a title conveying the imperative: *Returning the Mentally Disabled to the Community: Government Needs to Do More.*

In less than two years, Judy Turner had expanded the original ad hoc group at NIMH. She inspired a coalition that shared information about pilot programs, innovations, and challenges to community services. Folded into NIMH's Division of Mental Health Services, the CSP was a penniless stepchild. In 1977, fate or coincidence intervened when a residual of the community mental health centers, the Hospital Improvement Program, was about to sunset. The provision had been included to help states transition to local community care. But the program had been largely ineffectual. Now it was an oxymoron since the purpose of community centers was to move people out, not improve the hospitals. Time was now up, and nobody had thought about how to spend the money that would return to NIMH's budget. Bill TenHoor got the assignment to figure it out, which is what he told Turner and McCuan when he apologized for leaving early from their regularly scheduled meeting.[55] He needed to work on a proposal for spending five million dollars of NIMH-administered funds.

"FIVE MILLION DOLLARS?" they shouted as they leaped from their chairs.[56]

TenHoor recommended underwriting the CSP with the funds. It would benefit patients who left hospitals but didn't have the skills they needed to live independently in the community. Five million dollars could cement local and state partnerships and build accountability with contracts based on performance and meeting targets—not open-ended grants.

By government measures in 1978, five million dollars was meager. But it was a lot more than zero, and it opened the door to funding demonstration projects.[57] The first set of grants funded nineteen state projects.[58]

What began with Lucy Ozarin's brainstorming sessions with NIMH colleagues ended with a budget line, a small staff, and a strategic program in the NIMH Division of Mental Health Services. Its genius recognized that, since patients were not identical, neither should their treatment plans be. Paul Polak knew this when asked about exporting Denver's surrogate family alternative model to hospitals: "It would be arrogant to assume that any model of hospital alternatives . . . can be transplanted directly into any other area. . . . The client needs and the community characteristics of any area are unique."[59] Visionaries like Polak hoped services would become coordinated and mobile, informed by former patients or families, with both state and federal assistance to help clients conquer problems.

———————

After 1977, the Community Support Program became a catalyst and an incubator for services. Linking states to new ideas with resources took place at Turner's conferences, now called "learning communities." That's where historically ignored people—former patients, families, small service providers of self-help programs, and volunteers—gathered to talk about what approaches worked and what didn't.[60] There was no need to reinvent everything, but there was a need to share.

An analysis of clients in CSP-supported programs indicated that these initiatives were shaping change. Based on information from 150 people at eighteen different sites, one-half spent less time in hospitals than they had the year before. Turner was pleased. But this was not the full story. Roughly half of the clients also suffered from malnutrition, displayed side effects from medication, and showed impaired motor control.[61] But the new challenges were identifiable, and that meant they were also surmountable. Word spread, and thirty-three states applied for the new federal program for the fiscal year 1980–81.

Turner had cleared a path for collaboration despite professional and geographic differences, and she had influenced people who would implement and monitor innovation. Mary Ann Test quipped, "Judy has an incredible ability to ask impossible questions, and, worse than that, she has the nerve to expect an answer."[62] Praise came from many quarters, including the American Psychiatric Association's celebration of the CSP for its "major departure" and leadership "for securing not only mental health services, but also support and rehabilitation services in the community."[63]

———————

In the decade since Mary Ann Test finished graduate school, the field had expanded far beyond ameliorating chronicity, institutional neurosis, or social breakdown. A lot of that had to do with her and with Len Stein. They traveled to Montana, Colorado, North Dakota, New Hampshire, or Minnesota, laying out their vision for the benefits of bringing state and federal authority to community-based services. Michigan replicated their model for community living, resulting in lower costs, fewer hospital days, and greater independence.[64] In Chicago a nonprofit, Thresholds, used

PACT to provide support for its housing program. Thirteen of Indiana's thirty mental health centers incorporated PACT.[65] As far away as Australia, PACT confirmed that social supports to manage a crisis, engage in living and working relationships, and promote community success mattered. PACT was not without its critics. Activists charged paternalism, while others worried about burnout. But it was now possible to say that yes, opportunities for community care had proven successful. Unique services outside the state hospitals had shown they could work in the service of patients. And, yes, as it claimed, the CSP could provide a "national strategy that could introduce coordination and define responsibility."[66] But was any of this politically feasible on a larger scale? Would the CSP become a mere band-aid for vulnerable people discharged from state hospitals? Or would it become a foundation for widespread mental health reform?[67]

NIMH director Bert Brown liked to talk about the convening power of the federal government. In this regard, Brown embodied Robert Felix's public health ambitions when he gave Lucy Ozarin and Judy Turner a platform. Whether they would sustain change was, in the end, a question that politics, not mental health partisans, would answer.

CHAPTER 4

BECAUSE OF OUR SONS

A RT BOLTON BELIEVED THAT ONCE COURTS STOPPED SENDING PEOPLE TO HOSPITALS, California's families would need community services. With LPS a half-finished reform, and his goal for building after-care services unrealized, he feared the consequences for patients and their families. Eve Oliphant certainly lived with those consequences when her son Brett desperately needed help.

Brett was twenty and had just returned from travel abroad when everything seemed to collapse in 1971. He was jumpy, and the Oliphant family thought Brett was probably on drugs like so many other young people at the time. But when Brett hit his mother over the head with a chair, the family nightmare became urgent. He was hospitalized at Agnews State Mental Hospital in San Jose, California. For the next four months, he was heavily sedated and, because of his violent outburst, locked in and cut off from family.[1] As stressful as it was for Eve, she continued to hope that her son's health would be restored.

After Brett was discharged from Agnews, his first stop was Synanon, a drug treatment program that some considered a cult. When Brett was there Synanon focused on primal scream therapy, primarily patients shouting their hatred of their mothers. Eve was horrified. After a month, a new belligerence, paranoia, and auditory hallucinations took hold. Eve assumed it was due to stopping his medication. When he left Synanon, he lived on the streets. He returned to Agnews, and this time a conservator was assigned. When he left, for the next ten months Brett lived in an apartment complex in neighboring San Mateo. When his psychiatrist moved on, Brett ran out of medicine and became agitated. The manager kicked him out. He moved into a hotel for a month, during which he disappeared for five days. He then checked himself into Chope Hospital in San Mateo. After that, he went to the St. James Hotel in San Mateo and remained there for three days until medication misuse sent him back to Chope. He stayed for two weeks. Leaving Chope, he returned to the St. James Hotel but was barred from the restaurant for the meals for which his mother had prepaid. Angry, hostile, and again hearing voices, he slept on park benches, followed by another hospitalization, with hopes for admission to Tri-City Convalescent Home.

By now, Eve was depleted and fearful. She never stopped looking for help from psychiatrists, from mental health services, from anybody who knew something she didn't. Instead of actual help, Eve got a lot of advice from people who wanted only what was best for her. Live your own life, friends counseled; forget about such a nasty and ungrateful son. Keep the door locked and don't let him in, others advised. Doctors scolded her, "You caused it."

She already blamed herself for everything, starting with Brett's learning disorder in elementary school. She was confused as to where she'd gone wrong, because her other two children seemed to be just fine. But doctors insisted she was toxic, a schizophrenogenic mother who had caused his anxiety, agitation, and paranoia. Some professionals even recommended a "parentectomy," a complete break in their relationship.

Eve carried herself with the poise befitting someone with her theater experience. At one time, everything about her had sparkled—her glistening eyes, her vigor, her dangling pendant earrings. But three years of continuous struggle left her dulled. By then, in 1974, she was going through a divorce, managing two younger children, and handling Brett's problems without her ex-husband's help. She was desperate to know how other parents coped. One day, theorizing that some of the cars parked at a local general hospital belonged to people with a mentally ill relative, she tucked notes onto all the windshields inviting people to talk. She closed her note with a meeting time and said, "Looking forward to seeing you at my place."[2]

Ten people showed up at Eve's garden apartment in the San Carlos Hills, about twenty miles south of San Francisco. Among them was a couple whose son had sustained frontal-lobe brain damage from a car accident when he was twenty-two. They didn't want him to spend his life in a hospital where staff beat him black and blue. Another couple, Fran and Tony Hoffman, was livid because the staff at Napa State Hospital was no longer permitting them to see their son Ed, claiming that their calls and visits were causing trouble.[3] One mother, a widow, reported having been brushed off by doctors who doubted her son's mental health problems were more than grief over his father's death.

They had all been told to continue counseling after their kids' discharge, had been given a prescription for medication, and had received lists about aftercare in the county. But there were no vacancies in the county programs. Their children had housing only as long as the manager of a rooming house allowed them to stay. The one recreation center in their region, Friendship House, was remote and run by volunteers from a local mental health organization. And no public transportation traveled there. As far as these parents were concerned, they had been abandoned.

"At first all we could do was discuss our problems," Fran Hoffman said. "And cry a little bit."[4] They called themselves Parents of Adult Schizophrenics, or PAS, and they returned to Eve's apartment the first Wednesday of every month for "woe night." They shared information, supported one another, and welcomed new parents at each meeting. Within a year they numbered more than a hundred; in another two years, when their group doubled, they outgrew Eve's living room and met in the San Carlos city hall.

Marian Russell, part of the original group, didn't understand why psychiatrists said parents made their kids crazy. What had these people done? she asked herself, looking around the room at the moms and dads at Eve's. They all seemed pretty normal and nice to her as they pondered what might have happened had their kids not been consumed by symptoms of schizophrenia or manic depression, and what actually occurred because they had been. They felt guilty, revisiting what they had done and what they hadn't. Of course it was worse when one of the doctors said a mother had caused this. Russell didn't get it. She loved her son Kenny, thought she had been a good mother. She had tried, tried very hard.[5]

Kenny was one of those kids every parent admired. He was a gifted tennis player, an accomplished musician, a talented potter, and an honors student who had been invited to Annapolis for a college interview. He was lean and handsome and, according to Marian, the most gentle of her three children. Things changed during his senior year in high school. He started using street drugs and began showing an uncharacteristic defiance. Shortly after he turned nineteen, his father died while fishing near the Golden Gate Bridge. That was two years prior, and his body had not yet been found.

Until the night Kenny claimed the FBI was coming through the television, she hadn't worried about him. The next day he was okay, so Marian assumed it was a drug episode. Six months later, the voices started. At least that's when she knew of them. He even talked about hurting his best friend. To keep a watchful eye, Kenny's older brother hired him to work in his store.

Kenny's first hospitalization soon followed. There were several more, some as brief as a few nights, but a couple lasted two weeks and one, six months. He assaulted other patients, but medicine he received usually calmed him. That didn't reassure Marian. She told everybody—the doctors, counselors, social workers, emergency room nurses, and the local police—that her son "had a short fuse." She feared he was "going to blow any minute." One night, Marian had to summon the police. She called three times to say she feared for herself and her young daughter. But Kenny hadn't broken the law, they said, and there was nothing they could do. They told her that if she was afraid, she should leave the house.

Marian tried to convince his psychiatrist that smoking pot and mescaline had changed him. The psychiatrist didn't think so. But he had never read Kenny's medical history, he said later. If he had, he might not have prescribed a drug known to cause agitation. Once Kenny started saying he didn't want to harm anybody, Marian told his friends. "Be watchful," she said. They brushed her off, saying Kenny wasn't that kind of a guy. Again, she contacted his doctors. No, they said, his troubles came from his father's body being lost at sea.

At one of the woe nights in 1975, Marian arrived filled with grief. None of the parents sitting in Eve's living room had yet heard, or at least none said so before she blurted it out, that Kenny had killed his best friend. As Marian talked, she wiped her eyes, and the others did too. As she was telling her story, she became acutely aware of a newcomer, a mother sitting off to the side, fidgeting impatiently while Marian talked about Kenny's unspeakable violence and her indescribable shame and guilt. With Marian's words still hanging in the air, the newcomer could contain herself no longer and blurted out what had happened in her house that week: "My son killed himself."

As a place to share sorrows and fears, that evening was as intense as it ever got at Eve's.

———————

Parents realized they needed to do more than share their woes and channeled their anger into political action. The most appropriate target was the governor, Ronald Reagan, in his last year in office in 1975. Again he had announced he would cut funds for mental health and cancel programs already approved. Furious, one of the PAS regulars, Fran Hoffman, told parents, "Governor Reagan cut back funds last year for mental health, and we, along with many others, wrote, telephoned and marched with picket signs to get it restored."[6] Funds would be cut from patients traveling to aftercare programs, which would further deplete already understaffed programs. "All these programs are cancelled," she said. The meaning was clear: "It means," she said, "nothing is available for your family member, sorry."[7]

Like Eve Oliphant, Fran and Tony Hoffman came to political activism easily and naturally. Tony was a union leader, a shop steward at the International Association of Machinists and Aerospace Workers in San Francisco. When it came to grassroots organizing or negotiating with management, people described him as a "spark plug." They saw an open face and an easy smile, and when he spoke they heard the timbre of a baritone floating on air. But when he challenged politicians, he thundered. "We decided something had to be done," Tony Hoffman said.[8] He directed his anger at San Mateo's county advisory board, which, in California, made decisions about its local services.

In 1975, families learned that the advisory board had redirected funds previously allocated for mental health services to a vague category called "management or contingency."[9] This reduced programming and capped outpatient services at five hours a day, five days a week for a total of fifteen people. It turned out that what the county board termed "management or contingency" amounted to diverting $1.5 million from the $12 million budget to increase salaries for doctors working for the county.[10] That the board had ranked "consumer satisfaction" thirteenth on its list of priorities infuriated Tony. His son, Ed, had rotated in and out of hospitals for five years and had been denied outpatient services. This was just intolerable not only for Ed but for his parents and younger sister too.

Fran, Tony, and Eve started attending county board meetings with a list of problems needing attention. Their pleas impressed a psychiatrist named Richard Lamb, the head of San Mateo's rehabilitation programs, who thought they were eloquent, and he told the county supervisors not to ignore them. The county administration started treating him as an outcast, became hostile, and referred to the parents as "your people."[11]

PAS parents quickly realized that a living room conversation might bring comfort, but it didn't bring change. They needed focused action, and in 1976 they staged a sit-in—more of a sleepover—in Governor Jerry Brown's Sacramento office to publicize their demands for better hospitals. Eve Oliphant, Fran Hoffman, and Marian Russell unrolled sleeping bags on the floor next to other moms. Their action brought the press, but not the governor. Two years of lobbying, however, led to Tony Hoffman's appointment to San Mateo's mental health advisory board. Oliphant was appointed the next year.[12] Hoffman never lost sight of the goals, never let his anger derail him.

PAS parents had always made housing a priority. Within months of Eve's organizing meeting, their ranks had grown, and twenty-eight people signed a letter telling San Mateo's public health director that their kids needed supervised, community-based housing to replace the flophouses private operators ran.[13] Neither safe nor stable, and rarely employing professionals, these facilities existed only for profit. Roughly three new families a week called PAS in 1975 asking about housing. Taking matters in their own hands, PAS scouted for a residence substantial enough for round-the-clock live-in staff. Anticipating that a house was on the horizon, in May they applied for a county grant to cover staff salaries. Their request for $15,000 was denied, and when two private foundations provided $18,500 for operating funds in December 1975, the PAS newsletter was overjoyed: "Mateo Lodge Hits Jackpot."[14]

The following April, Mateo Lodge opened with donated furniture and equipment. Two women, four men, and two full-time live-in staff opened Mateo Lodge. It called itself a therapeutic residence for people "who need intensive, long term treatment outside of State hospitals and within a community setting with comfortable expectations." In contrast to the board-and-care facilities, Mateo Lodge focused on "increasing responsibility" and "independence in the community."[15] Residents could remain as long as they wished. Mateo Lodge would become the prototype for the family-like "low-cost alternative to institutionalization."[16] Two years later, members located a second house on the same street. This time the county financed treatment services, as it would again for a third family-style residence, Hawthorne House.

Meanwhile, Tony Hoffman spotted an empty TB sanitarium. Low-slung, it was boarded up where tree limbs didn't poke through windows. He cajoled county officials to let PAS fix it up for fifty residents living in the community houses who needed more direction in their daily living. When Cordillera House opened in 1978, Brett Oliphant became one of the first residents. California again cut budgets, however, and Cordillera lost the funding for thirty of the fifty promised beds.

In the meantime, Fran and Tony's son Ed was deteriorating in Napa State Hospital. The hospital responded to their queries first with threats they would discharge him "to a board and care home in the County." Then they actually did, to a day hospital, but Ed "did not conform" to their structured program and he didn't last long.[17] Nothing else was available, so the Hoffmans kept Ed at home. When PAS opened yet another house, Cassia House in 1979, Ed moved in with the lifetime guarantee his parents needed for him.

Responsibility for the county's rehabilitation services led Richard Lamb to fret that flawed housing would turn the board-and-care homes into community asylums.[18] "The long-term patient's survival, not to mention his rehabilitation," Lamb would later write, "begins with an appropriately supportive and structured living arrangement. Other treatment and rehabilitation are of little avail until the patient feels secure and is stabilized."[19] Lamb believed family concerns warranted attention. To help PAS reach a larger audience, he collaborated with the Hoffmans and Oliphant for an article about family grievances, which appeared in *Psychiatric Annals*. He arranged for Oliphant to appear at the 1976 meetings of the American Psychiatric Association in Miami.[20] The next year Lamb sponsored Oliphant at the World Health Association meetings in Hawaii. According to the *San Mateo Times*, she packed a "wallop."[21]

Across the country, in Wisconsin, Bev Young and Harriet Shetler also had sons diagnosed with schizophrenia. A mutual friend surmised they might want to talk. They did, for three hours nonstop. That was the beginning of a friendship that would grow for forty years to include dinners with their husbands, tennis games, and daily conversations.

Young and Shetler suspected other parents might also welcome sharing concerns and worries. In April 1977, they recruited a dozen other middle-class, well-educated mothers itching for connection with people who shared similar burdens and met for dinner at Madison's Cuba Club. That evening turned into a mutual support group they called AMI— French for "friend." Eventually it came to mean Alliance for the Mentally Ill. At Harriet Shetler's funeral service, Bev Young would say, "Because we loved our sons there was the AMI."[22]

Young and Shetler brought out the best in each other. Plainspoken, Young would blurt, "Let's just do it." Just as often Shetler wanted to pause, think, and wait for the right moment. A writer, a lover of books and words, Shetler was an editor working at the University of Wisconsin's extension division. She called herself a PK—a pastor's kid—and admirers spoke about her even-tempered gentleness and her systematic and analytic thinking. And of the afternoon cocktail she enjoyed each day.

Young preferred quick action. Living with her husband and three sons in a farmhouse in Verona, on the outskirts of Madison, she clocked twenty years volunteering with the Association for Retired Citizens, the League of Women Voters, the Democratic Party, and the United Congregational Church. Skill and confidence rewarded her, and she funneled those qualities into advocacy on behalf of her eldest son. By attending meetings of the National Mental Health Association, she learned that they didn't have family representatives; she joined. She heard that the Wisconsin legislature was conducting hearings on mental illness, and she testified about housing shortages, patchy public transportation, days her son spent with little structure and even less satisfaction. She learned that the United Way wanted to help people. But when she discovered that they only provided "some feel-good pamphlets about education and nutrition," she got mad. Advice about getting exercise or choosing foods from all the nutritional groups was worse than useless. "It bordered on invisibility. That was the same as not existing. . . . If a kid is sick and lonely with a mental illness you can't just wait."[23] She wrote proposals and soon the United Way was supporting their work in Madison's Dane County AMI.

In the fall of 1977, a psychiatrist named Ron Diamond moved to Madison. Fresh from training in California at Stanford University and Agnews State Hospital, he had learned of the aftercare needs of discharged patients while talking to social workers in San Jose County, where Agnews had dumped fifteen hundred patients onto the streets. A social worker had offered to show him where the discharged patients filled storefront clinics, lined up at soup kitchens, and idled in church basements. Diamond was struck, even shocked, and started rotating through these sites. The people he was meeting seemed less dull than the overmedicated hospitalized patients he'd known at Agnews. One day at a storefront, playing a game of chess with a patient in his twenties, their similarities struck him. He was the son of a doctor, the patient the son of a dentist. Diamond had gone to medical school, while his opponent had gone to dental school. From there, their lives had diverged dramatically. "But for a tiny curl in a gene," Diamond said to himself, "I realized I might have been sitting in his dental chair."[24] The image stayed with him for decades and helped shape his approach to doctoring.

Diamond invited the parents of these patients to come to a meeting where he could answer their questions. How could he, the well-trained doctor, one of Stanford's elite, help them understand their children's illnesses? To his surprise, he found himself learning from the parents instead. They talked about their difficulties, the obstacles and challenges of parenting men and women who had not been helped by a hospital, who were dumped in places like San Jose, which had no mental health services. He discovered parents had organized a network in San Jose, calling themselves Parents of Adult Mentally Ill (PAMI), and that others, such as PAS, existed farther north. They had newsletters, telephone lists, and brochures. He learned all this shortly before heading to Madison, where he had received an NIMH-funded training fellowship to work at the Mental Health Center for Dane County.

Wisconsin appealed to Diamond. He met fresh thinkers there, like Mary Ann Test and Leonard Stein, who were actively building the PACT program and spreading the word about assertive community treatments. He and Stein had a lengthy conversation, imagining the future, pondering how different treatments could be for people in the community with schizophrenia.

While settling in, Diamond realized he had taken cross country the phone lists of the names and addresses of the California families, along with a couple of newsletters.[25] After meeting Young and Shetler, whose sons received services at the mental health center, he knew they would want to have it.

The list made them giddy. Young wrote to Oliphant immediately about her PAS group. "A WOE night," she said. "We do need something like that . . . we may give it another name—our needs and our work are the same although state laws and available services seem very different." Young's letter twice referred to "a national agenda that will unite us." The patchwork clusters of parent advocacy resembled state-based patchwork approaches to mental health services. Young believed it was imperative to organize beyond local boundaries. She urged Oliphant to share whatever information she had about other family groups in the Midwest. "Soon we will be ready for regional meetings—or perhaps a national meeting," she said, ending with an affirmation: "Just knowing you are there is encouraging."[26]

Young and Shetler began to believe that their idea about a national meeting was more than wishful thinking. In just three years, news about families had spread and connections were being made. Richard Lamb contacted one of psychiatry's opinion leaders, Dr. Walter Menninger, urging him to mention PAS in his nationally syndicated newspaper column.[27] The professional journal *Hospital and Community Psychiatry* published an article submitted by a California parent, "The Patient as Seen by the Patient's Family."

Young and Shetler asked their group, AMI of Dane County, to host a national meeting of parents, and the membership agreed. In January 1979, Shetler enlisted a colleague at the University of Wisconsin, Roger Williams, to help them write grant applications and coordinate the logistics. They expected between thirty-five and fifty people, and to keep costs down for out-of-towners, they offered lodging.

Soon word of mouth spread and letters from around the country cluttered Young's kitchen table. That's about when Bev decided to change her name. Working every night to pound out letters on her manual typewriter, she never got to the bottom of the pile, and her hand ached when she went to bed. She figured she could write more letters, organize more parents, visit more cities where she would contact more people to grow a national organization if she had more time. "I didn't have time to write Beverly," she told me. "I had so many letters to write it was faster to call myself Bev."

Young was hearing remarkably similar stories about doctors who had claimed mental illness was a myth, a label society—not to mention author Thomas Szasz—gave to people who were different, creative, or unique. She knew parents saw nothing romantic about madness. It wasn't just an exaggeration of normal characteristics, as some therapists claimed. Nor was it something that bad parents did to their children, as other doctors said. She heard from those who had invested their hopes in the orthomolecular promise of vitamins, or in hemodialysis, which was then under scientific review for ridding the blood of psychosis-making toxins as a therapy for schizophrenia. Some spoke of their mission to bury stigma or of their desires to see mental illness receive attention equal to that of heart conditions or diabetes. Mostly Bev heard about shattered dreams or broken hearts, of having to juggle the emotions of admitting a daughter to the state hospital one day and celebrating a son's magna cum laude college graduation the next. She heard from parents who were forced to rescue a child from a so-called therapeutic school that used cattle prongs to change behavior. Others told about their grown children who were discharged from hospitals without a way to get home. She corresponded with mothers and fathers in Maryland, Illinois, Florida, Georgia, New York, and Colorado who were asking for advice about organizing in their communities. "Get yourself a church basement," she told them. "It's free of patronage. Meanwhile, tell local politicians to spend more money for seriously mentally ill people."[28]

The more she heard from parents whose kids were stuck in hospitals, or were in jail or homeless shelters, or had been kicked out of motels, hotels, or single-residence occupancy apartments, or from people whose children had overdosed on medicine or drugs, or whose voices returned because they had thrown their pills away, the more she knew they craved connection. She was determined that they should meet, talk, and build something to carry them together.

Exhaustive planning went into hosting a conference over Labor Day weekend 1979. In the end, 284 people registered, nearly nine times more than they expected. The gathering would be a summit for people who were desperate for information as well as affiliation. A father from St. Louis, George Hecker, came alone while his wife stayed home should their daughter, who had disappeared on the streets, return. A widowed mom from New Hampshire, Peggy Straw, came because the Alcohol, Drug Abuse, and Mental Health Administration, home to NIMH, knew nothing about finding groups or literature she needed to manage her son.[29] And from California, Tony Hoffman organized twenty-five parent groups who came under the banner of the California Alliance.

Labor Day weekend was idyllic on the shores of Madison's Lake Mendota. The conference took place at the Wisconsin Center, an auditorium with large windows overlooking the lake where boats were gliding under sail. It was a scene so perfect that Mary Ann Test worried that the emerald grass and the Dutch-blue sky might keep people outside. She needn't have fretted. Purpose filled the parents who carpooled to Madison, or came by bus or by plane. They came with anger but also hope, with knowledge but also curiosity, and as strangers linked by a common pain.

Friday afternoon at 5:00 p.m. Agnes Hatfield stood ready at the podium on the campus of the university to deliver her keynote address, "The Family and the Chronically Mentally Ill." She was sixty years old, an education professor at the University of Maryland, white-haired, practical, and resolute. This wasn't the lecture she usually delivered as a professor. On this day she wouldn't be yielding to academic research with footnotes informed by scholarship. She would be speaking as a mother who had struggled for seven years with her son's schizophrenia.

Every person in that room had a speech to give, a tale to tell, a burden to lighten. She could have dwelled on how families had been wronged, or what science or medicine hadn't done for them. But she left the disappointments on the margin and pivoted toward social justice, seeing her mission aligned with civil rights campaigns, the women's movement, or gay rights. "It's time to bring the handicapped into the central aspects of American life," she said.[30]

The people filling seats that evening were advocates as well as caregivers and mediators. They thought of themselves as consumers who purchased services and goods for their relatives. The metaphor of the marketplace was apt as far as Hatfield was concerned. "We are consumers of mental health services and are being recognized as people who should have a voice and a very real choice in the way that services are provided," she said.

As did all parents, Hatfield wanted better relationships with service providers, and she was particularly critical of doctors. She could have used her own words—she had certainly accumulated enough complaints—but she chose to quote from an article in *Schizophrenia Bulletin* in which a psychiatrist depicted his field's "insensitivity and dogmatism" and its attempts to "rescue itself from drowning . . . in competing schools of humbug" while hoping to save itself "with a little science."[31]

Hatfield knew her audience—she was one of them, the organizer of a family group called Threshold in Montgomery County, Maryland. They were unwilling to accept a flawed mental health system that accused her of causing her son's disorder. She knew which strategies brought attention: "You had to be pretty darned unpleasant before you got heard. Once you got heard, you didn't act quite that rambunctiously," she later said in her straitlaced style.[32]

The Madison conference turned out to be a pivotal weekend. Years later Hatfield, normally with little show of emotion, brightened when she reminisced, "It was just roaring in there. . . . Everybody [was] talking, everybody deciding what we were going to do."[33] Photos show a joyful, vivid, colorful crowd animated in conversation and line dancing under a tent. Primed to even poke fun at themselves, at one point a group burst into singing "The Last of the Red Hot Schizophrenogenic Mamas."

———————

Although the conference consisted mostly of parents, a handful of professionals also traveled to Madison that weekend. Only one was asked to play an advisory role, and that was Mary Ann Test. She had encouraged NIMH's Judy Turner to come, and Turner made sure that NIMH psychiatrists who could shape policy were there, especially Sam Keith, who was by now heading NIMH's center for the study of schizophrenia and had become editor of the *Schizophrenia Bulletin*.[34] Turner also asked the NIMH director, Herbert Pardes, to attend. It was his first year on the job—Bert Brown had been fired in a political shake-up—and this was an opportunity for him to see grassroots family and community groups in the making.

Mental patient liberation activists, calling themselves ex-inmates, learned of the conference and that they had not been invited. Judi Chamberlin phoned Bev Young. "What in the hell are you doing without us?" she asked. Young was puzzled by someone speaking to her that way. She had never heard of Judi Chamberlin or her book *On Our Own*, which had become the equivalent of the movement's manifesto by 1979. Nor had she ever heard of the Mental Patients Liberation Front. Young invited the patient-activists to the conference on the spot, and that is how Chamberlin came to chair a session, "Ex-Psychiatric Patients Speak Out," at what would become known as the first meeting of the National Alliance for the Mentally Ill.

Chamberlin was unimpressed with the people she met and the activities in Madison. Writing about the conference for *Madness Network News*, she exploded with anger that "ex-inmate activists" had not been initially invited. And being there wasn't so great either. "Being around so many straight people who spoke constantly about their 'sick' and 'schizophrenic' relatives was very depressing." She elaborated: "I felt like my main function at the conference was to make clear it was impossible to speak of being *the* national advocacy organization without involving the ex-inmates movements. . . . Over and over again, in informal discussion and in meetings, I made the point that our movement would not stand silent."[35]

These were not the only phrases offending former patients. They objected to being described as fragile or unfortunate, and they especially objected to being characterized as incapable of surviving on their own. They didn't see themselves as victims or vulnerable or mentally disabled, or as long-term psychiatric patients. They found the term "chronic" especially noxious. Just as words could shape protest, they could create inclusion. But the words parents used were hurtful, not inclusive.

The choice of words alone didn't explain the crackle in that room when Chamberlin spoke. Seeing how she conducted herself, how articulate and knowledgeable she was, led some participants to question whether she was, as one parent put it, "truly mentally ill." Her purpose and her goals, the way she carried herself with independence and self-assuredness, differed from most of their children. One mother, Vi Orr, recalled that before the conference began, none of the parents had heard of her. "But everyone left certainly knowing who she was!" Orr would later acknowledge that Chamberlin was "way ahead of our time." Young also reflected, "We were better because they came." During that weekend, however, parents noted

Chamberlin's outspoken style and the manifest contempt she and the three other former patients showed by their self-imposed exclusion, sitting on the floor, leaning against the wall and apart.[36]

Chamberlin knew that the ex-patients were disruptive; it was intentional. "All of us on the panel were to some extent alienated by the conference," she would later write. She believed families hadn't taken them seriously. "By speaking out, we showed that the constantly repeated theme of patients being unable to speak for themselves was a cynical fiction, although it was a message few audience members were open to hearing."

Nor did she accept pervasive claims about parents being legitimate consumers: "NAMI calls itself a 'consumer' organization, and its call is for more 'treatment' for people labeled 'mentally ill,' not for human rights and self-determination. On both the local and the national level, the true 'consumers'—present and former psychiatric inmates—must speak out even more forcefully for ourselves." Chamberlin belittled Leonard Stein's remarks about sustaining former patients in the community and ridiculed PACT, calling its work "repressive." She had contempt for Pardes's assertions that patients were unable to advocate for themselves, and she was angry that parents espoused a model leaving patients voiceless. It was imperative, she said, for ex-patients to confront the parent advocates who were calling for more treatment.[37]

Parents knew that the differences between themselves and the patients were oceanic. Writing to Chamberlin after the conference, Shetler expressed her frustration. "I do feel very discouraged that we seem to be so far apart on some important issues, such as the persons that our AMI advocates for are barely able to cope in the community, let alone go all out on the political front to get needed services. Would to God that my son had his head together the way you have!"[38]

———

At the end of the conference, Eve Oliphant introduced a resolution to form an organization with a name suggested by Bev Young, the National Alliance for the Mentally Ill. Shirley Starr, an Illinois parent, became the interim executive director. Chamberlin was nominated for the steering committee, and she declined.

Pardes, in his luncheon address, said that NIMH needed citizen advocates for many reasons: community supports, research, the destructive power of stigma, and Medicare and Medicaid restrictions. With a hat tip to Judy Turner for the CSP, he mentioned that NIMH had funded projects with the hopes they would demonstrate better treatment approaches. He lauded Rosalynn Carter, who was undertaking a national reform. He also challenged parents:

> The success of our efforts specifically on behalf of the chronically mentally ill will occur only in the context of a successful national mental health effort. . . . I would hope that the participants in this conference and your colleagues across the country will work with the NIMH and other mental health constituency groups. . . . I urge you to express your interests. . . . Collaboration may sometimes be difficult but it is an effort that must be undertaken on behalf of all mental health concerns.[39]

Seeking collaboration, Pardes pacified some parents. As a former educator, he knew that an entire generation of psychiatrists was woefully out of date and that doctors had treated families shabbily. They had blamed and dismissed legitimate concerns, and when they should have treated parents as allies, they treated them as culprits, dousing them with guilt bringing self-recrimination. Parents had been waiting for psychiatrists to come around. Now Pardes's words were soothing.

Before leaving Madison, Pardes gathered with the conference leaders to let them know he welcomed their activism. Young remembered he said they "belonged, they were needed, they were accepted." Standing in the crowded hall, he affirmed that they could make a difference as citizens, taxpayers, voters, people who were well spoken, well mannered, angry yet motivated. They agreed about wanting more research about what caused and eventually what would cure mental illnesses, and they wanted to affect federal agendas and policy. Pardes assured them that he knew they would, without doubt, provide the citizen voices that government desperately needed to hear. Brief though it was, for Bev Young it was an indelible affirmation, one she never forgot.[40]

Ten days after Madison, the new president of NAMI, Shirley Starr, and the new board chair, George Hecker, flew to Washington to meet with Pardes.[41] Pardes spent two and a half hours outlining Washington's playbook—committees, key members, hearings, appropriations, entitlement programs, important dates and deadlines. They were excited. "We didn't know the players," Starr said.[42] NAMI needed information and guidance, but members also needed access, and Pardes opened doors. His ample Rolodex included leaders of mental health organizations. If families were to have a voice, to influence national policy, they needed to know these people. NAMI also needed an office in Washington. Tom Bryant, then working with Rosalynn Carter on a major reform initiative, helped them with temporary office space while they settled. NAMI would also seek foundation funding, and Pardes was helpful with introductions to the MacArthur Foundation.

Starr left Washington with thirty pages of scribbled notes containing names and telephone numbers, and the "feeling of excitement and well-being about the challenge." It didn't take long to realize her enthusiasm was well placed. A grant from the MacArthur Foundation, the first of the annual grants, added $78,650 to their budget, a handsome addition to the $4,000 they had collected passing a hat in Madison. NAMI rented a studio apartment with a walk-in closet for the copy machine, which doubled as a desktop. Soon membership and finances augured expansion.[43]

Six weeks after leaving Madison, NAMI families were invited to attend an NIMH conference that Judy Turner had organized. Pardes welcomed them all, and he talked about the difficult economic times and the growing conservative political climate, which could potentially dampen new programs. It was also, he said, a time of opportunity. He pointed to a presidential commission on mental health; to recent collaborations with HUD, the federal housing agency, which had announced a new program for housing people with a serious mental illness; and to a newly established NIMH Office of Prevention.

Chief among the reasons he was optimistic, he said, was because of "a new association of families of people with mental health disorders—the National Association for the Mentally Ill."[44]

CHAPTER 5

A FIRST LADY'S LAW

THE ELECTION OF JIMMY CARTER and the passion of his wife Rosalynn turned the East Wing of the White House into a nerve center for mental health reform. There was never any doubt that Rosalynn Smith Carter was personally and deeply committed to helping people with a mental illness. She grew up in Plains, Georgia, a town of six hundred, where most everybody knew everybody, and all knew Jimmy Carter's cousin Tommy. They "would know [when] he was in trouble," she said, because that's when the police came. They would "unceremoniously lay him across the backseat of their car, give him a shot, sometimes even handcuff him or put him in a straitjacket, and take him back to the hospital." Tommy's erratic behavior, and the way he was treated, left an impression on her.[1]

After Jimmy and Rosalynn married in 1946, they would visit Tommy at Georgia Central State, which had opened as the Georgia Lunatic Asylum a decade before the Civil War. Located in Milledgeville, it spread across 3,772 acres. Eventually more than twelve thousand people would reside there, many in the original brick and wooden buildings in which the wind whistled through walls and windows. The signatures of two doctors and a local attorney were all that was needed to confine someone for years, or indefinitely. Black and white, male and female, patients lived in separate quarters where everything depended on the whims of superintendents or politicians.

Milledgeville boasted that it was the world's largest insane asylum. It had its own zip code, railroad stop, post office, chapel, mortuary, and rows of graves with numbered markers.[2] And it was synonymous with terror.

Treated as inmates, patients could be starved or sterilized, and many fell victim to pellagra, tuberculosis, malaria, or lobotomies. There were cold-bath treatments for "maniacal exhaustion"; escapees could be found dead in the swamps or on the riverbanks, and mere mention of its name lit fear in naughty children.[3]

Visiting Tommy taught Rosalynn Carter a lot. After Jimmy's election as governor of Georgia in 1970, she chose mental health advocacy as the project worthy of her attention as the state's First Lady. To learn more about the issue, she volunteered with the Georgia Mental Health Association, assisted children with developmental disabilities, worked with the elderly, and helped people wanting to become sober. Volunteering at Atlanta's Georgia Regional Hospital filled one day a week of her unofficial schedule. In her official capacity, she served on Georgia's mental health commission to improve services. In ten months, she visited all twelve of the state's community mental health centers as well as the regional state hospitals in Savannah and Augusta, and she returned to Milledgeville to tour Georgia Central State. When she was later asked about the high point of her years as a governor's wife, Mrs. Jimmy Carter replied, "My work with the mentally ill."[4]

Georgians appreciated Rosalynn Carter's efforts. The appearance of one local news story prompted Mrs. Amelia Barn to write Carter about her own experience as a patient in Milledgeville. "The rats and roaches are so bad it's unbelievable," she wrote. Once the lights dimmed, rats scampered across the floors, crawling over sleeping patients; one even chewed a hole in her roommate's nightgown. When she reported this, the doctor and social worker accused her of hallucinating. "The hospital was so bad" that she knew she "had to leave to 'get well.'"[5] Other letter writers wanted better treatment for a child or an elderly parent. Why, they asked the governor's wife, were treatments insufficient, so barren of hope? Rosalynn Carter knew there was really no good answer, not in Georgia, and not in the nation.

When stumping for Jimmy's presidential campaign, she drew from her experience and knowledge to lament the nation's failures to meet its obligations. Among Americans, 15 percent suffered with depression. Others went from a hospital's back wards to "dingy welfare hotels and boarding houses." She excoriated Presidents Nixon and Ford for their respective cuts to NIMH. "Health is one of the matters that public officials can do something about," she declared at a stop in California.[6] Just look at her husband's term as governor, when community mental health centers grew fivefold and the number of hospitalized people declined by about 30 percent.

Two weeks after Jimmy Carter defeated Gerald Ford, Rosalynn attended the annual meeting of the National Association for Mental Health in Philadelphia. She beamed while wearing two hats. One was for her work as an activist from Georgia; the other was as the wife of the president-elect who told people that her husband would soon announce a president's commission on mental health.[7]

Psychiatrist Peter Bourne, one of Carter's advisors, thought a presidential commission would allow Rosalynn Carter to maintain her involvement in mental health reform. Bourne had been running Atlanta's only federal community mental health center when Carter campaigned for governor and had remained a trusted advisor ever since.

Tactics mattered, and Bourne emphasized choosing the right procedure to authorize a commission. One option was an executive order, which at that time had been used only about a hundred times throughout American history. A benefit was that the commission could then be announced promptly. But it carried the risk of isolating Carter from congressional power brokers. They could ignore or compete with him, and natural allies would not be fighting the battle for him. The other option was to call on Congress to authorize a commission, which could result in favorable bipartisan support and cooperation.[8] That year alone, Congress had submitted fourteen bills relevant to mental health. That approach, however, required sharing power with ambitious politicians who might have earlier staked their ground.

Already on the scene with a muscular interest in health reform was the estimable senator from Massachusetts, Edward M. "Ted" Kennedy. Political differences on top of a personal animus bracketed Kennedy and Carter's relationship.[9] Tensions had started in 1974, when the Carters hosted Kennedy for dinner in Atlanta. The senator was heading to the University of Georgia to give the Law Day lecture. Guests remember Kennedy's entourage as rude, arrogant, condescending, and disrespectful. Carter's youthful advisors behaved equally badly, like self-styled bumpkins. Years later, when Bourne asked Carter's chief of staff, Hamilton Jordan, why he had ignored Kennedy's phone calls, Jordan pointed to that evening.[10]

Carter's prickly relationship with Kennedy illustrated why he preferred an executive order. He could keep power brokers at bay. His advisors tried to argue he would need people who met at the watercooler or in the cloakroom, people who would be as compelled to succeed as would he. But Carter dug in his heels.

It was a given that Rosalynn Carter would want to chair this commission. To guide her around Washington, Bourne recruited Thomas E. "Tom" Bryant, a doctor with a law degree who was heading the Drug Abuse Council. He had previously worked with Donald Rumsfeld on the War on Poverty, and with Sargent Shriver in the Office of Economic Opportunities. NIMH director Bert Brown had previously invited him to join policy committees, and he was being considered as an assistant surgeon general. That he was from Alabama, not far from Plains, and didn't look down on the Carters' southern manners made him even more attractive. Dapper and with a bounce in his step at the age of forty-one, he would become central to the first lady's strategy and agenda. He told Bourne, "Congress should be involved in this [commission] from the beginning. It will make for much easier implementation."[11] The president thought otherwise.

The Oval Office scheduled a mid-February announcement about the President's Commission on Mental Health (PCMH). A few weeks after the inauguration, it would be the administration's first official proclamation, and everything was in place when chaos erupted the day before: the Justice Department said nepotism rules prevented the first lady from chairing the commission. Acting quickly, the president elevated Bryant from his two-day-a week consulting role to that of chair of the President's Commission on Mental Health. As if this had always been planned, and before 150 guests and reporters, on February 17, 1977, the president kissed his wife on the cheek and named her the "honorary chair." But everybody knew, especially Rosalynn Carter, who was in charge.

The executive order was broad in scope, short on time, and capped at a frugal $100,000 for a volunteer-assisted staff. They had a year to figure out how to better serve people with a mental illness. What research should the federal government support? How should services be unified?

Mrs. Carter was in a hurry and a year was too long. She wanted a report sooner, in September 1977.

Fourteen hundred people vied for one of the twenty slots on the PCMH. Bryant didn't want to showcase only mental health professionals; he started a search to include people from public television, the judiciary, and Head Start educators. He personally championed "consumers of mental health services";[12] the first lady favored people interested in the elderly.[13]

The selection process sidelined Joseph Califano, secretary of the Department of Health, Education and Welfare (HEW), who had wanted to direct it.[14] It also marginalized NIMH staff from the Community Support Program. The final roster included twelve men and eight women from thirteen states. There were three psychiatrists and one former patient. Three were Black, one from Puerto Rico, one Native American, and the rest white, between thirty and eighty years old.[15] They would hold public hearings, and more than one hundred experts would be invited to join "task panels" delving into specific issues.

———

In many respects the PCMH hadn't a clue about what to expect when hearings opened in April, at Chicago's Institute of Psychiatry, at Northwestern Memorial Hospital. To focus and organize them, staff member and child psychiatrist Betty Hamburg prepared a short and succinct analysis of approaches they should consider. Consistent with Bourne's recommendations, she focused on the two million people diagnosed with a psychotic or mood disorder. She spoke about a second category of need for people whose emotional distress prevented them from carrying out daily activities. A third group, perhaps as many as ten million people, were at risk because of addiction to alcohol or other substances. While these groups seemed clear on paper, the "clientele are not always easily categorized," she cautioned, and "rigid boundaries cannot be established."[16]

Questions came quickly. Would their mission include, as Surgeon General Julius Richmond hoped, the overlap between general health and mental health? Not so fast, said Rev. Franklin E. Vilas Jr., an Episcopal minister and a Jungian therapist from Brooklyn. What was mental illness? To him the definition of "mental illness [was] fuzzy." Ruth Love, a school superintendent from Oakland, California, wanted to know whether they were going to focus on the causes of or treatments for these conditions. And Charles V. Willie, a sociologist from Harvard's education school, asked about "the groups along the edge, the young people or the old people, or the Indian people, or the black people, or the Chicano people, or the prisoners."

Priscilla Allen was the only former patient represented on the PCMH. A Phi Beta Kappa graduate of Stanford, she had been gainfully employed before her first hospitalization in 1960, but not since. Her unique contributions would come from having voluntarily hospitalized herself, written about "the consumer's point of view," and spoken at meetings for families, including Oliphant's PAS in San Mateo, California. She desperately wanted her perspective as a recovering patient to inform discussions about programs and policy. There were times, however, that Allen felt diminished, that her role on the commission was little more than a token. No one else had to hide a personal story to get a sink fixed or a wall painted, or invent a fictitious reference on a job application, or lie to rent an apartment because the building's manager didn't like people who had once been in Napa State. This was all the more reason she thought other commissioners had a lot to learn from her, and she sometimes adopted the role of the group's conscience.[17] When she joined the commission, she had no idea that she would be the only former patient along with psychiatrists, educators, ministers, nurses, and social workers. For this reason, she humbled herself with an apology to Judi Chamberlin.[18]

Allen fell easily into verbal combat with the other commissioners. The first instance followed the opening meeting in Chicago at the Institute of Psychiatry of Northwestern Memorial Hospital, which didn't bear the telltale sounds and odors of a typical mental health institution. Staff wore street clothes. Conversations weren't interrupted by the clangs or buzzers of locked doors. It was almost too nice, with brightly painted walls, modern furniture, and paintings. Even the reporter covering the meeting noted it was among the more handsomely appointed mental health centers.[19] Allen described it as "immaculate, highly decorous, [and] beautifully carpeted." It seemed staged to her, "more bureaucratic than friendly."

After commissioners concluded their scheduled conversation with officials running the center, they disbanded. Allen, on her own, also visited an off-site community treatment program, Sustaining Care. The commissioners had declined an earlier invitation to visit, and the staff was surprised to see her. Allen didn't need a formal tour. She knew the ropes and poured herself a cup of coffee before settling into a conversation with seven patients who shared their stories about looking for jobs or their fears about being sent to nursing homes. The commission needed to hear from these people who had persistent problems and viewpoints they hadn't heard from Institute of Psychiatry doctors. They were of the community, the "people who have been traditionally excluded," she said. And now the PCMH had ignored them. She crammed tiny script resembling ocean whitecaps onto two pages, writing to Bryant to ask, "How would you feel, especially when you had had similar experiences many times throughout your life?" Allen worried that behavior such as this might whitewash the very questions bringing her to the table: How were patients treated? What services were offered? She expressed her doubts about how the "commission has operated, and will operate in the future."[20]

In May, the commissioners went to Philadelphia and Nashville, and in June to Tucson and San Francisco. They found a few recurring themes. Shortages of doctors or other clinicians affected patients' access to treatment and services. Poor planning meant insufficient funds for community mental health centers. Families had become caregivers. Disparities based on race, class, gender, or ethnicity exacerbated everything. In rural areas, multiple problems overlapped. Ricardo Samaniego, a clinician from El Paso, Texas, described working with seventy families and the difficulties they had getting services. The closest hospital was 365 miles away. A shortage of Spanish-speaking therapists meant people went to Mexico for help from "curanderos" and "hereberos."[21] Speaking as a mom from Maryland, Agnes Hatfield confirmed the desperation of parents who sought services for their adolescent children. Joy Tuxford, director of Maricopa County's Mental Health Bureau, insisted that funds follow patients.[22] Clinicians, bureaucrats, and parents echoed the same story.

Activists from the patients liberation movement had a different set of concerns. Most of the services offered to people with a mental illness felt like impediments to the restoration of a full life. Bob Harris, from

Philadelphia's Alliance for the Liberation of Mental Patients, excoriated psychiatry, excessive drugs, and ECT. They just made him feel "more weak," and he had choice words for high-handed methods to promote "adjustment" and "conformity." Client-controlled alternatives were his choice. Commissioner Martha Mitchell, a psychiatric nurse at Yale, asked him about patients' rights groups. Could they work productively with mental health professionals? Although the National Commission on Patients' Rights consisted of mental health and legal professionals, he said that conflicts potentially threatened the ability to work together. When Rosalynn Carter asked for specific recommendations, he said to toss out "the whole vernacular of mental illness, mental disorders."[23]

Of the several former patients who testified, none was angrier than Judi Chamberlin. She arrived edgy, upset that her request to appear in Philadelphia had been denied, and unhappy that she had to travel to Nashville. Her opening statement succinctly focused her objections: "Recipients of mental health services traditionally had little or no input into planning, providing or evaluating those services." This had to end. Ex-patients deserved their own voices. She opposed coercion and discussed programs in Vancouver, New York, Oakland, and the Boston metropolitan area where noncoercive alternatives existed. A lively exchange followed her remarks.

"Did she see any role for mental health professionals at all in the management of people who—people who may need help?" asked Surgeon General Richmond, who was also the assistant secretary of the Department of Health and Human Services.

"I think people have to have choices," she said. "There have to be several systems, and one needs to be outside the mental health system. If they want to go to a professional, they have that choice," she said.

Summarizing her appearance before the commission for *Madness Network News*, Chamberlin said she challenged commissioners to take a strong position on patients' rights but doubted they would do so.[24]

Chamberlin resented having been overlooked to serve on the PCMH and considered Priscilla Allen a token. Allen's activism—she had campaigned for decent and permanent housing, vocational training to replace sheltered workshops, and nutritional education—mattered less than her willingness to work with professionals, especially psychiatrists. This invalidated her, according to Chamberlin, suggesting that Allen had disowned her peers in favor of the power elite.[25]

Each hearing struck a unique chord, and the fourth and last one opened in San Francisco, the epicenter of survivor activism where more than five hundred people had asked to testify. San Francisco's mayor, George Moscone, a stylish forty-eight-year-old Democrat, welcomed commissioners that June. A champion of helping people who were disadvantaged, he told them that he wanted services for "the most severely afflicted." Their needs, Moscone said, are "most often outside the scope of services traditionally provided in mental health settings." He took it one step further, asking for a redefinition of services "to properly distinguish between what can be accomplished by therapeutic intervention and what can be accomplished by providing life-support services."[26]

Moscone's words were energetic and controversial. He was followed by California's Republican assemblyman Frank Lanterman, now seventy-seven years old. While Lanterman and Moscone were different in many ways, they agreed that people with mental illness needed additional services. Even before working with Art Bolton to pass LPS, which bore his name, Lanterman was cherished by the mental health community. He didn't hide his regrets that LPS had fallen short of expectations. Certainly court commitments had been a disgrace—Lanterman called them a "greased chute" to "policies of neglect and preventive detention." But ending them hadn't fixed the problem. State hospitals continued to receive disproportionate funds despite the exodus of patients. "The state hospitals have disintegrated to the point where they're almost as bad as they were in the '40s," Lanterman said. Dollars didn't follow patients. "All I can say to you is, it was inadequate staff, inadequate funding, inadequate training care." He tipped his hat to "the President and his Lady on their appreciation for the great need for the emphasis on local care."

In an unusual alignment, family members and former patients spoke with one voice to indict hospitals. San Francisco was home to the Network Against Psychiatric Assault (NAPA), and ex-patients had a new platform to denounce forced treatments. A parent and a charter member of San Mateo's PAS described forty-one safety violations at Napa State Hospital.

California's hearings concluded the PCMH's information-gathering phase. The next step was to distill and "identify the mental health needs of the Nation." If they performed their duties well, the commissioners thought they could influence the next quarter century.[27] They enlisted task panels to review the testimony and write up the proposals for mental health reform.

———————

Selected commissioners and task panel leaders met at a conference center in Racine, Wisconsin, in January to answer the question: "What, as a nation, can we do to bring the right services to citizens afflicted with mental illness?" The discussion included the problems of one John M., whose sister had written to Carter. His menu of problems alternated between crossing busy streets with his eyes closed, sniffing transmission fluid, and returning to hospitals. He lived with their seventy-eight-year old father, and worry filled her letter.

Problems like John's had occupied the commissioners from the start. They knew that whatever they would say would bear on roughly two million people like him who had been diagnosed with depression, schizophrenia, anxiety, and phobias, and they were mindful of how the $114.5 billion spent for direct care for mental illnesses was divided. A little less than one-third went to nursing homes, and another quarter went to public mental hospitals. But only 3.1 percent of the total went to rehabilitative services or halfway houses to help people like John and his father.[28]

Keeping with the president's dislike of lengthy prose, they summarized 117 practical recommendations in a report, then appended 2,100 pages of exposition. This concluded the first stage of reform Peter Bourne wanted for the commission—reform that he expected would establish Rosalynn Carter's authoritative leadership of mental health reform.[29]

The *Report to the President* was released in April 1978, and the press noticed.[30] "Carter Backs a $500 Million Plan to Improve Mental Health Care," wrote the *New York Times*. Optimistically, the president called it an "investment in the future."[31] Big numbers filled stories: 15 percent of the population needed mental health services, two million people had schizophrenia, one-quarter of the population was depressed. And America was spending $17 billion. For what?

PBS news anchor Jim Lehrer opened the *News Hour* declaring that millions of Americans were "deplorably served." That evening's guests were Rosalynn Carter, Tom Bryant, and New York City's mental health commissioner, Dr. June Jackson Christmas. They explained the details:

There was a critical shortage of doctors, and the future looked bad with nearly four hundred fewer medical students intending to become psychiatrists in 1978 than five years before. Foreign medical graduates filled 40 percent of hospital jobs.[32] Rural America was particularly hard hit.[33] And too many federal dollars were funneled to states to be spent on their near-empty hospitals. Bryant wanted this to stop. The country needed accountability, which he wanted to achieve through contracts linked to performance, similar to what the Community Support Program was doing. This approach aligned with the austerity principles President Carter was implementing to control for inflation.[34]

About the time the PCMH released its *Report to the President*, ABC was building up the audience for *Good Morning America* and its host, David Hartman. A two-part interview with the first lady became a trophy for both. The Map Room of the White House set the stage for Rosalynn Carter's interview. Poised and reserved, she was the picture of spring in a teal-green shirtwaist dress, with a spray of yellow and purple flowers at her side.

The day before this interview, an ABC film crew followed while Rosalynn Carter toured the Green Door, a community service program in walking distance of the White House. It had opened the previous year in the basement of All Souls Church and provided services to people who, if provided with suitable support programs, could live outside of hospitals. The membership consisted of 150 former patients, who were honing skills for independent living and employment.

ABC filmed Mrs. Carter shopping with Green Door members at a nearby supermarket. They followed her into a used clothing store that Green Door operated. Returning to All Souls Church, they got her on camera as she popped into the clerical and maintenance units to see people at work. She attended a meeting where members discussed "how one gets and keeps a job," and she peeked into the kitchen where members were preparing lunch. Their menu that day was a macaroni casserole, with pears for dessert. At the appointed time, Rosalynn Carter walked through the dining room's green-trimmed doors and sat with members at a table where someone presented her with a lifetime membership to the Green Door.

With a toothy grin, Hartman noted her delight. "You actually seemed to be enjoying yourself," he said in a half question.

"Oh, very much," she affirmed.

"Were people in state hospitals really able to live in the community?" Hartman asked, voicing the concerns others harbored even if they had not uttered them.

She responded confidently, firmly explaining that people who didn't need to be in state hospitals were still confined to such institutions. Thanks to programs like the Green Door, they were able to renew their skills and rebuild confidence. This conversation probably answered a question in many a viewer's mind, and Hartman seemed earnest though dubious.

Rosalynn Carter understood that Hartman's questions were born of ignorance and a lingering stigma showing how much work they still had to do. Combating stigma was among her priorities. Some considered a diagnosis no more than a label for nonconformists, or people with deviant behavior. Others easily dismissed serious mental illness as little more than a character flaw, or something that better parenting could straighten out. But it was *Newsweek*'s article discussing the commission's work in May that angered her when it referred to patients as "inmates." "Inmates," she complained to *Newsweek*'s editor, "was a word for criminals, not mental patients."[35]

The *Report to the President* contained the commission's blueprint for a new system for delivering services, and Bryant needed Secretary Califano's help. The secretary's priority was insurance reform, not mental health, and after losing his bid to run the PCMH, he had become remote. His antismoking campaigns revealed an unwelcome independence complicating everything, especially the president's standing in the tobacco-growing South.[36]

By the fall of 1978, the secretary's aloof and sluggish manner irked Rosalynn Carter.[37] The budget he had submitted for the reform package made him an unreliable ally. The president had requested $500 million. His department estimated costs at $100 million less than that. Then Califano undercut his own department by asking Congress for only $82 million. Livid, Bryant told Rosalynn Carter, "We will have real problems on our hands." The larger community of advocates would accuse them of "mounting a rhetorical charade." Their credibility was at stake, as were the proposals they had spent more than a year crafting.[38]

Bryant needed help on all fronts. Since Peter Bourne had left in July, he'd lacked an ally on the president's domestic policy staff, and there was nobody who worked side by side with party leadership to move legislation through Congress. That's why he had opposed birthing the PCMH with an executive order, and now he was shouldering that decision's weight. Even the Office of Management and Budget posed a threat to the agenda by recommending cutting drug and alcohol programs to pay for mental health reform. "Given the close correlations between those programs and mental health," he snapped, "I fail to see much logic working." Cut elsewhere, he commanded.[39]

In the meantime, opinion polls showed the president's popularity slipping. His presidential campaign had promised reforms for health insurance, but in two years he hadn't delivered. It hung in the air when in December sixteen hundred Democrats went to Memphis for a midterm convention.

Senator Kennedy was closely associated with insurance reform, and he disagreed with Carter about many things, including the pace of change. Carter wanted a gradual policy. Kennedy wanted speed. Insurance reform had complicated the 1976 campaign, and Carter had struck a bargain for Kennedy's help delivering union support. After the election, it seemed to Kennedy that he had been shut out, and now he nursed wounds of betrayal. He wanted Carter to deliver immediately. And both were heading to Memphis.[40]

The conference already seemed tedious and lifeless when Carter stepped to the microphone with a speech described as bland yet balanced, and a delivery termed "super cool." Carter looked weak and White House staff knew he'd fallen flat. On day two, with the fifteen minutes allowed to him, Kennedy ignited the audience. "National health insurance is the great unfinished business on the agenda of the Democratic Party," he bellowed. People jumped to their feet. They cheered, whooped, stomped, and roared through twenty-one ovations. Kennedy said Carter's policies had balanced the budget "at the expense of the elderly, the poor, the black, the sick, the cities and the unemployed." With the exception of South Africa, he said, "no other industrial nation in the world leaves its citizens in fear of financial ruin because of illness." America stood virtually alone in the worldwide movement for social justice.[41]

Memphis was like a stink bomb at a garden party. Kennedy told the press their differences were "fundamental and rather basic."[42] Peter Bourne worried from a distance, and he urged Carter to do an end run, bundling insurance, mental illness, and hospital containment costs together in a "Presidential Commission on the Future of Health in America." Bourne told Hamilton Jordan to get Califano's help attacking Kennedy. Whatever you do, he said, "keep the battle away from the President."[43]

———————

In February 1979, three months after Memphis, Rosalynn Carter was due to appear before the Senate Subcommittee on Health and Scientific Research to discuss the *Report to the President*. Senator Kennedy was the chair. The president's staff was concerned and cautious. They knew the senator intended to introduce a bill for national health insurance, and they worried that he might treat Rosalynn Carter as a pawn to push spending the president didn't want. She disagreed, thinking an appearance would build momentum for the mental health reform bill she expected to reach Congress soon. Bryant and her aide, Kathy Cade, prepared her, reviewing details that she would later summon as the honorary chairperson of the PCMH. She wanted to glow under the spotlight on mental health reform, but the president's team feared a double-cross and worried that Kennedy's light might dim hers.

Not since Eleanor Roosevelt had a first lady appeared at a congressional hearing. That morning Rosalynn Carter would be on public display. She wore a crisp, long-sleeved blouse with pointed collars and sat at a table with a glass of water at her elbow, a pile of paper in plain view, and a tangle of microphones capturing every word. Opposite her sat Kennedy. He opened with a roster of facts and figures about people needing mental health services, and he cited the fragmentation and inefficiency of existing separate programs. "We have taken people out of institutions but we have failed to provide them the community support services they need," he said.[44] For solutions, he turned to the first lady. "There is no finer place to begin," Kennedy said, than with the PCMH's recommendations. He credited the "energy and skill, the dedication and compassion of its honorary chairperson, Rosalynn Carter."

For the next hour and a half, Rosalynn Carter fielded questions about the commission's work. Visibly nervous at first, with her soft voice quavering at times, she used her hands to emphasize what she had learned from citizens.[45] Americans sought services, longed for research, hoped for prevention, and demanded parity. The more she spoke, the more confident she became until she soared, showing she was clearly in command of her material.

Instead of unease, she found bipartisan sympathy. Pennsylvania's ranking Republican, Senator Richard Schweiker, punctuated his remarks with phrases like "we have failed," "appalling examples of neglect," "services are lacking." He referenced the *Philadelphia Inquirer's* exposé, "Movable Snakepits," and introduced it into the record. "The system of mental health remains a national disgrace," he said. Ohio's senator Howard Metzenbaum asked about helping the nation's families. Senator Jennings Randolph from West Virginia spoke about his next-door neighbors who were exhausted struggling to keep their disabled daughter at home.

Senator Kennedy revealed his own experience with stigma, speaking in tones that were deeply personal:

> I think of my sister and the difficulties in the very early years of her life being in a large family and trying to involve her in the activities with the other children of her family—the schools and other kinds of occasions. . . . We must take the issues of mental illness and mental retardation out of the closet and into the sunlight of discussion and hopefully lead to constructive recommendations and movement.[46]

This led Rosalynn Carter to recall something Priscilla Allen had said at the commission's first meeting. They'd been sitting around a table, introducing themselves. The press was present, and Allen was painfully self-conscious. She'd wanted her fellow commissioners to know she was a former patient. But she didn't know she "was going to have to tell everybody in the United States." Allen lived with stigma every day, Carter said. "It made a great impression on the whole commission."

Tactfully, she brushed aside problems associated with the viability of JFK's community mental health centers. They had not met the challenge. A recent NIMH survey reported that fewer than one person in five with a chronic mental illness had received services after leaving a state hospital; only one-third of the scheduled clinics had been built.[47] The menu of services seemed of dubious value to the "underserved citizens." But she didn't want to linger on the struggles of mental health centers at this hearing. Instead, she said, "We tried very hard to preserve that which is good, while at the same time developing a greater capacity to meet the needs of the unserved and underserved." That satisfied Kennedy. At a later date, at another hearing, he would dive into the community mental health centers. For now, he listened respectfully and attentively while Rosalynn Carter summarized the *Report to the President*—the status of research, finances, prevention, and education, plus necessary aspects of revamping state and federal responsibilities. "It is an excellent summary," he exclaimed. Twice he called her eloquent. He praised her "personal caring and concern." Later, posing for pictures, they appeared relaxed, not postured. That afternoon Kennedy called the president to praise the first lady's performance.

In her prepared statement, Rosalynn Carter said she hoped senators would help implement the *Report to the President*. She wanted 1979 to be "the year a new national commitment is made to the proper care and treatment of the mentally ill."

Drafting a mental health bill, however, would not be as easy as Rosalynn Carter had hoped.

Secretary Califano's agency, HEW, was responsible for turning policy ideas into bills, and the first draft of the mental health bill angered Bryant. HEW had ignored the recommendation for flexible funding for working cooperatively with states. It had overlooked prevention priorities. It seemed geared up to revise the Kennedy-era community mental health centers rather than following the commission's recommendations. And, incomprehensibly, it seemed to Bryant that it was consolidating Califano's power. The PCMH had intended to revamp the *federal* role in mental health, not the secretary's role. This was not the "bold new thrust" they had been promising. Bryant, beside himself, shouted they just rewrite it.[48]

Until then, the commission had ignored Judy Turner, Anne Drissel, and the NIMH staff working with the Community Support Program.

Their boss, Dr. Steven Sharfstein, had been meeting with Bryant. When Bryant told Sharfstein he was disappointed with the progress of the bill, Sharfstein phoned Drissel, asking for help to tighten a draft.

When the call came, Drissel leaped at the chance. Linking federal and state leadership was her playground. The proposed bill's weakness worried her. "Many of us at NIMH were appalled because we didn't feel it was going to advance anything," she later recalled. While still on the phone with Sharfstein, she meandered over to her dining room table where she rifled through a stack of papers. Yes, she could get it done, she told him as she turned the pages of reports she brought home every night. Hanging up, she grabbed her sewing shears to cut and paste a draft. The next day, a group from the CSP worked together revising a draft of the Mental Health Systems Act (MHSA), which she delivered to Sharfstein a week later. A month after Bryant's outrage had overflowed, the president forwarded a draft of the MHSA to Congress.[49] His message spoke of a "new partnership between the federal government and the states in the planning and provision of mental health services."

The American Psychiatric Association met in Chicago in May 1979. Rosalynn Carter had been invited months before, when no one would have thought the bill would still be in play. That it was meant the first lady would need to fire up her audience. She had become angry at the dismissive attitudes she saw around the topic of mental health. A journalist had said it was not a "sexy topic." A note to herself read, "We do not have the luxury of giving in to these views. The facts—the impact of m[ental] illnesses on the nation are too compelling to ignore."[50]

During the APA convention, NIMH was out in force to salute the first lady and applaud the commission. At one symposium, billed as "Implementing the President's Commission on Mental Health," Steven Sharfstein addressed the fiscal challenge to community mental health services; Lucy Ozarin championed twenty years of research explaining primary care for psychiatric patients; Judy Turner explained the federal government's work on behalf of chronic patients; and psychiatrist Tom Plaut linked state and federal collaboration for a comprehensive system. Others addressed community mental health centers, where services were located, the prevalence of mental illnesses, and strategies for reaching Spanish-speaking citizens. Director Pardes outlined the needs for an expanded workforce, on which everything depended. These policies were a spirited attempt to meet citizen needs.

On the outside, on the Hill, the bill crawled. In July 1979 Carter fired Califano and replaced him with a more sympathetic secretary, HUD's Patricia Harris. They renamed the agency the Department of Health and Human Services. The next month, she directed a national plan to integrate programs with financing of initiatives. It was part of the PCMH's earlier essential recommendations, and to spearhead this yearlong project, Sharfstein turned to Anne Drissel.[51]

The first lady's East Wing staff and the president's West Wing had worked independently and unaligned until now. But Rosalynn Carter knew she needed to engage Congress. She agreed to keynote Representative Claude Pepper's conference on aging and mental health. She courted Henry Waxman, a new congressman from California, and invited his entire health subcommittee to bring their wives to a reception in the State Dining Room to learn about mental health initiatives.[52] Two more White House briefings invited nearly two hundred organizations representing thousands of minorities, children, women, and the elderly.[53]

In the months since Rosalynn Carter had testified in Congress, the White House had been bracing for Ted Kennedy's challenge to the president's reelection bid. When the Kennedy family invited President Carter to speak at a dedication of the JFK Library in Boston in October 1979, all knew this would be a tense and very public encounter. Keep the speech gracious and warm, cautioned the president's advisors. Avoid concealed digs at the senator. Ignore, even pretend there is no such person as Edward Kennedy.[54]

Carter agreed, but he couldn't deliver. He even joked about Kennedy launching a presidential bid. Bearing his discomfort with more humor than malice, the audience roared. Two weeks later Kennedy announced he would seek the Democratic Party's nomination for president.

By early fall, the MHSA seemed off course when political allies and professional supporters sought a slew of changes.[55] The Mental Health Association, the National Council of Community Mental Health Centers, and State Mental Health Administrators were dissatisfied. Power contests aggravated the governors. The National Mental Health Association threatened to withdraw support of the bill, endorsing instead Kennedy's formula for Medicaid and Medicare.[56] Bryant had voiced concern that the "painfully constructed coalition" might come apart, and his fears appeared to be coming true.[57]

Early in the new year, January 1980, Rosalynn Carter learned of another blow to the law on which she had her heart set. It seemed that the West Wing's list of legislative priorities had omitted mental health. This was unspeakable, and she shot over a note that this had to be "Highest Presidential Priority."[58]

With a ticking clock, travel obligations for the entire month of February, and political trickery threatening to upend agreements, worry about meeting a new deadline in May consumed her.[59] Everybody went into overdrive with meetings and phone calls, arm-twisting and pleas, yet three days before the deadline to vote a bill out of subcommittee, Cade warned Carter that they were still on the brink of disaster.

Although the House subcommittee managed to squeak out a bill in time, a junior senator from North Carolina was holding things up in the Senate. He didn't like the federal government maintaining authority for protecting civil rights, something he believed was a responsibility for the states.[60] They were the authority, he said, to make decisions about imposing involuntary mechanical restraints, or monitoring treatments in isolation and seclusion rooms. He threatened to filibuster.

This was unanticipated, and it became personal for Kennedy, a leader in the Senate's campaign for federal protections of patients' rights.[61] A filibuster could kill the entire bill. There was no time, no breathing space, and this latest obstacle could smother reforms based on four years of hearings listening to America's citizens. It would erase the added dollars for research. It would dishonor and discredit frontline service providers. All was at risk, and the filibuster additionally threatened protecting rights of persons deemed mentally ill.

For Rosalynn Carter, Ted Kennedy would blink. This was more than a partisan fight, more than disappointment with the president, more than his thwarted ambition to become president. This was as much a fulfilment of his late brother's last public pledge as it was his own deeply held commitment about better health for all. He alone could change the bill's fate, but it required withdrawing federal oversight of patient rights. This he did, allowing the Senate to vote on the MHSA in August, with a passing vote of 97 to 3. The House followed in September, with a vote of 277 to 15. Congress then left for the campaign trails.

This decision cost Kennedy the goodwill of activists, who felt betrayed. But there was too much to lose. The MHSA embedded many of the principles Rosalynn Carter, Tom Bryant, and Peter Bourne had wanted. Grants funded services for a broad group of people with a chronic mental illness; performance contracts required planning, assessments, and evaluations. The MHSA recognized patients' rights even if states, rather than the federal government, handled enforcement. It tweaked the community mental health centers. Labor would be protected, even if it meant people were working in obsolete facilities that should have been shut. NIMH would establish an administrator for minority concerns. It would open a prevention center. The bill exemplified the sausage making of legislation, and it hadn't passed nearly as fast as the first lady had hoped, but it was now the law of the land.

President Carter intended to sign this legislation immediately, and they chose a community mental health center in Annandale, Virginia, a Washington suburb, for the signing ceremony a week later. On the afternoon of October 7, 1980, President and Mrs. Carter, along with HHS secretary Patricia Harris, Congressman Henry Waxman, and four aides, boarded Marine One. Senator Kennedy drove from his home in Virginia, along with his advisor, Dr. Stuart Shapiro. NAMI's new president, Shirley Starr, attended, as did Mental Health Law Project attorneys Leslie Scallet and Paul Friedman.[62]

The event lasted barely twenty minutes. The *New York Times* reported the attendees predictably "all praised each other." The first lady beamed, the president flashed his smile, and between them, on the platform, was Senator Kennedy appearing pensive, preoccupied, perhaps even perplexed. Despite obvious tensions between Kennedy and the president, Peter Bourne and Rosalynn Carter believed he had worked very hard on behalf of the MHSA. The president was unconvinced, and he would remain stubbornly so.

Peter Bourne, by then an assistant secretary-general of the United Nations, regretted that an event in Sweden kept him away. In a note to his friend Rosalynn, he said she deserved "the most special congratulations for this accomplishment." He continued,

> You have made years of hard work and dedicated investment in the problems of the mentally ill pay off in a way that will touch positively the lives of every mentally ill person in the country. It is only because you cared. . . . Few people will appreciate how much you have contributed to this field over the last ten years and how tough it has been to get *any* legislation through the Congress. . . . We all owe you a very great debt.[63]

PART 2

THE CHALLENGES

CHAPTER 6

WITH BLINDERS ON

W HEN ROSALYNN CARTER TOOK TO THE STUMP to campaign for her husband's reelection, the polls had the president trailing California's former governor, Ronald Reagan, by seven points. While President Carter visited battleground states, she swept through seven cities in a desperate but futile effort to hold the White House. On November 4, 1980, Reagan scored one of history's biggest landslides. For Rosalynn Carter, it was a profound disappointment.[1]

Reagan's election punctured optimism for many in the mental health community. Steven Sharfstein recalled that barely a month before, he had luxuriated in Eunice Kennedy's phone call congratulating him about the Mental Health Systems Act (MHSA). Now, feeling emptied of hope, he resigned from the mental health services section of NIMH.[2]

One of Sharfstein's most effective deputies was Anne Drissel (formerly McCuan), who also asked herself whether she could serve the new administration. She didn't have Sharfstein's options. She was in the middle of a divorce, raising four school-aged children, and feeling clobbered by the double-digit inflation that had blanketed the country. Needing the job, she put her reservations out of mind while she turned to an assignment from Secretary Patricia Harris to finish writing a national plan to accompany the MHSA. It would provide guidance to states and local governments about implementing the complex law. Her deadline was December 31, 1980.

Drissel was better suited than almost anybody in Washington to explain the MHSA's goals and how local authorities could understand them. She knew the importance of finishing the national plan by year's end to preserve the work that had already gone into the draft and make it possible for states to follow up. Otherwise, a lot of people would suffer.

Immediately after the election she assembled a team from the eleventh-floor offices at NIMH headquarters in Rockville, Maryland. She had previously engaged the White House Domestic Council and would eventually count more than a hundred people who helped identify which funding streams could provide legally authorized services—food stamps, rental assistance, and loans for community shelters. It was essential that new financing work with the delicate balance between state and federal jurisdictions, and clarifying the process for fifty different state bureaucracies was a mammoth undertaking.

Night after night people stacked typewritten chapters, hundreds of pages with detailed graphs, on all the chairs, tables, and desks—every flat surface. Late one night in December a hard-hat demolition crew arrived to reconfigure the offices, which had been abandoned to make way for the new administration. Drissel was stunned. She hadn't received notice about a demolition crew, yet there they were, stacking chairs and desks, tearing down walls and destroying the very furniture that she and her team were using. There was no stopping them. Staff were able to rescue completed pages from the debris for what turned into a five-hundred-page blueprint for implementing the MHSA.[3]

Toward a National Plan was written with a master chef's understanding of mixing the ingredients of government to correct "poorly coordinated, inappropriate, or ineffective services."[4] It wasn't intuitive to look for housing in the Department of Education's special program called "Independent Living Services." Yet it had been authorized in 1978 to "assist persons so severely disabled by mental illness that they are unlikely to be able to participate in gainful employment." Through the matching of programs with needs, *Toward a National Plan* could direct state offices to the federal resources within the Department of Education's existing initiatives.

Toward a National Plan also explained how to gain access to programs for people with addiction. Although statistics were spotty, experts estimated that 60 percent of the men and women with a chronic mental illness also struggled with alcohol or drug addictions, and they accounted for four of every ten patients in state mental hospitals. After they were discharged, patients needed coherent services. But unaligned government programs, each with its own requirements for services, complicated that.

Cora was a prime example. She was forty years old, a mother of four, divorced, living alone, and she had been hospitalized four times after suicide attempts. She needed mental health services and counseling for alcohol addiction, which usually existed in separate sectors. *Toward a National Plan* showed providers how to get Cora help.

That Drissel's team completed *Toward a National Plan* before the new year was an accomplishment on its own. Only time would tell whether printing two thousand copies in the closing days of 1980 would accomplish the goal of helping states understand how to knit services together. But nothing could have been further from the incoming president's ambitions, or those of the team he assembled to implement his vision.

David Stockman, thirty-four years old with boyish looks and a former two-term congressman from Michigan, was a rising star on the new Reagan team. After Christmas, he rolled into Washington to assume one of government's most powerful jobs—head of the Office of Management and Budget—to further Reagan's campaign promise to reshape government. It required trimming $40 billion from Carter's $650 billion budget. As a candidate Reagan said he would balance the budget, cut taxes, increase military spending, control inflation, and bring government to a manageable size. Historian Garry Wills says Stockman saw this transition from an elected politician to a fiscal czar as an opportunity, "an economic Dunkirk."[5] With a bite to match Reagan's bark about ending waste, fraud, and mismanagement, he ripped into social services with what *Washington Post* reporter Walter Shapiro called a "frontal attack."[6]

Early in January 1981, the transition team took a victory lap at NIMH headquarters where they grilled its director, Herbert Pardes, about the MHSA. How did NIMH intend to implement this new law? How many people would it take? How much would it cost? Overestimating the team's interest and curiosity, and underestimating its intentions, Pardes planned the next year's budget. He earmarked money to continue underwriting professional education and to maintain staff for the community programs and mental health centers.[7]

Late on a Friday afternoon in February—Pardes never forgot that it was Friday the Thirteenth—Stockman phoned to say that the MHSA would be dismantled. That is where the bad news started: community mental health centers would be cut the next year. After that, the Community Support Programs would be purged. Research for social programs would end. There would be million-dollar cuts to basic research. And one of Pardes's special priorities, training the next generation of mental health professionals, was also in the crosshairs. When added together, the cuts amounted to half of NIMH's budget.

Stockman gave Pardes the weekend, which happened to be a regularly scheduled three-day federal holiday for Lincoln's birthday, to respond. He had given NIMH staff an early dismissal to spend time with their families. But he recalled them at once to prepare a counterproposal restoring half of the cuts.[8] It helped, but losing one-quarter of the budget was substantial.

The administration, meanwhile, was speeding ahead. The following Wednesday, February 18, in a televised joint session of Congress, Reagan gave a thirty-five-minute speech about the economy. He said there would be a "day of reckoning" and stunned members of his own Republican Party saying there would be cuts amounting to $41.4 billion for eighty-three programs. He boasted about a theory "for legitimate" government and vowed to implement tax cuts. But there would be cuts to measures he considered illegitimate government activities, such as spending for health and social programs.

The following day, February 19, capped three days of Senate hearings about health programs. It had been one week since Stockman told Pardes about the administration's intention to destroy NIMH services. Saying that four million people would be denied community services still stung Director Pardes like pepper spray in the face.

The administration's catchall phrase was "austerity," but nobody knew how much austerity was enough for the cuts they'd floated. New Hampshire's Republican senator, Warren Rudman, opened the hearings with flat-footed humor.[9] "Nobody looks too shell-shocked after last night," he said, and he proceeded to pose questions "in light of developments of the last several days." In the witness chair, Pardes told senators about current research, new discoveries, the accumulated knowledge about mental illness and how many Americans struggled with it. He referenced the benefits of the MHSA twenty times, how it worked with states and with their constituents to maximize mental health programs and extend opportunities to those who had been underserved or unserved because of where they lived or how much money they made.[10]

Reagan's plans to harness government by cutting discretionary spending stupefied Pennsylvania's Republican senator, Arlen Specter, as did the fact that none of the administrators of the nation's major health programs had been consulted about these decisions that had been rushed directly to the American people under the guise of a new legislative budgeting system called reconciliation. Ostensibly quick action was intended to tame out-of-control inflation, but a lot of legislators were dumbfounded. Specter didn't mask his surprise when he asked for a detailed evaluation of the Alcohol, Drug Abuse and Mental Health Administration (ADAMHA). Without such details, Specter said he was working "with blinders on."[11]

Stockman had warned Pardes not to discuss NIMH's role in providing services. "That was the dictate," he remembered. "They told us don't argue with it, it's policy." Pardes wanted to study the impact of service programs. No, no, they said, "We're not going to evaluate it because we're no longer involved in it."[12]

In March the NIMH advisory council met for the first time since Stockman's call. Pardes reported that something the administration was calling "block grants" would apply to "all services previously supported by NIMH." Should anybody ask about the MHSA, however, the institute was told not to reply, not to discuss services. To the long-term civil servants, government scientists, even casual observers, being muzzled this way seemed dystopic.

At the same March meeting, Pardes reported that two thousand copies of Drissel's work *Toward a National Plan* had been printed for distribution. They would go to community mental health centers and other local providers. How that might inform local reform or how that would survive new policies was left unsaid. Perhaps it could not even be imagined.

Ronald Reagan signed the Omnibus Budget Reconciliation Act, which officially repealed community mental health legislation, on August 13, 1981. Less than a year after Jimmy Carter signed the MHSA, it was gone. If there had been any doubts about what Stockman meant when he boasted, "We destroyed the system,"[13] this made it clear.

Earlier congressional hearings about block grants foreshadowed the vast reach of the Omnibus Budget Reconciliation Act. In the future, funds would go to states in the form of health blocks. Mental health was grouped with addiction disorders, and they were part of the block for black lung disease, migrant health needs, blood pressure reduction programs, lead abatement, and rodent control. When the budget was final, the block had 25 percent less funding than the prior year.

"This proposal would profoundly restructure Federal support for vital health and prevention services," roared Ted Kennedy in April 1981, when the Senate Finance Committee met. The cuts were "unfair and unequal," he said, aghast at what they would mean to poor, urban, and rural communities, and for maternal and child health programs, which had been a federal priority for fifty years. At that same hearing, on behalf of 850 cities, the Conference of Mayors cried foul. Block grants would "irreparably damage the structure and intent of this nation's public health service," said those at the conference.[14]

Hearings throughout 1981 and 1982 routinely explored the impact of block grants. Democratic representative Ron Dellums of California explained how his state had deteriorated under Governor Ronald Reagan. It was "disastrous," he said. There were budget cuts, hospital overcrowding, service shortages, and staff reductions. Now Dellums feared a nationwide repeat of California's decline.[15]

The administration portrayed the federal government as bloated and idealized block grants as sensitive to local needs, practically a symbol of democracy. Utah's Republican senator Orrin Hatch accused skeptics of lacking "faith in the American people and in democracy itself." Block grants, he maintained, were evidence of "a new Federal spirit," one that countered a "homogeneous welfare state."[16] Somehow it fulfilled Reagan's goal to "get the government off the backs of the people." Partisans celebrated block grants as the "new federalism." Opponents called them "a wishful riot of contradictory slogans."[17]

Rolling out ideas for the most vulnerable citizens who were homeless, the administration presumed that local plans of cities and small towns would succeed. For nearly two million homeless people in America, local planning seemed a cruel joke. Mary Ellen Hombs, with the Community for Creative Nonviolence, told members of the House of Representatives that the homeless crisis could be traced to "cutbacks in social services budgets, elimination of entire programs on which people depend, unemployment and the abysmal failure of Reaganomics." She reported the grim truth about a thirty-four-year-old homeless man, asleep in a broken dumpster, who had been compacted along with the garbage.[18] Others told of people sleeping in cars, train stations, or bus depots. From New York City, one witness described people dying from hypothermia. He accused authorities of abandoning former patients.[19]

The Reagan administration worsened the existing housing crisis, which had emerged alongside shuttered hospitals before his election. Block grants, with proposed budget cuts, would only intensify the problem. With nine thousand spaces in halfway houses, and nine hundred thousand people diagnosed with schizophrenia alone, it was inevitable that most ended up on the streets, observed one psychiatrist.[20] Yet the administration intended to reduce housing supports by $9.1 billion. New York, Detroit, Cleveland, Seattle, Salt Lake City—or any of the cities the Conference of Mayors represented—would be affected. By April 1981, it was evident that Republican senator John Chafee's bipartisan effort to restore $1 billion for the next fiscal year, 1982, had failed. Reductions would continue to put education, community health, mass transit, and numerous programs benefiting poor urban Americans in peril.

After a particularly brutal Senate debate failed to restore funds to education, another Republican senator, Connecticut's Lowell Weicker, lamented that Reagan had hijacked the message of his campaign. The election, he said, was a rejection of President Carter, who was "perceived to be incompetent. It was not a rejection of education, the cities, or people who are in need."[21]

When Ronald Reagan arrived at the White House in January 1981, roughly 4.4 million people received Social Security Disability Insurance (SSDI). Within two months, his administration changed federal policies for reviewing disability claims. At its heart was the intention of weeding out people the administration didn't think were sufficiently disabled to warrant $851 a month to support a family, or $419 for an individual.[22] To bolster its cost-cutting campaign, the administration spread defamatory rumors saying that disabled citizens were unwilling to work and that disability claims had been fabricated or exaggerated. Surrogates for the president called people freeloaders. The word stuck and the press repeated "freeloader" as if it were legitimate.[23]

During his first month in office, Reagan announced a "stepped-up" review of eligibility for SSDI. Kathleen McGovern of Pennsylvania was typical of the beneficiaries. She was forty years old and variously diagnosed with depression and paranoid schizophrenia. Since 1975 she had been receiving disability insurance; she had enrolled in a day hospital program and had undergone several hospitalizations as a result of suicide attempts. Anxiety and nervousness made it impossible for her to remain employed; her work history amounted to about four months as a waitress. Her eligibility was denied in August 1981. For the next seven months she tried to get it reinstated. The idea of returning to Bayberry State Hospital in Philadelphia terrified her. Before that could happen, in June 1982, she took her own life.

McGovern's case horrified Pennsylvania senator John Heinz. She was a constituent whose story exposed the Social Security Administration's failures, including a shoddy review and a cursory examination, twice from an incompetent doctor. The new rules were punishing. People were asked to display their specific disability. Unlike citizens who had lost limbs or sight, people could only describe, not manifest, the hallucinations, delusions, depression, or social anxieties interrupting their gainful lives.[24] Added to the difficulty of being asked to exhibit their disabling symptoms at the time of the interview, only people with an established work history qualified, thus penalizing people with a serious mental illness who had never worked. Heinz called the review process "a virtual holocaust committed against the most vulnerable group of beneficiaries."[25]

He hoped McGovern's story, which he told at two different congressional hearings, would provide the rationale needed to halt the terminations. One Wisconsin official believed the reviews were designed to "deny, deny, deny."[26] A shortage of examiners had built up a backlog of cases. On top of that, doctors who were performing the exams were unfamiliar with the psychiatric lexicon of diagnosis. Complaining about the unfairness of criteria, Melvin Sabshin, the medical director of the American Psychiatric Association, wrote to John Svahn, the commissioner of Social Security.

Svahn delayed replying to Sabshin for more than a year, and when he did, he dismissed Sabshin's concerns as "political diatribe."[27]

———————————

Lawmakers expressed outrage about the disability reviews in the two dozen hearings they held in Washington and cities nationwide. Three months into the Reagan administration, litigation began with *Mental Health Association of Minnesota v. Schweiker*. When he handed down his decision in December 1982, US District Court judge Earl Larson called the terminations "arbitrary, capricious, irrational." He was particularly concerned about the unrealistic assessment of an applicant's ability to work, saying the very process was "an abuse of discretion."[28]

Of the 310,000 mentally ill people whose eligibility for SSDI was reviewed during that first year of Ronald Reagan's presidency, half were terminated; roughly two-thirds of those were reinstated on appeal. Ten states, including Pennsylvania, didn't have even one psychiatrist assigned to the task. It would later be said that this was a crisis created by the federal government.[29]

At the same time, the American Psychiatric Association, under the leadership of a psychiatrist in New York City, John Talbott, was studying policies affecting homeless people. Speaking on behalf of seventeen organizations, he pointed out the paradox that hospitalization cost ten times more than continuing a person's disability benefit.[30] It made no sense to him to deny services such as housing for people who would otherwise end up on the streets, in hospitals, or in prisons. It was apparent that social values, not financial crisis, influenced decisions denying promised support to people with a disabling mental illness while earmarking $6.6 million for "storefront centers to counsel against promiscuity."[31]

———————————

Hits to mental health came from several directions simultaneously. A hiring freeze in 1981 would cost NIMH 22 percent of its full-time staff (from 1,575 down to 1,228) the next year.[32] Fleeing or retiring colleagues contributed to some of the decline, but a mandated reduction in force (RIF) terminated fifty-five others. Reassignments shuffled people from department to department where vacancies existed. Salaries were locked in for each position, even for people who were reassigned to roles far below their typical duties or their pay grade. A science writer, Jules Asher, who also edited the institute's newsletter, was deployed to a typing pool at St. Elizabeths. Anne Drissel became number twenty-eight in line for the job she had been doing since creating it five years before.[33] RIF's consequences could be profound, as in the case of an NIH scientist, formerly a branch chief, who ended his life after he was reassigned to a laboratory to decapitate rats. With the force of an urban legend, rumors spread about someone leaping from an NIMH window at the Parklawn building. Morale plunged. One of NIMH's scientific leaders sarcastically remarked, "The business school method of evaluating productivity in an automobile factory has not been usefully adapted to the evaluation of creativity in a biomedical research institute."[34]

The next year, 1982, the NIMH budget lost another $73.7 million. Of the staff positions eliminated, attrition accounted for about half. The total number of staff fell to 745, and 1983 was just as bad when full-time staff dropped to 313 people.[35] At NIMH, the Office of Rights Protection was extinguished.[36] The federal workforce braced for periodic waves of layoffs. In the meantime, disability reviews continued to terminate people disabled by a mental illness, and criticisms grew more intense. The American Psychiatric Association complained that the restrictive criteria did not conform to medical standards as outlined in the revised *DSM-III.*[37] By 1983 it seemed that slashing NIMH might appear a political liability, and Secretary of Health and Human Services Margaret Heckler proposed a moratorium on disability terminations until after the presidential election of 1984.[38]

———————

Shortly after the RIFs were implemented, Anne Drissel was reassigned. She was placed in the office of the assistant secretary of health, and her new duties included explaining federal block grants, including how Medicaid and Medicare programs would operate, to state officials. She needed a background check for this work. It showed that one summer, as a college student, she had volunteered to work in the office of a county supervisor in Virginia. He happened to have been a Democrat. That summer job disqualified her for employment in the Reagan administration. It mattered not that she had an exemplary history of service. In 1988, with Steve Sharfstein's help (he had moved to head Shepherd Pratt Hospital in Baltimore), she got a job with a general hospital in Amarillo, Texas, intending to revamp its psychiatric wing. Poking around the hospital library, she was delighted and amazed to discover a copy of *Toward a National Plan for the Chronically Mentally Ill*. She later found another copy at the county reference library. Now she could answer, at least partially, the nagging question about the fate of the two thousand copies she had rushed into print. Two of them ended up in the Texas Panhandle.[39]

CHAPTER 7

FINDING A
STRATEGIC VISION

RONALD REAGAN MIGHT HAVE CALLED HIS PROPOSALS "MORNING IN AMERICA," but mental health advocates saw them as storm clouds, and a dark humor hung over the Community Support Program. In June 1981, Judy Turner convened people she called "Doers and Thinkers," and the next January she announced "The Last CSP Project Directors Meeting As We Know It."

In public, Turner projected a guarded confidence. At that year's NAMI convention in Arlington, Virginia, she described the fiscal magicians and policy sleuths in Washington who helped trickle additional funds to the CSP. She had in mind Wisconsin representative David Obey, a member of the Appropriations Committee. He estimated that the Pentagon could spend in just two days, one hour, and thirty-seven minutes the same amount that Social Security Disability Insurance spent in an entire year.[1] For the 1982 fiscal year, he quietly restored $5 million to CSP's budget, something he would repeat in subsequent years. Of course, Turner could have also been referring to Pete Domenici, a Republican senator from New Mexico and a member of NAMI, solid in his support.

It was evident that the money hadn't followed the patients into the community but instead was spent on the brick-and-mortar hospitals housing 133,000 patients, a quarter of its peak number in the 1950s.[2] Now, a new kind of patient was showing up on the streets—young adult males, needing food, or housing, or both. For Turner, the challenge was keeping the vision sharply defined and nimble. She organized a meeting for state project directors to answer what to do "when the well runs dry."[3]

Turner knew that CSP must do more than pay lip service to the recipients of services. Some had avoided taking any government funding, equating it with ceding their authority to an external source. Yet great needs existed as evidenced by professionals who still used the metaphor of a "sick mind" and equated emotional problems with someone's capabilities. Su Budd came from Kansas for that meeting, and she spoke about needing "support for our hope for ourselves" while overcoming and growing beyond mental illness. Joe Rogers, an ex-patient attending his first CSP conference, took it one step further. "Support of consumer self-help groups," he said, "can lead to support of a patient-run alternative program."[4]

Rogers had come from New Jersey bearing a reputation as a lefty with flair. His job at a community mental health center was winding down before he moved to Philadelphia for a job with the Mental Health Association of Southeastern Pennsylvania. At one time he liked to raise a ruckus, he told me, chaining himself to other former patients or to outdoor fences. He was reenacting the victimization he felt during the seven years he was hospitalized, starting when he was nineteen years old. After he decided he wanted to see results in the human rights movement, he became practical. He stopped getting arrested. He got a job.[5] In 1978, in his late twenties, he worked at a community mental health center in New Jersey helping recently discharged people develop skills they would need in the community after leaving a hospital. His streetwise smarts made it easy for him to work with homeless people. He assured them that he had once been there and still remembered what it was like. That he could also negotiate with administrators contributed to his climb to management positions in public and nonprofit agencies, and to his ability to found Project SHARE to develop self-help advocacy for former patients in Philadelphia.

At the Learning Community Conference, Rogers cochaired a workshop about the relationship between professionals and consumers. He knew doctors and social workers were ambivalent about self-help and autonomy. Self-help was a nice idea, they would tell him, but naive. And then they would elaborate and list all the reasons self-help wouldn't work for their own clients among the "chronic population." These patients, they said, needed "tightly structured, professionally run programs."[6]

Rogers thought tightly structured and professionally run sounded condescending—and wrong. Service providers valued punctuality for appointments and compliance with doctors' orders. But that was often off the mark of what people needed, which was a personal connection. He countered them by saying a shared experience, common ground, listening, and respecting a client's wishes could be more important than arriving on time only to sit in an overcrowded and overheated waiting room before a cursory conversation to satisfy an oblique rule. There might be a reason, he thought, people were "no-shows" for professionally run programs.

Rogers seemed equally comfortable when he was talking to a homeless person in a back alley as when he was testifying at congressional hearings. He displayed a jocular grit and a polished charm talking to politicians.[7] Shrewdly he flattered senators like Connecticut's Lowell Weicker or New Mexico's Pete Domenici, with greetings from former patients in their home states.[8] A well-pruned beard and a sliver of hair sculpting his shiny dome-shaped head bespoke conventionality: Rogers looked like a civil servant when sitting at the witness table, and many found it hard to believe that he had had to sell his blood to buy food, or that he had struggled with hallucinations, fears, and anxieties so severe he couldn't attend college.

When Turner closed that year's Learning Community Conference, she noted that "patient-run programs are the wave of the future." It would be up to them, she said, to "reconceive our purpose, recreate a shared vision, and undertake strategic planning in the light of our changed world."[9] Just what was contained in that "changed world" could not even be fully imagined. Parents representing the burgeoning NAMI wondered when the light of a changed world would shine on their sons and daughters on the back wards or in the prisons. Consumer activists wanted that light of a changed world to include self-help and choice.

———————

Self-help, with its person-centered practices, differed from the anti-psychiatry movement. Judi Chamberlin explained the differences this way: anti-psychiatry was a reified abstraction with "academics and dissident mental health professionals" discussing the existential nature of psychosis, or the social and emotional boundaries separating therapists and patients. This was not people-centered, she said. It wasn't helpful, and its adherents had shown "little attempt within anti-psychiatry to reach out to struggling ex-patients or to include their perspective."[10]

Howie the Harp had been preaching self-help principles in Oakland and New York City for more than a decade. These values guided Project Release, a New York City project he had organized in 1975 to help people fight for their rights, whether as tenants hoping to stave off eviction in substandard apartments on the Upper West Side, or with a lawsuit such as the one Project Release launched to get Carrie Greene released from Creedmoor Hospital, where her voluntary admission was converted to an involuntary hospitalization in 1979.[11] There were plenty of health problems for which doctors did not forcibly send people to hospitals. Nobody would round up someone with heart disease, Parkinson's disease, diabetes, gout, or cancer, or use a police escort and insist that they take medicine and remain for as many as seventy-two hours.

Like the Black Power and women's liberation movements, former patients rejected identities others had imposed. Choice started with what to call oneself. When *Nightline* asked Minnesota activist Marcia Lovejoy if she wanted to be introduced as "a schizophrenic," she replied, "I was not a practicing schizophrenic."[12] Former patients spent countless hours discussing preferred terms for themselves and their campaigns. Some objected to "ex-patient" because it derived from a sociomedical model. *Madness Network News* activists endorsed "ex-psychiatric inmate," which conveyed having been pressed into an unwanted role. "Survivor" seemed as militant as inmate, and for some, it was a good fit. Still others preferred "consumer," implying a marketplace of options. Chamberlin, for one, disliked this implication: "I deeply resent the constant use of the terms 'consumer' and 'consumer movement.'"[13] She explained that, when shopping for a refrigerator, she could choose between models, costs, colors, and style. "I was *not* a consumer in the mental health system—I had no power and no choices," she said.[14] "Consumer" seemed like window dressing, and it did nothing to challenge the professional norm invoking "involuntary commitment and treatment."[15] Despite her objections, and her alternating description of herself as an inmate or a survivor, the word "consumer" stuck.

Howie the Harp had a different approach. If you were poor, he said, psychiatry called you "nuts"; if rich, you were "eccentric." He preferred "just 'crazy' folks." He didn't care whether people called themselves "ex, or former mental or psychiatric patient/inmate/consumer/survivor/ client/

recipient/prisoner/mentally disabled/differently disabled/psychiatric his-toried."[16] He cared about rights and independence. That's what had led him to escape from Creedmoor Psychiatric Hospital in Queens at the age of sixteen. After hearing doctors discuss keeping him for another two years of treatment, he jumped out a window, became a self-proclaimed "street dweller," and disavowed the arbitrary rules of a board-and-care program. A decade later, in California, he would set up the Oakland Independence Support Center for people who needed housing or a place to ride out a short-term crisis. Whatever activists chose to call themselves, they loathed "chronically mentally ill." Peter Breggin, one of the few doctors support-ing their movement, agreed. The language of medicine, he told readers of *Madness Network News*, "allows us to treat so-called 'mentally ill' people as if they're non-responsible."[17]

Self-help advocates opposed forcing former patients to accept services that were now in the community. PCMH commissioner Priscilla Allen posed the ultimate challenge to choice when she asked whether, given so many unsavory housing operators, some people were better off in hospi-tals. The quality of housing was as necessary as its supply, and the federal housing agency, HUD, like NIMH, didn't directly operate programs. It could draw up guidelines and regulations about eligibility and disability, then subsidize private housing operators. Until 1974, when Congress ex-panded the definition, individuals whose disability came from a mental illness did not even qualify for HUD-supported housing. Allen had seen California's landlords, as they did nationwide, exploit former patients and take advantage of inadequate regulations. Even under the best of circum-stances, housing programs resembled hospitals with staff rooms, nursing stations, hours for medication compliance, rules dictating phone usage, hours restricting access to the living room, curfews, and mandatory bed-times. Nobody said it more directly than Chamberlin when she insisted, "Former patients must be able to choose where to live and what kind of living arrangement they want."[18]

Hearing of these concerns, the CSP encouraged grassroots activists the only way it could: providing grants to promote innovations.[19] It supported a telecommunication system built by an ex-patient with a master's degree in communications, Paul (Dorfner) Engel, for the Vermont Liberation Organization to link hospitalized patients in Vermont, New Hampshire, and Maine.[20] Engel had curly, shoulder-length blond hair parted down the middle and an interviewer's smooth, calm, even-tempered voice. He expanded within a year to enable teleconferencing for former patients in twenty-eight states, allowing monthly conversations stretching from California to Maine.

CSP funded the project, which became a nerve center for ex-patients. A different moderator chaired each conversation, reflecting the ideals of shared responsibilities and the democratic principles they wanted to perpetuate. The group was decentralized, reflecting its pursuit of a nonhierarchical membership. Anybody could request the call's transcripts, and Judi Chamberlin mailed them out. Talking, even just once a month, provided an immediacy beyond *Madness Network News*. When Kansas introduced a bill for involuntary commitment based on hearsay evidence about danger, Vermont former patients shared information about a similar battle they had fought and won.

Interest expanded beyond decrying injustice and abuse of involuntary hospitalization with forced treatments. Conference participants now talked about preferred community services commensurate with autonomy, collaboration, and self-help. When the CSP requested proposals to develop tools, the California Network of Mental Health Clients got the green light to write a self-help "how-to" manual. Howie the Harp, Sally Zinman, and Su Budd collaborated and solicited practical information. Fourteen people replied, and their answers became the basis of a book, *Reaching Across*, with detailed and specific guidance for "mental health client controlled/self-help groups."[21]

In 1985, CSP granted $65,000 to On Our Own, a four-year-old drop-in center in Baltimore, for the purpose of organizing a consumer-run conference. On Our Own, an homage to Chamberlin's book with that title, was open evenings and weekends, when mental health programs typically were not. Cofounder Mike Finkle called it atmospheric with "old pine paneling and [a] fake fireplace" in the basement of an old house. With mutual support groups, picnics, hikes, and movie screenings, as well as tickets to Baltimore Orioles games donated by the chamber of commerce, it pulsed with activities. Members also invited speakers, including the superintendent of a local state hospital, someone from the attorney general's office, and counselors from the vocational rehabilitation program. "It's these people coming to our turf. That's a neat thing to do," Finkle would later tell a group of psychiatrists.[22] By the time he and cofounder Peg Mc-Cusker applied for a CSP grant to host a conference four years later, they had become seasoned organizers.

The idea of CSP funding consumer-run conferences had come up earlier, when, in 1983, Joe Rogers mused about a "patient-run alternative project in every CSP state." Paul Carling, a psychology professor in Vermont, then completing a review of the CSP, endorsed funding ex-patient conferences, perhaps one that addressed patient-run alternatives.[23] On Our Own planned a conference about alternatives to standard medical clinics and treatment options. Alternatives were more than allowing former patients decisions about what time the bowling club should start. Alternatives validated self-determination and collaboration, and activists didn't want service providers who controlled agendas to attend.[24] It was time to be on their own. Might that include organizing a national organization carrying the consumer voice?

Coincidentally, key grassroots leaders were hearing from establishment organizations inviting them to appear at conferences. The Mental Health Law Project had asked Zinman and Chamberlin to speak. CSP regional offices had invited Joe Rogers to address their local meetings. John Talbott, APA's president, had contacted Su Budd and invited other consumers to discuss the "journey through mental illness" and debate whether psychiatry was oppressive.[25] Former patients worried. Might they be confronting a Faustian bargain that would co-opt and silence them? Were they being used if CSP funded a conference about alternatives? Ridiculous, said Joe Rogers, who thought their fears close to self-censorship. He pointed out that On Our Own had requested the CSP grant, and the ex-patient community would ultimately control the content.[26] Not all agreed, and splintering resulted.

Teleconference callers formed a steering committee to draft a statement outlining the mission, vision, goals, and structure of a national organization. Membership would be key. Who, in the final analysis, could participate in and actually speak at a conference? Or, more importantly, do so on behalf of a national organization? Reminiscent of earlier days, defining the essence of legitimacy was vague.

———————

Four hundred people had registered for Alternatives '85, a three-day conference at the College of Notre Dame, in Baltimore, starting Wednesday, June 19, 1985. CSP funded travel so that former patients could attend, and they came from forty-three states and territories as far away as Hawaii, Alaska, and Puerto Rico. They would discuss stigma, ECT, writing grants, developing newsletters, working broadly with oppressed groups, organizing ex-patients, building a network based on empowerment of members, and rights, most notably the right to refuse treatments. Wednesday evening included dinner and conversation with CSP staff member Neal Brown.

A consensus about the need for patient-run alternative programs and ending stigma was palpable. But it was around the internal struggles, nearly as combustible as conflicts with families, where opinions flared. The air was thick during the second-day plenary session, "How a National Ex-Patient Organization Could Work with Other Advocacy Groups," which gave equal billing to nonconsumers sitting on the stage of LeClerc Auditorium. There was Leslie Scallet, a longtime activist, now an attorney with the National Association for Rights Protection and Advocacy (NARPA); Jim Howe, a family activist and NAMI's president; and Preston Garrison, a family member and the head of the nation's oldest advocacy association, the National Mental Health Association. Each spoke about building coalitions and collaborating. It started smoothly, with a few bursts of applause following Garrison's opposition to "not in my backyard" (NIMBY) efforts to ghettoize former patients. Moderator Su Budd acknowledged the complexities, saying there were "no easy solutions." Fearful of being swallowed up, she cautioned watchfulness that "professionals do not end up organizing ex-patient groups." It was important, she said, "for each group to keep its own integrity."[27]

Alternatives '85 attendees voted to create a group called the National Mental Health Consumers Association. Conference participants became charter members, and a new cycle of debates began. Not all of the former patients wanted to be called consumers, a term that didn't convey objections to psychiatry. Was anti-psychiatry the same as self-help? One person asked whether dupes had been planted to declare themselves "mentally ill" during debates.

The sharpest disagreements came from parsing the term "forced treatment." What exactly did it mean? Look at the paradox: debates about euthanasia asked whether patients had the right to decide when to die but psychiatric patients couldn't refuse medication. Discussions exceeded the time limit, only to start up again, and again, and still without a consensus. Rogers lived up to his reputation as charismatic yet ornery, flamboyant, and overbearing. In one session, he took off his shoe to pound on a table, in much the way Nikita Khrushchev had done at the United Nations during the Cold War. Rogers's talent as a community organizer generally served him well, but some thought he used *Robert's Rules of Order* to control sessions he chaired by calling participants out of order.

It seemed imperative that they arrive at a position about tolerating or opposing forced treatments, and it wasn't happening.

The closing session of Alternatives '85 voted for a reprise the next year. They discounted their earlier objections to government funding and asked for another CSP grant. Closing ceremonies included renditions of "We Shall Not Be Moved," "We Shall Overcome," and other anti-war and civil rights favorites. Tears and emotions flowed. "The energy in the room had an unusual presence, a reality all its own . . . sharing pain and sharing beauty," wrote two observers.[28] The 131 participants who returned evaluations of the conference were generally appreciative of the event, their confidence and sense of empowerment renewed. But none of that replaced the lingering discontent about what this new national organization might look like, and the debate precipitated differences. Those calling themselves psychiatric survivors left unsatisfied.[29] "We must have a voice of our own as strong as that of our enemies who claim to speak 'for' us and in our 'best interests.'"[30] Everybody knew that meant the families comprising NAMI, the psychiatrists affiliated with the APA, and the volunteers from the National Mental Health Association.

Hoping to see their futures enshrined in a national body, representatives of the newly affirmed steering committee headed to Burlington, Vermont, in August where they intended to complete the job.

An almost unanimous consensus had opposed forced hospitalization. It had been axiomatic to the Mental Patients Liberation Front. Condemnations of ECT, seclusion, four-point restraint, insulin treatments, and forced medication followed, not exactly in that order. When leaders met again in Vermont for the scheduled Thirteenth International Conference on Human Rights and Psychiatric Oppression, many were surprised to learn there were differing opinions about this salient principle. For Judi Chamberlin, forced treatment unequivocally denied the essence of personhood. She equated involuntary treatment with a police state. The feminist author and activist Kate Millet proclaimed that involuntary psychiatric treatment was "at odds with the spirit and ethics of medicine itself."[31] Many former patients still harbored scars from sexual abuse, trauma, or isolation they'd experienced in hospitals. For them, ending involuntary treatments was the sine qua non of activism.

Joe Rogers disagreed that involuntary treatment was the primary evil they faced. He wasn't oblivious to the problem of force, having once been chained for three days in an emergency room before an injection brought him down. Was he not the person who would shackle himself to other former patients in hotel lobbies to vividly portray imprisonment from psychiatry? He was, after all, a spokesperson for self-help. But he could imagine instances when a patient's self-harm, or harm to another, complicated the blanket objections to forced treatment.

When the Vermont meeting opened, even if uneasily, everybody stood under the banner of the National Alliance of Mental Health Consumers, which Alternatives '85 had anointed the month before. Two camps, however, quickly emerged because the group could not agree on an irrevocable condemnation of forced treatments. Judi Chamberlin, Sally Zinman, Rae Unzicker, Su Budd, George Ebert, and Paul Engel stormed out, protesting and rejecting Rogers and those with him.

That was in August. In December, Rogers tried to mend the fray and bring everybody together in Pottstown, Pennsylvania. All agreed to embrace self-help alternatives and empower people receiving services.[32] That was, alas, the extent of their reconciliation before conflicts boiled over again. With solidarity eclipsed, Joe Rogers led the National Mental Health Consumers Alliance, and Judi Chamberlin and Rae Unzicker led their new creation, the National Alliance of Mental Patients (NAMP). Separately, but destructively, they would continue their work.

————————

Rogers's charisma and the timeliness of his focus on self-help appealed to CSP staff. Rogers was spreading the gospel, believing that consumers "can organize themselves on local and state levels, develop independent support systems, tie into national networks, [and] develop client-run programs."[33] In dealing with state bureaucrats, he wanted to show them formerly hospitalized patients "participating in the management of their own programs in developing self-help alternatives."[34] His critics saw this as a transparent betrayal, with self-serving ambitions, hardly healing internal divides. They pointed to his affiliation with the Mental Health Association of Southeastern Pennsylvania, an emblem of the status quo, which housed his work for Project SHARE. That a mental health association could host an organization to promote self-help seemed to belie the independence some thought paramount and was, by implication, an indictment of Rogers.

For those in the NAMP orbit, lack of character attached to people who would work with other groups, notably Rogers, whom Chamberlin considered "cynical and unprincipled." Others said he had been co-opted. In a five-page, single-spaced, even-tempered letter, a fellow activist, Patrick Irick, let him know just how they felt: "Joe, I don't know what you're doing, but I can count the people who don't trust you easier than I can those who do. . . . I have no wish to play favorites here, but neither do I desire to see loads of needs neglected or replaced by needs that a few people in positions of power and control perceive to be 'important.'"[35]

Charges of naked ambition stalked Rogers. As the special projects director at the Mental Health Association of Southeastern Pennsylvania, and with invitations to testify at congressional hearings, his influence seemed locked in. Profiles in the *Philadelphia Inquirer* and *New York Times* anointed him a formidable leader. Barely in jest, Rae Unzicker, NAMP's coordinator, proposed a penalty box for people who uttered his name during one of their meetings. When she and Rogers appeared on the same episode of *The Oprah Winfrey Show* in April 1987, she used it as a platform to broadcast their differences. "I was able to state NAMP's clear and unequivocal position against forced treatment," she would later say. Meanwhile, "Joe Rogers for NMHCA [National Mental Health Consumers Association] made clear his organization's clear desire to 'cooperate' with APA and NAMI."[36]

Howie the Harp worried, one might say anguished, about festering public disagreements. Avoid schism, he pleaded in an anguished open letter.[37] Join both organizations, as he had done. Patrick Irick agreed, and he served on the boards of each. But he was unusual. Howie feared that two groups vying for national prominence threatened membership and influence. Public denigration would surely follow and had actually already started. One faction accused Rogers and his allies of being in cahoots with the "Mental Health Empire." After a disagreement at a NARPA meeting, Rogers led a walkout.

Rogers was not the only person they disdained for working with external organizations. Former patients on NAMI's client council were considered suspect. Chamberlin questioned anybody's independence working with NAMI, which she believed paternalistic. And she had grave doubts about Jim Howe, who had previously dissed ex-patients, privately saying, "The militants are not a majority of the functional consumers."[38] That, she thought, spoke to why former patients needed their own national body. Others concurred. "If we don't form an organization, groups like them will gain more power."

As for Howe, he didn't believe Chamberlin's orbit represented two of his four children challenged by schizophrenia. Similar doubts chafed many NAMI parents, especially those whose adult children still lived at home and depended on family for basic survival.

Positions about involuntary treatments remained key to disagreements in the community. Howie the Harp said he wanted everybody to oppose forced treatment. "But as long as there are such bad feelings between these groups, I am afraid that the National M[ental] H[ealth] Consumers Assoc. will never be exposed to our liberating views."[39] It proved impossible to heal the breach. If anything, positions hardened. It had started earlier, Su Budd said, when the "liberation movement was betrayed in Baltimore."[40]

Howie's plea for unity puzzled Chamberlin. She reminded him that most of the four hundred people in Baltimore had taken "a stand against forced treatment." She didn't understand how he could tolerate what seemed a betrayal to her.

If people who consider themselves "mentally ill consumers" want to have an organization to work for "better treatment" (whatever that may be), don't want to take a stand against forced treatment, and refuse even to condemn ECT and psychosurgery, that's one thing. But why you, as a prominent spokesperson over the years for freedom and self-determination, want to join such an organization and to urge the National Alliance to enter into negotiations for "unity" with it, is quite another.

For nearly two years, each group perseverated about the loss of unity. Guilt-inducing lamentations of disloyalty rippled. Charges and counter-charges appeared in three consecutive issues of *Madness Network News*.

In the meantime, CSP hoped it might coordinate all groups—former patients as well as family organizations—seeking to influence mental health policy. It seemed as if one deafened the other. Harriet Lefly, a psychologist on the faculty of the University of Miami School of Medicine who chaired NAMI's curriculum and training program, described the intensity of their differences as a reflection of "the differential weighting of patients' rights and patients' needs."[41] Parents thought of themselves as equally justified standing on the front line, ready to spear stigma and demand services, and that justified having a voice. Perhaps Lefly summarized the conflicts best by saying, "Many families feel that the rights of patients have taken primacy over their needs to such an extent that a vicious and irrational circle has developed." Paul Carling saw it differently. The conflict, he thought, was about the former patients' "need for a fundamental shift of authority and autonomy" at the same time families were seeking "greater responsiveness by professionals."[42]

Looking back at these years when internal conflicts rivaled external, Su Budd said people lined up either as consumers or as psychiatric survivors. "Consumers," she said, "were satisfied with the mental health system."[43] Judi Chamberlin thought them weak, people who "may have seen the liberation perspective as a threat." Chamberlin characterized her own faction of psychiatric survivors as the self-declared "extreme radicals" who opposed organization and embraced "a totally decentralized and unstructured movement."[44] Sally Zinman's viewpoint, like Sally herself, was cerebral, strong, and without accusations. She described this period as a transition from a separatist militancy to "re-entering the world that had so hurt us."[45] In retrospect, she believed that insisting on purity might have been a mistake because the fighting diverted them from the reforms they sought.[46] "The schism proved fatal to both organizations . . . and both are now defunct," she later recalled."[47] Growth tested goodwill, and struggle wasted time and energy for the vast number of consumers, ex-patients, or psychiatric survivors seeking help, self-help, autonomy, the pursuit of self-determination, and the benefit of whatever services they could access.

CSP's pivot to embrace consumers did not surprise observers. But CSP hadn't been able to stem the internal bickering between the representatives for former patients and families. The conflict reflected essential disagreements about the role of psychiatry, models of medical authority, the benefits of rehabilitation programs, and perceptions of choice and autonomy. Ultimately, it was about power.

Diverging perceptions would influence how parents and ex-patients got along for years. It nearly contaminated the CSP's ability to work impartially after NAMI leaders attempted to have Jackie Parrish, the adored champion of former patients, fired. She survived with her job intact, but the incident left a lingering scent she remembered years later.[48]

By the middle of the 1980s, CSP's mission to enlist consumers on their own behalf seemed rather audacious, said CSP staff member Neal Brown. So too was imagining that they could change a hardened system with a budget never more than $10 million or $12 million. That is what turned everybody into opportunists, Brown joked. They needed to make their own opportunities.[49]

Judy Turner had left NIMH after the CSP convention in 1983, when her husband, a diplomat, was reassigned to Bern, Switzerland. Nobody was surprised that it took two people, Neal Brown and Jackie Parrish, to replace her. In 1987, on the tenth anniversary of CSP's first distribution of monies to launch innovation, Jackie Parrish paid tribute to Judy

Turner-Crowson, as she was then known. The moment celebrated their accomplishments, and Parrish credited Turner-Crowson with having changed attitudes to build a new delivery system. She was the same person who had initially wanted, some thought naively, to create a Fountain House on every corner. People laughed and told her it couldn't be done. But as midwife to grassroots coalitions, she didn't abide received wisdom or conventional orthodoxy. Neither pugnacious nor self-aggrandizing, she supported mavericks giving voice to different people to assure rehabilitation, recovery, and autonomy.

From Mauritius, an island nation in the Indian Ocean where her husband had been assigned after Bern, Turner-Crowson reminisced.[50] She thought about the former patients and the families who inspired her, people who had stoked her hopes for change. Of the "patient organizations," she wrote, they "vary greatly in ideology, structure and goals. In addition to groups sharing the ideology of the patients' liberation movement, I was impressed to learn that organizations for mental sufferers . . . have demonstrated considerable effectiveness for people with extensive hospitalization history." She ended her musing for this anniversary celebration by urging coalitions to transcend differences, work together, and look for a strategic vision. "I pray that as the CSP network matures," she wrote, "we will move beyond CSP—to create healing communities, within which, through the grace of God, suffering and despair will be transformed to hope, joy, and peace."

CHAPTER 8

THIS IS AMERICA'S SHAME

T HE DEPARTMENT OF JUSTICE HADN'T BROUGHT A SINGLE CIVIL RIGHTS CASE during Ronald Reagan's first two and a half years in office. The deaths of institutionalized adults in hospitals, disabled children in schools, elderly citizens in nursing homes, or incarcerated prisoners had been ignored. When Tim Cook, a lawyer in the Civil Rights Division, could no longer tolerate what he considered the "meager enforcement of the nation's civil rights laws," he resigned with a public letter. He said investigations in his division had failed to prosecute institutions receiving federal funds, and investigations begun in the Carter administration were still unresolved.

Writing to Attorney General William French Smith, Cook implicated the assistant attorney general, Bradford Reynolds, head of the Civil Rights Division, saying he had raided civil liberties. Cook was thirty-two years old, had worked for DOJ for four years, and spoke with firsthand knowledge of a disability stemming from a childhood illness leaving him with fused knee joints. He knew that kids with disabilities, then called "retarded" or "handicapped," had been neglected in state psychiatric hospitals. Whether their needs came from a physical, developmental, or a psychiatric condition, they were at risk. He accused Reynolds of emasculating the laws protecting them.

Cook didn't think it was a problem of insufficient proof of institutional deficiencies. There was proof aplenty, some of it had come from his own investigations, and a lot was documented in a backlog of cases carried over from the Carter administration. For Cook and the staff attorneys the issue came down to penalties and remedies. He said this in pleading memos as well as during face-to-face meetings with Reynolds. Tools at the department's disposal included the Rehabilitation Act of 1973, and the more recent 1980 Civil Rights of Institutionalized Persons Act (CRIPA). The Carter administration had used CRIPA twenty-five times, but the Reagan administration had not used it once. Infuriated, Cook decided to quit and go public.

On the day he resigned, October 18, 1983, Cook released a thirty-three-page whistleblower's letter and appended 150 pages of documentation. He alleged that the DOJ had diverted funds, hired special assistants to "keep career attorneys in line," and used political appointees to strip career investigators of their authority to supervise cases. He got an advance copy to Carlton Sherwood, a Peabody Award–winning investigative journalist then working for the local television station in Washington, WDVM. He aired the story that day on the 6:00 p.m. news.

Sherwood had previously exposed the sordid conditions leading to five deaths in Oklahoma's state schools for developmentally disabled and mentally ill youngsters. In one instance, the coroner had falsified the death certificate. "Oklahoma Shame" aired in 1981, and it was sufficiently stomach-churning that 20/20 followed up with an independent, equally disturbing documentary, "Throwaway Kids."

Two years later, working for WDVM, Sherwood understood the implications of charging that the head of the DOJ's civil rights division had "ignored court decisions which provide legal remedies for discrimination." Sherwood independently verified Cook's accounts; he interviewed advocates; he spoke to attorneys. Four high-ranking civil rights attorneys who had served in Republican and Democratic administrations had recently left the department because political appointees had also upended their professional work. Another hundred staff lawyers had fled public service. Policies strangling vigorous law enforcement led to plummeting morale, and budget cuts had recently thinned staff from the Legal Services Corporation, whose sole purpose was to help poor people.

Disability rights lawyers called the department's work "dismal." Sherwood had obtained a never-before-seen video about one of the schools in question in Grafton, North Dakota, which was the subject of a pending lawsuit, *Association for Mentally Retarded Citizens v. Olsen*. The school had been accused of whipping disabled youngsters with steel-headed leather belts. Sherwood described a state hospital in Blackfoot, Idaho, that placed "emotionally ill" children on the same hall as predatory adults with a history of child molestation. He interviewed Cook about a school he had investigated in Missouri where staff tolerated fecal matter in showers and cockroaches in food, and injured children dressed in diapers or underwear. Every month, someone died in custody. Had Sherwood chosen to, he could have discussed similar schools in Utah, Pennsylvania, or Oregon.

In a Q&A following the broadcast, Sherwood told fellow journalists that he had confidence in Cook's assertions about Reynolds's failure to prosecute. The federal government was letting states monitor themselves. In Michigan, Reynolds had swapped negotiated improvements for weak voluntary plans for prisons. Ditto for psychiatric hospitals. Cook would later explain that complaints to the deputy assistant attorney general, J. Harvie Wilkinson, were fruitless. Wilkinson seemed as supine as Reynolds, dismissing Cook's concerns by saying, "Brad prefers not to intervene in ongoing cases."[1]

Cook had gotten nowhere lodging internal complaints. He hoped that by turning to the press, he could prevent further weakening of DOJ's oversight responsibilities and prevent more abuse and more deaths. Sherwood was his last hope.

———————

Connecticut senator Lowell Weicker happened to be watching WDVM's evening news when Sherwood's story aired. Weicker was a liberal Republican with a track record of advocating for the rights of institutionalized children. He had burnished a prosecutorial, if not pugnacious, image on the Senate's Watergate hearing committee a decade before. And since his earliest days in state politics, when he toured two Connecticut institutions, one in Southbury, the other in Mansfield, the memory of youngsters dressed in diapers and ill-fitting clothes had remained vivid to him. These kids had been parked in front of televisions they weren't watching and locked away where nobody could see. In 1975, after his election to the US Senate, he sponsored the Education for All Handicapped Children Act, guaranteeing that all children receive an education.

Protecting children had become a passion in his public life. Three years later, his own son, Sonny, was born with Down syndrome. From the day of Sonny's birth in 1978, Lowell and Camille Weicker fought stigma and misunderstanding with the same boldness he displayed as a senator. It started with a visit from a priest who said they didn't have to take their baby home. Camille had had a normal pregnancy and was still stunned, processing the news. But not her husband. He was indignant. He told the priest, "Absolutely not." He wasn't going to hide his baby. When Sonny was a few months old, Weicker wrapped him tenderly in a blanket and, breaking with the tradition that didn't permit children in the Senate chambers, brought him to meet everybody. "If you bring all this out into the open," he later said, "you'll all understand that everybody's in the same boat to some extent or another."[2]

Weicker had fought the Reagan administration's efforts to rob special education of funding and rollbacks for disabled children and adults. Now, as chair of the Senate Labor and Human Resources Subcommittee on the Handicapped, the combination of Cook's allegations and Sherwood's investigations, combined with his own deep sense of moral outrage, fed Weicker's appetite to rekindle the fight.

On November 17, 1983, he gaveled a subcommittee's hearings to learn, he said, how the DOJ had "retreated from its role as defender" of children. As much as any of the witnesses filing into the Russell Senate building on that Thursday morning, five-year-old Sonny Weicker informed his purpose and understanding.[3]

The first witness Weicker called was Assistant Attorney General William Bradford Reynolds, who opened his remarks with fierce criticism of the WDVM story. The broadcast was a circus with factual errors, he said, the "most distorted" he had ever seen.

No, Weicker said, it was journalism at its best.

The hearings bristled with mutual contempt neither Cook nor Reynolds attempted to hide. For three years they had exchanged memos about tactics, conflicting legal interpretations, and their opposite viewpoints about state versus federal authorities. Reynolds had once said their relationship was bound for a collision. Now the wreck was on display.

Reynolds called Cook a hothead, saying he was biased against the Reagan administration's "tripartite system of government." Cook accused

Reynolds of massacring civil rights. It was nothing less, he said, than perverting the will of Congress. Each stood his ground, punching and counterpunching with attacks and defenses, while disagreeing about the DOJ's role determining the government's rights and responsibilities for protecting children.[4]

<hr>

Lowell Weicker and Bradford Reynolds each hailed from power and privilege, alike in many ways. Weicker's grandfather had founded E. R. Squibb, and his father ran it; Reynolds was a DuPont on his mother's side. Both attended Yale College. Both had law degrees. Each was a Republican, in his prime, and working in the nation's capital. That's about where their similarities ended. As a law student at the University of Virginia, Weicker was sluggish, finishing in the middle of his class. Reynolds was editor-in-chief of the *Vanderbilt Law Review*. Weicker leaned toward chunky, with full jowls and a thick neck, and could be exuberant, even bombastic. Reynolds was lean, athletic, properly postured, and graying where he wasn't bald. Weicker too was graying, but with a shock of slowly thinning hair. Most important, however, were their opposite views about how laws could promote a just and fair society.

Weicker had heard that the DOJ's current practice of nullifying settlements had sabotaged cases. Particularly bothersome was Reynolds's preference for delaying and using negotiation rather than the more rapid tools of litigation. He wanted to know why cases that the DOJ had opened under the Carter administration, in 1980, were still unresolved in 1983. They involved threats to physical safety, or cruelty of institutionalized children in Oklahoma or Maryland. Reynolds explained he didn't want to rush the court. "Maryland has tremendous promise," he said.

Weicker didn't agree. He thought Maryland's record was thick with violations needing immediate action, and his interrogation boiled with the passion of a parent and the indignation of a prosecutor. He read into the record a partial inventory of Maryland's worst practices, details from the correspondence between Reynolds and Governor Harry Hughes. It seemed that of the 1,125 children resident at the Rosewood Center in Owings Mills, nine hundred had received only half of the services to which they were entitled; 777 had not gotten occupational therapy; the second floor of a building housing sixty-five patients had no emergency exits; six female residents had been raped by an intruder and subsequently suffered throat gonorrhea; one resident had eloped and had been missing for nine days before a passerby in the adjoining woods found the frozen body.[5] Reynolds ended his letter to Hughes offering to discuss this "at your convenience." Horrified, Weicker wanted to know why this case remained open three years later.

Reynolds explained his reluctance to trespass on a governor's authority. He preferred to allow states to police themselves. Weicker nearly exploded. One can imagine that, as he often did, he spoke with his hands as much as his words, cupping his fingers to emphasize his main points, jabbing the air with one finger before he bellowed, "Mr. Attorney General, you can move in on a situation like that tomorrow. Now let us not sit and play games." Reynolds insisted he wasn't. Weicker held firm. "You mean to tell me that if someone's life is threatened, in this Nation, they cannot expect immediate help from the Department of Justice of the United States of America? Now, do not tell me that, because it is not so."

Weicker was unforgiving. He wanted to know what protections had been established after the one-year investigation. What had happened in the next two years while waiting for Hughes to reply? "How would you like your son or daughter to be undergoing this kind of treatment, and have those that are responsible for her safety take 3 years?" he shot at Reynolds. Without waiting for Reynolds to reply, Weicker blasted forth: "I would not stand for it for 3 minutes, and neither would you."

This match went back and forth until noon when they neared adjournment. Weicker asked Reynolds what would happen if the DOJ learned someone's life was going to be snuffed out. "Do you have the authority right now to save that life?"[6] Reynolds thought before answering. It is likely that he appeared pensive, behind a crease-lined forehead. As he often did, he might have folded his hands, and he showed no sign of emotion.

Weicker waited in silence. One minute passed, perhaps two. Cook thought it might have been three minutes before Reynolds spoke. He said he needed to refer to the criminal code to know "whether the Federal Government is in a position to go in in advance of that."

Stunned, Cook thought Reynolds should have replied, "You should call the superintendent immediately." If that doesn't work, you can have the FBI in there, you can have HHS investigators in there.[7]

Had Reynolds ever visited a facility? Weicker asked. No, he hadn't. Weicker offered to give him a tour.

A reporter once asked Reynolds what he had learned after heading the Civil Rights Division for four years. Through a spokesperson, he said, "He didn't realize civil rights is such an emotional subject for so many people." To some this might have been a shocking admission about the person charged with protecting vulnerable people whose exploitation and mistreatment had not been in doubt. But not to his first wife. She told the *Washington Post* she didn't think he felt a lot—"the feeling component is missing. . . . Brad doesn't feel at home with that emotional side of life." Reynolds thought he was color-blind, but observers called him cold.[8]

Throughout the hearings, Weicker's obligatory politeness turned terse before his palpable distrust became evident. Weicker noted that Reynolds's record was rather "sparse," which was, he said, "the politest term." Reynolds's inability to answer questions satisfactorily, plus the disappointment that flowed from the answers themselves, triggered his fury. Weicker did not intend to back down, and he announced he would invite Secretary of Health and Human Services Margaret Heckler to future hearings to ask her about the accountability of institutions receiving federal funds. And with brisk authority, he dispatched the committee staff to undertake a field study and "personally visit as many of the institutions as is possible, and report back immediately." Adamant that "this is not a one-day hearing," he promised that "Congress will act to assure that those whose lives are in any way threatened, or endangered will receive the advocacy and the help of the Federal Government."[9]

––––––––––––––

The Reynolds fiasco convinced Weicker he needed another round of hearings, so he scheduled three days in 1985 to discuss "issues related to the care and treatment of the nation's institutionalized mentally disabled persons." Although abuses to children had whetted his interest initially, people with developmental disabilities and those with a mental illness often resided in the same public spaces. Conversation as well as policy often linked them. Weicker believed that federal oversight should, accordingly, concern threats to everybody under the same roof. Learning about the upcoming hearings, former patients were pleased about the potential publicity. More people will be telling their stories in a sympathetic way, said Judi Chamberlin on one of the routinely scheduled teleconferences ex-patients held. This opened the door "to get some favorable publicity." She asked participants to forward material that would be useful.[10]

This round of Senate hearings benefited from the investigative report Weicker had authorized. Three of the committee's employed staff interviewed six hundred witnesses from thirty-one public facilities in twelve states. Throughout its 250 pages, the report contained a torrent of criticism, documenting practices that had been condemned since *Life* magazine had first exposed them after World War II. Senate investigators confirmed neglect of urine-soaked or feces-stained patients. They reported how hand or ankle cuffs immobilized some people shackled to beds. In one facility, staff observed "a woman in 4-point restraint in a chair mounted to a wooden platform. Although the platform was in the middle of the dayroom, sheets were hung around the platform so the woman could not observe any part of the room."[11] To modify behavior with interventions dubiously called therapy, some patients had been restrained or isolated for years. There was the thirty-two-year-old man locked in a cubicle for eight years in a Massachusetts hospital. One man had been confined to a seclusion room for thirteen years at Chestnut Lodge, the exclusive psychiatric hospital in Maryland.[12]

For three consecutive days in April, mothers, fathers, and former patients testified. Their stories described drugged kids infected with bedsores, girls who had been held down with four-point restraints and raped, others whose underlying fears of more abuse had silenced them.[13] One witness, a South Carolina state senator who was also a parent, had been petitioning the DOJ for two years to investigate laws protecting the civil rights of institutionalized persons. Three hundred complaints in three years indicated widespread abuse in South Carolina. He described complacency in the face of "outrageous and abominable practices. . . . Our mental health facility is simply a warehouse for our mentally ill citizens in South Carolina. Through neglect and mismanagement, it is being run more like a penal institution than therapeutic."[14]

Weicker was horrified but not surprised when a witness described harsh, ill-conceived, punitive treatments. He would reply that people with disabilities were not guilty of anything, that they were not prisoners and shouldn't be treated like criminals. "Protection for these frailest of our society exists largely on paper," he said regretfully, calling these situations "our shame, our shame."[15] Former patients, and readers of *Madness Network News*, knew these stories well. To have a senator confirm that the conditions warranted investigation brightened ex-patients' confidence.[16]

Of the thirty-one institutions the senate staff visited, the Pennhurst School in Pennsylvania was of special interest. It had opened in 1908 as the Eastern Pennsylvania State Institution for the Feeble-Minded and Epileptic. Instead of helping youngsters develop to their full capacity and then return home, it had become a hellhole, a human warehouse with staff inflicting incalculable emotional, psychological, physical, and sadistic damage. Nobody knew more about the Pennhurst School than David Ferleger, who in 1974, on behalf of fourteen hundred youngsters and their families, had filed a class action lawsuit, *Halderman v. Pennhurst*. He charged violations of the First, Eighth, Ninth, and Fourteenth Amendments, and eighty witnesses filled thirty-two days with stories about assaults, abandonment, and caged children. The school was irredeemable, leading one of Pennsylvania's defense attorneys to refuse to testify. Another did, saying, "There is no way that Pennhurst could be made into an adequate facility."[17]

The challenge before Congress was far more extensive than Pennhurst, whose name alone evoked the shame of America. Ferleger's expertise was legendary. By the age of thirty, he had influenced changes in six sections of Pennsylvania's mental health law. Most litigators don't appear before the US Supreme Court even once, but he had already done so five times before he was thirty-seven. Three of his Supreme Court appearances involved US district judge Raymond Broderick's Pennhurst decision. The judge had declared Pennhurst "a monumental example of unconstitutionality with respect to the habilitation of the retarded."[18] None of the challenges overturned Broderick's decision. That alone made Ferleger newsworthy. He was a colorful figure, easy to describe with his "thick eyebrows over soft eyes," his "billowing black hair and lumberjack beard." It was said that he avoided lawyerly suits, except when he came to court wearing something wrinkled.[19] By the time he appeared before the Senate Labor and Human Resources Subcommittee, he had been dubbed the "Ralph Nader of the mental hospital circuit." His billowing hair had thinned, his beard was trimmed, and his suit was pressed.

Two of his clients, youngsters with disabilities, flanked Ferleger that November morning in the Senate hearing. Before he testified, their parents summarized the neglect and mistreatment that nearly killed their respective sons in state schools. When Ferleger spoke in his characteristically soft tone, he started with a paradox. It was both "an honor and almost a disgrace" to be present, he said. "One would have thought that the 50 States of the United States would long ago have remedied the abuse that goes on every day in institutions."[20] Although he had massive information about clients who died, or had nearly died, or had suffered additional injuries leading to a worse quality of life, he left senators with remedies.

Three low-cost suggestions could correct for DOJ's culpability keeping errant institutions open: criminalize those who abuse residents in state institutions; establish a special prosecutor who would be independent of the DOJ; and award triple damages in settlements against state officials who violated the civil rights of patients.[21] In other words, create accountability to disallow individuals with political appointments to bypass enforcement and ignore the law.

Hearings had laid bare, and Bradford Reynolds had personified, how powerful individuals could thwart laws, bend or break established policies, and interfere with departmental norms. The issue was power, and recipients of mental health services didn't have it. When Weicker opened the hearings in April 1985, he lamented the lack of protection for America's most vulnerable citizens. On April 23 he introduced the Protection and Advocacy for Mentally Ill Individuals Act of 1985. It would take a year and a month, with hearings in both chambers, to realize the extent to which support existed for protecting the rights of citizens with disabilities. And when it was passed, it paid homage to the Mental Health Systems Act, once heralded by Rosalynn Carter, signed by her husband, President Jimmy Carter, and repealed under President Ronald Reagan.

Protection and Advocacy for Individuals with Mental Illness, or PAIMI, ended Reynolds's preferred strategy of allowing institutions to police themselves. That made it too easy to draw the curtain between their closed doors and the public's need to know. Accountability and oversight, along with new visions, and the authority to regulate would become bedrock. PAIMI empowered independent advisory boards that each state would employ to investigate complaints. It confirmed, as one psychiatrist said, the need for external supervision to guarantee that the mental health system offered appropriate care.[22]

One of PAIMI's most significant achievements aimed to rebalance how policies were made. Families and former patients, previously kept at arm's length in agenda-setting deliberations, represented new voices. They might not have always agreed, but they both wanted a role, and going forward they were now entitled to half of the seats on advisory panels.

Consumers applauded giving them and family representatives an oversight role on policy panels.[23] It might lessen involuntary treatments. Judi Chamberlin cheered. Participating in the planning process, she said, might "help us to become true consumers, who 'shop' for services we want and reject those that do not meet our self-defined needs. Then we will see real, fundamental change—not just new names for old institutions and programs, but a true revolution challenging the very basis of paternalism and control."

Including consumers and families in the planning process turned something ad hoc into a requirement. When Congress considered renewing PAIMI, two years later, NAMI's Bill Snavely pleaded to extend protection to "mentally ill persons [who] are being inappropriately incarcerated in jails simply because there are not adequate treatment facilities." Joseph Rogers, who served on the Pennsylvania protection and advocacy oversight committee, collected statements from consumers in Washington, Ohio, and Michigan, all of whom reported instances in which consumers were generally ignored or bypassed. Steven Schwartz, from Massachusetts, reported on the recent deaths of six people in hospitals the DOJ had condemned as unconstitutional. He had visited Georgia where a hospital with three thousand patients had a half-time paralegal. He said at one time he wanted to focus on the people who had died. "Then we realized that that was not really the right place where we ought to start; it is preventing people from dying that we need to be attentive to."[24]

When Lowell Weicker opened initial hearings, he noted that Congress wanted a policy "of support and protection for the mentally retarded and all disabled Americans." PAIMI affirmed the importance of maintaining vigilance. But investigations and accountability were only a start. "I wish I could report that the deplorable conditions uncovered during the investigation . . . had been totally eradicated as a result of the passage of this law," Weicker said. But he couldn't. "Despite the valiant efforts of the Protection and Advocacy System, their services are needed as much as ever. . . . There is still a great deal of work to be done."[25]

———————

At the same time Congress considered PAIMI, the Senate held hearings on the nomination of William Bradford Reynolds for the DOJ's third-highest position, associate attorney general. A parade of mental health champions, civil rights activists, and former colleagues spoke against him, condemning his nomination. A score of written complaints outlined errant behaviors and questionable judgment, decisions, and performance. During his hearings, Senator Paul Simon, a Democrat from Illinois, asked about the mass resignations of lawyers in his division. Reynolds's memory failed him. He remembered only one notable resignation. The departure of others, he claimed, reflected a natural turnover. Simon could barely contain his doubts about Reynolds. His intelligence was undeniable, but his honesty and the political interpretations of the law bothered the senators. Some even questioned his heart. Said one reporter, "His head-over-heart persona is amplified by his demeanor, described by many who have met him as emotionless, meticulous, unfeeling and cold."[26] His public service career ended when he returned to private practice in 1988. He would remain, in the words of the *Washington Post*'s Juan Williams, a "living symbol of Ronald Reagan's assault on civil rights enforcement."

It was ironic that Reynolds, who challenged the federal government's moral responsibility and the practicality of holding states accountable, became a bystander when the government granted consumers the authority, and $10 million, to enact PAIMI and maintain supervision.

CHAPTER 9

THE GENTLEMEN
FROM KENTUCKY

I N 1975, WHEN JOAN AND BOSWELL "BOS" TODD'S nineteen-year old son, Sam, was hospitalized at Norton Children's Hospital in Louisville, Kentucky, his psychiatrist was optimistic.[1] He described a promising hypothesis linking schizophrenia to excessive amounts of dopamine. Some people didn't have enough dopamine, he explained, and they developed Parkinson's disease. That wasn't Sam's problem. He had too much dopamine, said the doctor, which produced a chemical imbalance and flooded the communication of neurotransmitters. But he said medicine could affect that and told Joan and Bos to have hope, to have courage while praying for their troubled son's future.

Joan and Bos knew that Sam had struggled since he was in nursery school when his teachers said he isolated himself. They had turned to a psychologist who helped Sam then, and over the years when his anxieties bubbled up. But by his last year at Ballard High School, it seemed that Sam was on a collision course. Six weeks before graduation, he quit school and moved in with a religious cult in downtown Louisville, where he remained for six months. Over the next few years, Sam alternated between getting jobs and getting fired. He returned home to live with his parents and two younger brothers. He became fearful of everyday things. When his mother went grocery shopping, staying home alone unnerved him. In six months he'd had six car accidents. After his parents found him walking barefoot through the neighborhood one morning at 6:00 a.m., Sam agreed to go to a hospital.

While the hypothesis about dopamine's influence on schizophrenia had once sounded promising, the medicine Sam's psychiatrist prescribed, Prolixin, hadn't helped him. Hearing about orthomolecular treatments, Bos took his son to the Brain Bio Center in New Jersey, for two consultations about megavitamin therapy. There he was diagnosed as "high histamine paranoid schizophrenia." The center recommended a boatload of changes consistent with orthomolecular theories. They increased his intake of ascorbic acid, stopped folic acid, and altered his intake of zinc, niacin, and the B-complex vitamins. But none of that helped Sam.

In the forty-four months after Sam's first hospitalization, there would be another half dozen. Throughout those years, his parents sought advice from experts in New York, considered residential treatments in Vermont, and attended meetings of the Schizophrenia Association of Louisville, a family group that sponsored lectures. One lecture in 1979, by the director of Fellowship House in South Miami, discussed a unique housing program consisting of three levels of services. One level enrolled fifteen people who, in addition to giving them a place to live, provided meals, counseling services, a recreation program, and vocational rehabilitation services. Another program, for twenty-eight people with less intense needs, offered supervised apartments but fewer services. A third was organized for fifty-two people with fewer needs who qualified for living in satellite apartments.

Nothing like that existed in Louisville; in fact, there were no opportunities for housing in Louisville at all. If there had been, things might have differed for Sam. He'd tried to live independently four different times, and each ended in disaster. He became malnourished, developed pneumonia, and stopped taking his medicine. He spent too much time with people his parents thought exerted a bad influence, fellows who spent their money on street drugs, cigars, coffee, and records. But living at home didn't work either. Bos Todd's success as a financial consultant, his problem-solving tenacity commensurate with a Harvard business school education, or his love and care for his family were not enough to turn things around. Joan and their other children never felt they were adequately vigilant. Their guilt grew, along with a palpable stress in the family.

The Fellowship House model impressed Todd. When Kentucky congressman William Natcher, chair of the House Appropriations Subcommittee, held hearings in April 1980 about the budget for the next fiscal year, three members of the Schizophrenia Association of Louisville went to Washington to testify. One father, Sheldon Rein, spoke about the federal government's responsibility to underwrite research and housing. Todd also spoke about housing, and with Fellowship House fresh in his mind, he made what he considered a passionate "plea for halfway houses . . . a haven, hopefully temporary, between hospital and home."[2]

Not much changed for Sam in the years after he was discharged from Norton Children's Hospital. He rotated between home, hospital, back home, return to a hospital, then home again. About a year after Bos testified in Washington, he bumped into his neighbor Phil Ardery as each was leaving a meeting at St. Matthew's Episcopal Church.

Ardery, now in his sixties, was a World War II hero and part of Kentucky's aristocracy whose family had arrived before statehood. He had flirted with politics but never got elected, so he practiced law while dedicating himself to philanthropy. He supported the church, the ballet, the American Heart Association, and Kentucky's signature horse derby. He knew it wasn't enough to speak only about justice or merit when campaigning for a cause such as heart disease, for which he had raised millions of dollars. The same applied to mental illness, which now affected his neighbor's son. Wanting to help spur change and expand the network of concerned citizens, Ardery called his friend Barry Bingham Sr., the publisher of the *Louisville Times and Courier-Journal.*

Having served on one of Robert Felix's advisory groups in the formative days of NIMH, Bingham had some familiarity with the field. At Ardery's urging, he reviewed Todd's story and studied his testimony before Natcher's subcommittee. Only then did he agree to help their campaign on behalf of research and community housing. In this way, the three gentlemen from Kentucky, as they would be called, got to work.

Ardery and Todd looked for a house, and when they found a fixer-upper in Old Louisville, they leased it. Wellspring House would open in March 1982 as a way station on the journey between a hospital and independence. New York, California, and Florida had similar programs. And soon Louisville would have its first.

A week before the ribbon-cutting event, with announcements out to the press and the community, a gunman dressed up as Abraham Lincoln entered the Lincoln Federal Savings and shot customers in the lobby. He killed two patrons, injured another, then turned the gun on himself. He had schizophrenia. A series of neighborhood meetings followed, and one culminated with several hundred people protesting Wellspring House. Neither Todd, nor Ardery, nor a psychiatrist named Dr. Herbert Wagemaker could calm them. Only Barry Bingham Sr., who cherished having grown up in Old Louisville, had any effect. He described his devotion to the community and his personal commitment to Wellspring. He told the crowd about his late son Jonathan, who had once volunteered at Central State Hospital, after which he wanted to become a psychiatrist and study schizophrenia. Then a freak electrical accident ended his life.[3] "Wellspring would be a memorial to him," Bingham said. And that alone affected his neighbors.[4]

In the spring of 1982, Sam and two other men moved into Wellspring House. Social workers provided twenty-four-hour supervision, and residents began to learn how to manage their medicines. Vocational rehabilitation counselors helped them develop job-ready skills, starting with volunteering their time. Weekly outings enabled leisure activities. Wellspring House was built to be transitional, and therapeutic building blocks helped residents move toward independent living. Rotating chores—preparing meals, cleaning the bathrooms, emptying ashtrays, along with reviving skills that might have become dormant—kept residents busy when they weren't involved elsewhere. After several months, the local community mental health system contracted for a portion of Wellspring's costs. Expenses amounted to twenty-eight dollars a day compared to three hundred dollars a day for psychiatric patients at the local Humana University Hospital covered by Medicaid. By year's end, discharged hospital patients filled all fifteen spaces.

After Wellspring's launch, Todd and Ardery turned their attention to the research gaps. Todd asked his senator, Walter Huddleston, what the

federal government was doing about schizophrenia research. Huddleston
sent them to speak to people at NIMH, where two-thirds of the nation's
research about mental illness occurred. Under the NIMH budget in 1982,
roughly $18.6 million, or 10 percent, funded research about schizophre-
nia.[5] Had the federal investment for NIMH kept up with inflation, it
would have been closer to the $290 million budgeted for heart disease,
but still short of the $693 million invested in cancer research. That seemed
reason enough to set up an organization dedicated to research. Ardery, a
seasoned and successful fundraiser, had once been president of the American Heart Association, and he agreed to chair the American Schizophrenia Foundation. When the men from Kentucky met with NIMH director
Herb Pardes and Sam Keith, head of the Center for Schizophrenia Research, there was a lot to discuss.

Keith was a Yellow Beret, a doctor who joined the Public Health Service during the Vietnam War era and had subsequently found a better
reason to stay. He was dapper, round-faced, "cherubic," said Todd, someone who also had a commanding knowledge of the state of the field. As
the head of the NIMH office funding schizophrenia research in the community, he processed research grants directed to university laboratories.
He edited the *Schizophrenia Bulletin*, part of NIMH's drive to disseminate
information about current research to professionals and the public, and
word on the street considered him trustworthy when it came to speaking
to families. They appreciated that he could recite the most recent biological research findings, didn't activate guilt, treated them with respect, and
could be reached at home anytime. He was among the rare psychiatrists
who openly listed his home number in the public phone directory. At their
first meeting, Keith, though only in his mid-thirties, seemed authoritative
in his starched white Public Health Service uniform. Subsequent conversations took place at NIMH headquarters.

Todd's interest in privately funding research came amid the uncertain
and demoralizing days early in the Reagan administration. Pardes was
looking to universities and pharmaceutical companies to develop research
relationships. They were growing in capacity, largely due to federal grants,
and the future of NIMH research was uncertain despite the new celebrity of the Nobel Prize winners it had produced. In 1981, a psychologist
with ties to NIMH, Roger Sperry, shared a Nobel Prize in physiology and
medicine for his discoveries about the differing functions of the brain's

hemispheric lobes. Pardes made sure Todd realized that Sperry had gotten his start in the 1950s and that NIMH had remained committed to his work even after he relocated to Cal Tech.

The most recent acknowledgments of psychiatry's research endeavors came when Dr. Louis Sokoloff won the Lasker Award. His basic research led to the PET scan, making it possible to view a living human brain in real time using a nonlethal radioactive agent to track activity. Pardes could hardly contain his joy describing this discovery's potential for understanding the brain. The Albert Lasker Clinical Research Award committee had described Sokoloff as brilliant, and Pardes wanted Todd to understand that they said it was a "prime example of a bridge that leads from basic laboratory research to clinical application that can benefit millions of people everywhere."[6] *Newsweek* would headline its February 7, 1983, story about the brain and the PET scan by referring to it as a "human computer."

NIMH didn't oblige its researchers to publish a certain number of articles to advance a career. Nor did it force competition among the research staff to get results or impose strict timetables for discovery. Sokoloff's story represented a model of research and discovery that could vanish if NIMH didn't support the searching curiosity that allowed him to range widely from question to question. Along with three others, he cofounded the International Society for Cerebral Blood Flow and Metabolism (1965); he spent four years as the editor-in-chief of the *Journal of Neurochemistry* in the 1970s and served on the editorial boards of other scientific journals. After a year in France studying the biosynthesis of thyroid hormones, he returned to NIMH where, between 1969 and 1978, he revisited his interest in 2-deoxyglucose. He had paused his work on this before, always telling himself, "I'll get back to that."[7]

NIMH pioneers viewed scientific discovery with a long lens. Scientists like Sokoloff could allow his ideas to marinate, whether it was the chemistry of blood flow, the physics of radioactivity, the properties of a radioactive isotope, carbon-14, or the derivative of a glucose molecule, 2-deoxyglocose. This is what discovery was all about, and Sokoloff's was transformative. Colleagues were astonished, awestruck seeing the brain's different centers actively working when a person was listening, thinking, seeing, creating, anticipating, planning, reading, or computing.[8] Initially, PET scans were intended to study epilepsy. But presumably benefits would include understanding Alzheimer's disease, stroke, and cerebral tumors. And, perhaps at a later date, they would even benefit psychiatric diagnosis.[9]

Soon NIMH scientists were using the new PET scan to probe vastly different questions: Could they compare the frontal lobe of patients diagnosed with depression to that of those with seizures? What about the frontal lobe of children with attention deficit disorder? Others could learn about dyslexia, autism, or the four million people with obsessive-compulsive disorder. It also provided a way to examine a drug that was gathering interest, clozapine, which was seemingly without the twitchy or frozen muscles, known as tardive dyskinesia, that were a side effect of several other drugs, called neuroleptics, prescribed for schizophrenia.[10] The possibilities were immense. Sokoloff pinned the earliest digital printouts of bold blues, pale yellows, splattered reds, and thick black lines, configured within an oval-shaped brain, to his office walls. His colleagues pinned them to their doors the way teens plastered posters of the Beatles or John Denver on their bedroom walls. Pardes carried copies rolled up in the crook of his arm and stopped colleagues in the hall, where he unrolled the printouts and together they stood and marveled.[11]

Pardes wanted to make sure Todd appreciated that this was the best of what science could deliver. Sokoloff's thinking wasn't confined to a laboratory. He bent the ear of colleagues at professional meetings, sought out their differing opinions on ski slopes, or tested ideas with chemists in the NIH wine-tasting club. He spoke to pharmacologists, nuclear medicine specialists, neurologists, and neurosurgeons throughout the National Institutes of Health, in the halls at NIMH, and at universities including UCLA and the University of Pennsylvania.[12] Even so, he was modest, and generous in attributing much of his success to serendipity. "There was a lot of steps in here which is luck," he said, "just luck, or serendipity."[13]

Sokoloff's pathbreaking research was one of many NIMH initiatives Pardes spun when bringing Todd up to date. At that time in the early 1980s, NIMH scientists were also pinpointing neurons and the chemical conductors activating memory, experience, emotions, and images.[14] On the grounds of St. Elizabeths Hospital, research in laboratories examined new classes of drugs, benzodiazepines. On the patient wards, clinical research was underway. Psychiatrists tapped patients for central spinal fluids searching for clues to human behavior, information about dopamine, or metabolites suspected to hold clues about cognitive deficits and abstract thinking. People diagnosed with schizophrenia had abnormally high amounts of norepinephrine, and patients diagnosed with depression had increased levels of a metabolite of norepinephrine. Some labs stockpiled urine, while others searched for markers found in saliva, blood, or the excretions of sweat to correlate with the behavioral symptoms of specific diagnoses. Meanwhile, pharmacological research explored drugs for people diagnosed with several mental illnesses, including schizophrenia, depression, or manic depression.[15]

Todd realized that NIMH buzzed with activity. And that was good. But none of the tracking, tapping, testing, weighing, and measuring had produced a cure. Six years earlier, in 1975, Sam's doctors had expected the dopamine hypothesis to bring success by the end of the decade. That was clearly premature, and while Todd had not entirely abandoned hope, he was impatient on his son's behalf. Despite brilliant NIMH scientists racking up prizes, it was no longer the institute it had been when flexibility prompted spontaneity into journeys unknown. Now a lengthy award process for research, inside and outside the institute, had slowed everything. The first step depended on accepting a candidate's proposal. The second step hinged on congressionally appropriated funds, and that could happen at the last minute or take up to a year. While waiting for news, young professionals who were poised to launch a career in clinical medicine or academic research could be lost to other opportunities. In 1979, of the 60 percent of 533 applications that were approved, only 30 percent actually received funds. The process was maddening, and for the next year the numbers were again down. About half of the 414 applications got approved.[16]

The current administration dampened optimism, and NIMH veterans complained about paperwork and bureaucratic reports piling high. Dr. Robert Cohen remembered the days researchers could swing by Sears and Roebuck to pick up store-bought equipment—fishing weights and hooks, band saws, cow dehorners—to complete a lab experiment. No more. He felt like a bookkeeper, following instructions about how to file, document, and certify meetings. The administrative culture belied the vitality of science.[17]

NIMH's shrinking research capacity had frustrated Pardes even before Reagan's election. When Jimmy Carter was still president, in 1980, Pardes had considered increasing awards to young clinical researchers, doubling grants, making stipends competitive with industry or universities.[18] Reagan's policies ended that, implementing aggressive competition for scarce funds. Where NIMH had once built knowledge by piling discovery on discovery, it was now plugging the holes from budget cuts, a smaller staff, and diminished morale.

This was the state of affairs the NIMH director described when Bos Todd broached his ideas for funding the future of research. No message, no person, no proposal could have interested him more.

———————

Had Todd, Ardery, and Bingham not created the American Schizophrenia Foundation to promote research, the pending crisis might have seemed even more dire. Pardes and Keith introduced them to two experienced psychiatrists, William T. "Will" Carpenter (University of Maryland) and John Strauss (Yale University), who were longtime collaborators on schizophrenia research from their earlier work at NIMH in the 1970s. Each had moved into an academic environment, but their probing work continued to differentiate between types of symptoms, subtypes of schizophrenia, or range of outcomes. They could provide leadership for a foundation and help Todd and Ardery engage research-oriented psychiatrists. They too found it unthinkable that a future generation of clinical researchers might be lost at the very same time the current generation was explosively generating knowledge. To address this threat, they imagined how a private foundation could nurture talent. Much of their work started with correcting the faults they saw hobbling NIMH.

Carpenter and Strauss proposed streamlining the application process. Simplicity and speed of response would benefit candidates who could start their work immediately. There would be no official delays, no restrictions stemming from congressional appropriations, political whim, House or

Senate subcommittee hearings, public opinion, caprice, or favor—or political elections. Formidable scientists, those with a track record, would volunteer to oversee the process without remuneration. The unpaid cadre of experts would form a decision-making scientific council. They would rely on the hint of genius, and the promise of discovery, to identify future leading scientists.

Carpenter and Strauss introduced them to notable psychiatrists, people heading academic departments or working in laboratories, who refined this idea over several lunch meetings with the gentlemen from Kentucky. Without financial underpinning, however, their outline was more utopian than real.

Todd and Ardery were discussing this alternative model from Carpenter and Strauss at the same time that Barry Bingham turned to Katharine Graham, publisher of the *Washington Post*, for help raising funds. Carpenter's earlier efforts to gain her attention had failed. But Bingham was a dear and trusted family friend. To him, Graham's support of research on mental illness seemed a logical extension of her family's philanthropic activities. Her father, Eugene Meyer, represented the National Committee for Mental Hygiene when he testified at the congressional hearings in 1946 authorizing NIMH. Her parents' foundation, the Eugene and Agnes Meyer Foundation, had contributed to Woodley House, an eleven-bed community residence in Maryland; later the family foundation supported Washington's Green Door, then in its eighth year. Graham also had a personal story, and that came from her late husband's mental illnesses.[19]

Philip Graham had been the formidable and dashing editor of the *Washington Post* and *Newsweek*, a confidant of presidents and power brokers. In 1957, he was hit with a debilitating depression leading to "overwhelming doubts about himself and his abilities, a desire to seclude himself from the world and from people." Graham would write about this in her autobiography, *Personal History*. The next seven years found her hiding her constant concern about her husband's declining health. His dysfunction alternated with energy-spawning manic outbursts of grandiosity tinged with frantic irrationality. As difficult as this was for him, she was pained and humiliated, especially when he tamed his elevated moods with women and drink. Aside from needing to guard her privacy as a player among Washington's power brokers, moments of crisis raised the same questions as for other families. What was known about this murky diagnosis? Would a hospitalization be needed? Did treatments help? Then came his suicide in 1963.

Bingham hoped that her personal experience, alongside her family's historic role in mental health advocacy, would be enough to encourage her patronage.

———————

Katharine Graham invited seventy people to have lunch at the *Washington Post* on July 5, 1984. Her invitation referenced a somber occasion, appropriate to discussing schizophrenia, which she termed a "strange and baffling" illness affecting two million people.[20] It would also be a hopeful event, she predicted, to discuss an issue with towering consequences.

As publisher of the *Washington Post*, Graham was widely esteemed for her courage during the Nixon-Watergate years. It was an opinion not just held by the public but treasured by her as well. The only historic memento on display in her office, in addition to pictures of family or travels, was a gift from reporters Bob Woodward and Carl Bernstein, "a tiny wooden wringer," symbolizing Attorney General John Mitchell's crude attempt to silence reporting about Watergate.[21] Now she escorted Bos Todd into the boardroom, where they would have lunch. He was touched by her warmth and grace, and reminded why he admired the woman who fought the intimidation of the Nixon White House and had the courage to say no. And he hoped similar courage would say yes to them.

Thirty-three people accepted her invitation. Guests included chairpersons of university psychiatry departments, including John Romano from Syracuse University, who had mentored some of the doctors present that day. The industry sent representatives. A new class of drugs hadn't been marketed since Thorazine, for schizophrenia, in the 1950s and lithium, for bipolar depression, in the 1970s. Chuck Miles, NAMI's board chair and himself a doctor, considered this such an important meeting that he skipped NAMI's fifth annual conference in San Diego to attend.

Chairing that meeting was Gwill Newman, whom Todd, Ardery, and Bingham had hired to head the foundation when they changed the name to the Schizophrenia Research Foundation. She came from her home in Chicago, still grieving her son's death in a state psychiatric hospital two years earlier.[22] Finding a cure for paranoid schizophrenia, the disorder from which he'd suffered, would forever guide her life's ambition. While they ate lunch, Newman had Pardes explain why a private foundation was needed to underwrite psychiatric research. Pardes had left NIMH a few months before, and now he spoke as the chairman of Columbia University's Department of Psychiatry. He described the field as "hotter" than it had ever been, pointed to the benefits lithium had brought to millions of people with symptoms of manic depression, and estimated that the savings since the 1970s approached $6 billion. He noted that brain tissue could regenerate. As he had been doing at practically every gathering of new faces, he explained the importance of the brain imaging techniques Sokoloff introduced. There was the urgency of training the next generation of scientists. His new role as a private citizen allowed for this unfettered leadership.[23]

Newman had Carpenter and Strauss explain the scientific council, their new model. It had undergone little revision since they had first proposed its mechanisms and operations. They announced that of the stellar candidates to head the scientific council, Pardes would carry it forward. Then came the pitch for money—half a million dollars for the next three years.[24]

Two hours later, they adjourned. Before they left, Katharine Graham pulled Todd and Pardes aside. The meeting had been called to discuss schizophrenia, but bipolar disorders mattered too, she said. The whole field needed funding, discovery, and scientific leadership. She asked that their mission be broadened to include the depressive disorders. That is how, when the foundation's new leadership coined yet another name, they became the National Alliance for Research on Schizophrenia and Depression (NARSAD).

Graham declined further involvement, pointing to the many worthwhile projects already compelling her attention. Still, Sam Keith believed the meeting at the offices of the *Washington Post* had anointed their cause, and Todd thought the meeting was fantastic.[25] It justified establishing an alternative to the federal government's mechanisms funding research. Other health conditions raised research dollars privately, up to 60 percent from citizen donors.[26] Models existed: Phil Ardery supported the American

Heart Association, the March of Dimes worked for polio, and telethons raised money for muscular dystrophy. They knew it could be done. After lunch at the *Post* offices, goodwill infused talks about a merger for research purposes between NARSAD and NAMI. Over the next four years, the respective leaders tried to hammer out an agreement despite tensions about power sharing. Eventually personalities, priorities, and differing policies muddied the likelihood of success over their shared concerns, and the relationship ended.[27]

It took another couple of years to structure NARSAD. Meanwhile, they searched for a pot of gold. Local communities held "Pass the Bucket" events, and in New York Leonard Bernstein dedicated a concert at Lincoln Center. In California, the actress Jennifer Jones Simon hosted a benefit in Pasadena at the Norton Simon art gallery. Meetings in Chicago included the MacArthur Foundation. By 1986, contributions were coming in. Barry Bingham and the Pew Foundation had each committed $150,000; NAMI— by then there were about 750 affiliates—raised more than $300,000. Most contributions were smaller.

In April 1986, Columbia University's Department of Psychiatry sponsored a one-day symposium about "Recent Advances in Schizophrenia Research." Families were invited from NAMI affiliates in New York, New Jersey, and Connecticut. It turned out to be a dreary day after a week of intermittent rain, so thinking optimistically, Pardes hoped twenty families and mental health professionals would be willing to travel to Columbia's medical school campus in Washington Heights to discover the latest research. Advertisements put a spotlight on diagnostic techniques, the biology of schizophrenia, community housing, social supports, and family coping methods. Stories about homelessness and schizophrenia were appearing often in the news, and in a laudatory letter to the editor of the *New York Times* he commended their March 16–19 three-day series about schizophrenia.[28] But he noted sadly that "the day after the series ended you reported that the Administration was backing cuts for research at universities."[29] He could not have been more pleased to see roughly seven hundred people fill the auditorium of the College of Physicians and Surgeons.[30] It took some of the sting out of the announcement that came from the federal government saying there would be further funding cuts to universities for scientific research.[31]

Of the people in the audience that day, a middle-aged couple, Stephen and Connie Lieber, approached Pardes before returning to Great Neck, Long Island. Stephen Lieber was a person of means. He had built a fortune as an investment counselor with a mutual fund, Evergreen. Like other parents, an urgent desire to improve their daughter's life propelled them. They intended nothing less than to conquer mental illnesses.

Soon the Liebers were involved in NARSAD. Their sizable financial contributions helped NARSAD fulfill its goal of supporting young investigators. Their commitment of $200,000 annually for ten years put NARSAD on a different footing. Key to their commitment was the guarantee that every cent of every dollar, 100 percent of everything raised, would support research.

NARSAD's scientific council had finally raised enough money to start awarding research grants. It was a first step toward meeting the pressing concerns about training a new generation of research psychiatrists, which had permeated the field for more than a decade. In 1987, ten young investigators, chosen from twenty-eight applicants, received prizes for research as wide-ranging as a study about the emotions expressed within families of a person struggling with schizophrenia, to tracking neurological damage from a psychotic episode, to a molecular analysis of amino acids affecting mood disorders.[32] Six of the recipients had doctorates, four were medical doctors, and they came from nine different universities. Of them, six would later receive additional grant funding. In addition to underwriting the funding for young investigators, the Liebers endowed a prize in their name for a senior investigator, the Lieber Prize, starting that year. The first recipient was Dr. Benjamin Bunney, a Yale University professor researching dopamine.

The numbers of applications for NARSAD grants, as well as the number of recipients, jumped the next year. In 1988, of the sixty-eight applicants, twenty-four received grants. Having raised $900,000 the previous year, NARSAD was well on its way. Optimistic, they set a goal of $10 million over three years. When Gwill Newman fell ill in 1987, Connie Lieber replaced her to oversee the organization.

Barry Bingham died in 1988. Writing an obituary, Bos Todd paid homage to Bingham's "personal actions on behalf of those in need." He reminisced about Bingham's heroic role quelling neighbors' fears about living near people with schizophrenia in the week before Wellspring House opened. Since then four additional homes had opened and were serving forty-four people with serious mental illness. The house Sam Todd had moved into as a charter resident had been renamed Ardery House. Todd also honored Bingham's importance as a founder of NARSAD. Both aspects of his support had been key, Todd wrote, "at pivotal movements [that] enabled Wellspring and NARSAD to surge forward and succeed."[33]

CHAPTER 10

DUELING DIAGNOSES

W HEN RESEARCH PSYCHOLOGIST COURTENAY HARDING LECTURES ABOUT MENTAL ILLNESS, she often opens her presentation showing classical Greek statues we've all seen in museums, inviting her audience to consider how blues, yellows, reds, or browns once decorated these figures, now bleached white by light and air. Technology has discovered layers of pigment deeper than the naked eye can see. In an easy conversational style she tells a Yale audience, "We thought we knew all about them."[1] It's a brilliant introduction to one of her lectures about recovery from schizophrenia, a talk she has given more than five hundred times. Recovery has become her signature, and it is her legacy.

Harding's work began in 1976, when she needed a job. She was a recently divorced mom with three young children, and studying at the University of Vermont to become a research psychologist to add to her qualifications as a registered nurse. Dr. George Brooks, the superintendent of the Vermont State Hospital, was nearing retirement, and, looking back, he was in the process of reconnecting to patients he'd discharged twenty years earlier. What did they do after leaving the hospital? How had they been managing? He hired her that spring for what appeared to be an uncomplicated task of reviewing letters from them. It was a job she could easily do at home.

His question was warm and friendly, but he also had a research interest. Of the 269 patients he wanted to reach, many had been part of his early study of chlorpromazine (Thorazine) soon after interest in the drug swept through America in the 1950s. It was a powerfully sedating tranquilizing drug spreading hope with excitement for treating psycho-sis in patients diagnosed with mania, depression, and schizophrenia. It had been discovered at Sainte-Anne Hospital in Paris and was used to calm surgical patients. Word spread quickly from Paris to Heinz Lehmann in Montreal, at Douglas Hospital, and then to the United States.[2] Chlor-promazine, it seemed, could quell agitation and induce quiet, even apathy, which contributed mightily to ending lobotomies. But it packed a wal-lop from blocking dopamine. Dosage and how long someone was tak-ing it mattered when it came to side effects. Heart problems ("adverse cardiac events"), dizziness, sluggishness, and enlarged breasts, even for men, were common.[3] The most significant and predictable side effect was tardive dyskinesia (TD), which affected about one patient in seven.[4] Its symptoms were rigid limbs, tremors, muscle spasms, and Parkinsonian-like stiff facial masks. The uncontrollable movement of the tongue and lips, as if rolling around a hard candy, was called "bon-bon mouth."

Patients who responded well to the new drug got a ticket out of the state institutions. But not everybody had a favorable response, and they were thought to be chronic, hopeless, and were assigned to back wards where they and their demons existed in dreary isolation.

Conventional wisdom in the 1940s and 1950s subscribed to the belief that one-third of those diagnosed with psychosis, then synonymous with schizophrenia, got better; one-third stayed the same; and one-third de-teriorated. Knowing that the very word schizophrenia invoked fear, and might even lead to lifelong institutionalization, Brooks would have been cautious. He would have assessed how a patient had functioned in an ev-eryday environment, and he would have wanted to understand the ten-sions someone lived with. Were their lives complicated by social isolation? Family struggles? Problems on the job? Could there be a brain injury? A venereal disease? Arriving at a diagnosis was amorphous, subjective, and he might have looked through a Freudian lens to ask himself whether the patient's ego seemed intact. As impressionistic as this process was, he knew—everybody knew—that the very word schizophrenia could shatter a life and crush the family of the unlucky patients for whom there seemed to be no way out.

That unlucky group comprised 269 profoundly ill and disabled souls whom Brooks now wanted to understand retrospectively. In the hospital they had had few visitors and received little mail. "Hopeless" was scattered throughout their medical records. They could be retiring and withdrawn, or delusional, boldly hallucinating, expressly paranoid, or markedly dysfunctional in uneven ways. Emil Kraepelin would have recognized a description of them in *The Vermont Story*, published in 1961, because it sounded similar to his description of people diagnosed with schizophrenia in the 1890s. *The Vermont Story* said these patients were

> touchy, suspicious, temperamental, unpredictable, and over dependent on others to make minor day-to-day decisions for them. They had many peculiarities of appearance, speech, behavior, and a very constricted sense of time, space, and other people so that their social judgment was inadequate. Very often they seemed to be goalless or, if they had goals, they were quite unrealistic. They seemed to lack initiative or concern about anything beyond their immediate surroundings. Because of their very low socioeconomic level and prolonged illness, they suffered from profound poverty, inadequate educational opportunities, and a very limited experience in the world.[5]

Brooks would later reflect that "if nothing could be done, little or nothing was done, so that deterioration did indeed take place."[6]

If Vermont's health authorities hadn't noticed hospital overcrowding, these patients might have remained institutionalized indefinitely. But Vermont's rehabilitation department wanted to know whether life outside the hospital was possible. A collaboration between the hospital staff and state officials resulted in the discharge of a group of patients in 1956, and they were moved into a house in Montpelier, about fifteen miles away. Two years later, another two houses, one for men and another for women, were opened in Burlington. Plans for discharging patients were simple: people needed housing, and they needed help getting jobs. That became the work for staff.

Not much changed for the patients in the first few years after their discharge. They certainly showed nothing to warrant optimism. Brooks encouraged patients to stay on their medicines, but at the lowest levels possible. As an early researcher of chlorpromazine, he knew the side effects risked neurological and muscular damage, called "extrapyramidal," and he cautioned people less they develop side effects that could threaten their participation in vocational training or other activities.[7] The last group of patients left the hospital in April 1959.[8] He continued to see them in the community, where they lived in one of the houses. There they participated in group therapy sessions, something of a holdover from the hospital, where group sessions had become a fad.

Over time, it was apparent that even among the patients for whom there had been little hope, there were improvements. After about four years, Brooks noticed the people living in these houses starting "to blossom."[9] It was remarkable, the antithesis of what psychiatry defined as schizophrenia's key feature. Although he would later say it was "beyond all expectations of anyone in the rehabilitation team," their blossoming was palpable.[10] They had started paying more attention to grooming, walked with more authority, and seemed less afraid.

When asked what they thought had helped them get better, half answered it was medication or jobs; the other half attributed their improvement to a relationship with a specific person or group of people.[11] It makes sense, therefore, that they wanted to help others and organized a club, Helping Hands, for activities such as picnics, bowling, and dancing. Helping Hands also returned to the hospital to dispel the concerns and anxieties of patients who worried about leaving a place where they had received food, clothes, and shelter for years.[12]

Brooks started to think about the "natural history" of a disease process, the course of symptoms and their duration. With this in mind, he asked NIMH to support a "detailed and precise delineation of the community care concept for chronic patients."[13]

A hopefulness about rehabilitation infused Brooks's approach, but he was also mystified about what made the program successful. "There [was] no magic," he would later say, unable to explain what diverted their perpetual and irreversible deterioration.[14] Nothing theoretical explained the six people in ten who had become integrated in the local community.[15] But he did boast that schizophrenia no longer attached to roughly half of the previously described "chronic group of patients." They appeared to have recovered. How did this happen?

To help him understand the process, in 1976 Brooks asked Harding to interview thirty-eight of the most disabled 269 people. With a robust curiosity and newly sharpened pencils, she contacted former patients. They had been between sixteen and sixty years old when they were discharged, making them somewhere between thirty-six and eighty years old at the time she began. They had averaged six years in the Vermont State Hospital. A few had completed high school. She intended to learn, quite simply, what they did after leaving Vermont's only public psychiatric hospital. She didn't pose questions about their failures or their deficits, but about their struggles and even their successes. Harding writes, "We endeavored to identify the variety of elements and their importance in the social support system which have enabled [them] to remain in the community for twenty years."[16] Where did they live? For how long? How did they support themselves? Amuse themselves? Survive? Her field notes went into a cardboard box.[17] How they managed, that they even *had* managed, would later figure in fundamental questions about the diagnosis itself. For now, it was just apparent that they had managed.

At the same time, in New York, Robert L. "Bob" Spitzer was tackling another of psychiatry's challenges: diagnosis. For the next two decades, Spitzer and Harding moved in different directions, each marking guideposts still felt today.

———————

The same year *The Vermont Story* appeared in print, 1961, Bob Spitzer finished his residency at the New York State Psychiatric Institute and started psychoanalytic training. He was clean-cut, with short dark hair parted neatly to one side of his high forehead, and a reluctant smile as if he were sitting in a straight-backed chair. Psychoanalysis did not agree with him, nor did he much like working with patients. For him the sweet spot was psychometric research: questions social scientists considered when they talked about methodology, statistical validity, and the reliability of measurement.[18] He was barely out of training when he collaborated with Columbia University's biostatistician, Joseph Fleiss, about eliciting patient information needed by doctors. This was as important for research questions as it was for a basic diagnosis. Vast methodological differences hindered both. One study of the standard questionnaire, the mental status schedule, that psychiatrists used to assess a patient's disorder indicated that Kentucky's psychiatrists didn't agree with those in New York about diagnosing schizophrenia.[19] Thus began Spitzer's lifelong journey compiling, scrutinizing, counting, and categorizing information to standardize a psychiatric diagnosis.

Bob Spitzer was an impatient person. He disliked how clinical interviews meandered through the mind's caverns with nonspecific subjective questions to decide whether someone was neurotic or psychotic, or had an organic brain disorder.[20] That put him in the company of many who thought the 1952 edition of the American Psychiatric Association's diagnostic manual (later called the *DSM-I*) needed revision, and he became the official notetaker during the association's meetings for what, in 1968, would become the *DSM-II*. By then he'd designed a computer program for scoring observable symptoms. Foreshadowing a posture that would become his trademark pursuit of specificity, he expressed confidence in computers. They could override error-prone and fickle human judgments. Computers could eliminate unreliability because, he said, it "will always arrive at the same diagnosis when given the raw data describing a subject." Of course this overrode the veracity of the data. With his longtime collaborator Jean Endicott, he created a computer program, DIAGNO, to simulate clinical judgment.[21]

Diagnosis was a vexing problem professionals discussed in journals and conferences. Then, in 1973, *Science* printed "On Being Sane in Insane Places." David Rosenhan, a Stanford University professor of law and psychology, tested the premise of diagnosis by disguising patient surrogates, *pseudopatients*, to seek admission to psychiatric hospitals. They were told to feign auditory hallucinations and report voices repeating the words "empty," "hollow," and "thud." Would hospitals admit them? How would they diagnose the problem?

Twelve different hospitals admitted nine pseudopatients. Eleven diagnosed them with schizophrenia. Rosenhan asked whether this was warranted. "Some behaviors are deviant or odd," he admitted. But he maintained that diagnoses are in the minds of the observers and not valid summaries of characteristics displayed by the observed. Only a small group of dissident psychiatrists shared his belief. Importantly, each of the pseudopatients who had received a diagnosis of schizophrenia was discharged because they were ostensibly "in remission." This alone undercut the prevailing model that schizophrenia didn't allow for remission.[22]

Critics pounced on Rosenhan's study. They disparaged the methodology, the intent of upending a medical model, and the flimsy ruse of behavior to trick careless clinicians. Spitzer couldn't imagine that someone with schizophrenia could actually be in remission, and his fury spilled over in an article for the *Journal of Abnormal Psychology*.[23] Grave doubts led him to conduct his own study using the records of three hundred patients discharged from the New York State Psychiatric Institute. Not one, he reported, had received the diagnosis "in remission." Calls to other hospitals confirmed his supposition, and he denounced reports about why patients had been discharged, saying they were illogical.

Since chronicity was part of the diagnosis, a diagnosis of schizophrenia nullified any possibility of remission. Spitzer maintained that any chance to recover could only be explained by a psychiatrist's error, not a disease process. "If a diagnostic condition, by definition, is always chronic and never remits," Spitzer wrote, "it would be irrational not to question the original diagnosis."[24]

This debate played out during another revision of the diagnostic manual, which the APA asked Spitzer to chair in 1974, under the heading of the Taskforce on Nomenclature and Statistics. He had previously earned respect for having shepherded psychiatry through a tangled controversy removing homosexuality from the designation of "sociopathic personality disturbance."[25] Now he could create a terminology more appropriate to current practice and understanding, not just for one flawed diagnosis but for many.

Had Spitzer's colleagues expected the *DSM-III* to reshape psychiatry's foundations, he might have been overlooked. "When Bob was appointed to the *DSM-III*, the job was of no consequence," Columbia University's prominent research psychiatrist, Donald Klein, told the *New Yorker*. "In fact, one of the reasons Bob got the job," Klein said, "was that it wasn't considered that important. The vast majority of psychiatrists, or for that matter the A.P.A., didn't expect anything to come from it."[26]

Spitzer's compulsion to untangle the reliability of the terms used in diagnosis was paying off. With a data-hungry appetite and his antipathy to psychoanalysis, at the age of forty he stood at the door of the inner kingdom to remake its keys.

Bob Spitzer once told a reporter, "Not every problem of living is for us." He was interested in what caused distress, the "generalized impairment in social effectiveness of functioning." For this, he wanted his work revising the diagnostic manual to "remain four-square within the medical model in our approach to the classifications."[27] He wanted to focus on pathology, not on a psychoanalyst's preoccupation with psychodynamics or the infantile conflicts influencing personality and causing distress. This had led psychiatry to a near crisis, he thought, and he would turn to a different model, one that was more rooted in contemporary medicine and more likely to issue the clarity that accountability demanded. He enlisted trusted colleagues searching biology to provide a roadmap for the future.[28] On this journey, nothing was more important than how an accurate diagnosis could bring psychiatry into the fold of accepted medical practice.

"Diagnosis has functions as important in psychiatry as elsewhere in medicine," wrote a six-author team of psychiatrists at Washington University in what would become a pivotal article influencing Spitzer's work.[29] They developed a list of criteria, called Feighner criteria after the first author, to diagnose depression, schizophrenia, bipolar disorder, and eleven other conditions.[30] Starting with Feighner's list of symptoms, Spitzer recruited like-minded adherents who would purge psychoanalytic terms and principles to build a diagnostic manual marking diseases based on empirically observed or reported behavior. The resulting diagnosis would emphasize the course of illness, with specific time lines for its onset, course, and resolution.

For each of the Washington group's diagnoses, Spitzer intended to establish "reliability," a statistical concept conferring authenticity.[31] It meant everybody was talking about the same thing, a first step to building consensus about a diagnosis. This wasn't the case when Dr. Gaye Carlson, a young clinical associate at NIMH in 1972, admitted a nineteen-year-old male with a history of psychotic episodes. His psychosis resolved between episodes and he resumed his otherwise normal life. But this didn't align with theories about patients under forty-five. Recoveries between episodes didn't make sense, so his hometown psychiatrist referred him to NIMH for further study.

Carlson suspected this teenager suffered from bipolar disorder and was perhaps nearing the end of a manic episode. Her supervisor, Fred Goodwin, didn't agree and asked for a consultation with an expert in schizophrenia. When the expert arrived, the patient was naked, dancing, and smearing feces on walls of a seclusion room. Classic schizophrenia, he said instantly and definitively. Carlson disagreed and told Goodwin of her theory. Convince me with research, he insisted.

Carlson reviewed twenty previous patients who had been admitted consecutively to NIMH's metabolic ward; fourteen showed similar patterns. Goodwin remained dubious but wanted to be agreeable, so he submitted an article she had written to the *Archives of General Psychiatry.* The esteemed editor, Daniel X. Freedman, was impressed and immediately accepted "Stages of Mania" for publication in the April 1973 edition.[32]

Clinical observations clearly could remake psychiatry. So could intrigue, chaos, and power vacuums, John "Mickey" Nardo would later write. Reflecting on the culture he found when he trained at Columbia University in the late 1970s, he acknowledged, "I knew next to nothing about medical politics, or Insurance Companies, or the Pharmaceutical Industry." He continued: "I had come into Psychiatry at a time of enormous change. The Mental Hospitals were emptying with the coming of the anti-psychotic medications. The Community Mental Health movement was dying out. Psychoanalysis was no longer the dominant force in Psychiatry. It was the era of Managed Care. And a lot of those things came together with the publication of the *DSM-III*."[33]

The need for better vernacular, and for precision in diagnosis and research, concerned all of medicine. It mattered especially in psychiatry, where consensus, not laboratory findings, defined diagnosis. None could say with certainty whether active psychosis, or the sounds and voices of auditory hallucinations, or social eccentricities such as Leonard Frank's long hair and beard got assigned to one diagnosis or another. Some patients received a different diagnosis from every clinician and hence acquired three, five, or more, each with a cocktail of drugs to abate symptoms. Rooting out these complications excited Spitzer; they demonstrated the importance of his ambition.

To begin reforming the *DSM-II*, Spitzer enlisted colleagues at Columbia University, the University of Iowa, Harvard College, and Washington University where Feighner and his coauthors were faculty. He knew they would agree with the goal of refashioning a field often mocked in cartoons with patients or doctors reclining on chaise lounges.[34] Categories of pathology would replace idiosyncratic hunches about the process of despair or an existential loneliness. They would come from consensus-driven criteria. In this way, the *DSM-III* would revise and stamp anew the intellectual framework of psychiatry.[35]

———————

Writing a manual changing psychiatry's paradigm was bold and controversial. Psychoanalysts feared the *DSM-III* would become a Trojan horse undermining their iconic treatments of nonpsychotic conditions.[36] A case in point was the *DSM-III's* elimination of neurosis. Some psychiatrists worried that the pursuit of observable, group-endorsed objective criteria simplified the complexities of patients' lives. Clinical judgments that psychoanalysts had spent years fine-tuning could be nullified with a list of criteria resembling a takeout menu. The *DSM-III* diagnosis for panic attacks required the presence of four out of twelve possibilities, including palpitations, sweating, faintness, vertigo, dizziness, or unsteady feelings. A major depressive diagnosis required four out of eight specific conditions; melancholia, a classification of major depression, required three of the six criteria. There were plenty of objections that with this specificity of symptoms, biological psychiatrists would be able to outmaneuver the diagnoses. Spitzer would later be accused of trying "to cram psychological suffering into faux medical categories."[37]

Christopher Lane's book *Shyness: How Normal Behavior Became a Sickness* shows how the *DSM-III* turned shy and quiet people, sometimes called introverts, into a diagnostic category. Did introverts have internal mental processes promoting morbid qualities such as withdrawal, isolation, self-absorption, absentmindedness, detachment, daydreaming? Were extreme introverts "asocial," flirting with antisocial personality disorders? Or were they "schizoid," which previous manuals had linked, along with "schizotypal," to schizophrenia? "Introverted," "withdrawn," and "eccentric" were on the checklist of characteristics of people who developed schizophrenia, and they were also criteria for paranoid, schizoid, schizotypal, or borderline personality disorder.[38]

Throughout 1978, the seven-person *DSM-III* Advisory Committee on Personality Disorders debated what to call shy people. Objections came from data-driven psychologists, educators, Freudian and Jungian analysts, and a few biological psychiatrists. They debated and attempted to package new disease categories. Spitzer polled the committee, but there was no consensus. He then bypassed his committee and created a new condition, the schizoid personality disorder. That is how attributes of "shy" became pathological "introversion," or in the words of Lane's subtitle, "how normal behavior became a sickness," describing "eccentricities of communication or behavior" compatible with personality disorders. The new diagnostic category listed people who were "loners," "humorless or dull," and lacked "affect in situations in which an emotional response would be appropriate." In short, they appear "cold" and aloof." As with other disorders in the *DSM-III*, as a unique medical condition, it qualified for Medicaid and Medicare benefits, commercial insurance reimbursement, research, and anyplace where diagnosis had to be specified.

Stereotypes about gender, race, and class riddled the process despite intentions of making diagnosis comport with empirical observations reflecting scientific methodology. Introversion, considered a negative in Western culture, was a positive attribute in Japan.[39] Gender-prescribed courtship accompanied a diagnosis of introversion, now part of schizoid personality disorder: "Because of a lack of social skills, males with this disorder are usually incapable of dating and rarely marry. Females may passively accept courtship and marry." Class stereotypes informed a diagnosis about people "working in jobs that involve little or no contact with others, or living in skid-row sections of cities."[40]

When it came to schizophrenia, the *DSM-III* noted that "diagnosis is made more commonly among the lower socioeconomic groups." Spitzer acknowledged that "the interpretation of the evidence supporting these hypotheses is controversial."[41] That a racial diagnosis also accompanied schizophrenia was apparent, as historian and psychiatrist Jonathan Metzl writes in *Protest Psychosis: How Schizophrenia Became a Black Disease.* Metzl's analysis of medical charts in a hospital in Michigan in the 1960s and 1970s shows that the fearsome qualities of aggression, hostility, and violence were more often attributed to Black patients whose classification was paranoid schizophrenia. Their white counterparts similarly diagnosed were more often described as depressed, cooperative, or withdrawn.[42] It was nonbiological, impressionistic, and in some instances tautological.

The *DSM-III* perpetuated the impression that remission for schizophrenia was rare. Reluctant to foreclose miracles in medicine, the *DSM-III* conceded, "There is always the possibility of full remission or recovery, although its frequency is unknown."[43] Under the best of circumstances, symptom remediation was all that could be hoped for, and with psychiatry's dependence on drugs, pharma became inextricably linked to diagnosis in the *DSM-III*, otherwise called "the bible."

Spitzer and the *DSM-III* advisory committee may have aimed for rigor, but despite the billions of dollars NIMH had invested in basic research, psychiatric diagnosis did not have a scientific foundation. The reliability of the diagnostic categories outweighed the validity, and uncertainty remained about whether the term actually fit the categories the new manual prescribed. Anne Harrington, author of *Mind Fixers*, writes that, in the 1970s, "psychiatrists had rallied around biology and the 'medical model' as a way of exorcising the specters of psychoanalysis, antipsychiatry, and radical social science. In the 1980s, they continued to rally around that model, but largely for a different reason: to assert guild privilege."[44]

Spitzer's teams of advisors, with their spin-off committees, spent five years reconfiguring disorders to arrive at 285, up from the *DSM-II*'s 182.[45] The committee spent another two years preparing for a rollout with field testing before 1980, when the *DSM-III* was finally published.

The project baffled colleagues who saw it claim unjustified authority to put its stamp on, even create, trenchant controversies. Watching this unfold at conferences, or in publications and newsletters, one of psychiatry's leaders, Paul Fink, mused in 1978, "I do not know who determined that this small group of people should try to reorganize psychiatric thinking in the United States, but I am somewhat concerned that they have such an arrogant view of their mission and are not willing to incorporate some of the things which we have learned over the past 70 years."[46]

The consequences would be lasting. Scholars Allan Horwitz and Gerald Grob describe how "the need for medical legitimacy, compatibility with a biomedical model, and conditions that third parties would reimburse, led psychiatry to replace the psychodynamically oriented *DSM-I* and *DSM-II* with the radically empiricist *DSM-III*."[47] With the clarity of a generation's experience, and the insights of retirement, Mickey Nardo reflected in his blog *1 Boring Old Man*, "Maybe the framers of the DSM-III had no intention of ushering in an era of increasingly corrupt and/ or trivial science." But "they facilitated that development by restricting the psychiatric paradigm to biology and counting on a steady stream of scientific discoveries to carry the day."[48] The University of Iowa's Nancy Andreasen, a member of Spitzer's advisory committee, initially praised the work, believing it was revolutionary and a "massive reorganization and modernization of psychiatric diagnosis."[49] Later, almost apologetically, she would say it also had a "dehumanizing impact on the practice of psychiatry."[50]

While the revisions that led to the *DSM-III* were under way, and outside the field's power centers, Courtenay Harding started tracking thirty-eight of Brooks's former patients in the summer of 1976. They had originally been diagnosed according to the *DSM-II*'s profile of symptoms for schizophrenia. In addition to difficult personalities, dysfunctional emotional states, and the likelihood of "misinterpretation of reality," they had behavioral oddities. Harding knew that as many as 80 percent had shed the peculiar, even life-threatening behaviors bringing them into the hospital. By the time she started to speak to them, about one-third had moved from the rehabilitation houses to boarding or nursing homes. Two-thirds held jobs in hospitals, hotels, or small businesses. Even though they participated in senior citizen centers or church groups, they remained pretty much on the community's social fringe. But more than half had shed the reasons they had been classified as "schizophrenic."

Harding's task that summer would be to explain what accounted for this improvement. She had replies from 87 percent of the people Brooks had asked for an update. George Albee, one of Brooks's colleagues and the chairman of the Department of Psychology, recognized the importance of such a powerful response rate. Suspecting there was something more to be learned by plumbing the material, he urged Harding to pursue a grant from NIMH. He even called his friend, Loren Mosher, the psychiatrist then heading the NIMH Center for Studies of Schizophrenia, to pave the way for Harding's continued study.[51]

NIMH usually funded university investigators with thick résumés, not young nurses who had just received a bachelor's degree in psychology. The same year that NIMH funded Harding for what was basically a feasibility study to see whether there was something meriting more research, it awarded grants steeped in biology examining pathology, family studies, psychopharmacology, and a host of chemical and neurological processes. Fewer social scientists found schizophrenia a compelling subject of study.

But of those who applied that year, Alma Menn, in Palo Alto, intended to learn how patients fared after leaving Soteria House, a homelike, non-drug treatment alternative to hospitalization; Dolores Kreisman, a social psychologist, wanted to further her research about families who were responsible for a discharged relative; and Steven Segal, in Berkeley, got a grant to understand the reintegration of patients into the community.

That Mosher responded favorably to Harding's query about initial NIMH funding doesn't surprise. As the progenitor of Soteria House, and having worked with Menn, he would be inclined to welcome deeper understanding of the post-hospital lives of an exceptionally responsive 87 percent of the entire cohort. He had been a coauthor of a 1976 *Schizophrenia Bulletin* special report about schizophrenia and cautioned that prognostic indicators should not be constructed to create a dichotomy but rather should describe a patient along a continuum. He had already sparred with Spitzer about the lingering impact of a diagnosis that would stay with a person for life. Shouldn't someone be able to shed the trappings of illness at discharge? he asked.[52] He would be inclined to think favorably about Harding's proposal to NIMH. But to cover the essential bases, he sent a team of experts to Vermont for a site visit. John Strauss was on that team.

Strauss had worked at NIMH for eight years before moving to Rochester University in 1972 to become the Psychiatry Department's director of clinical research. Study with Piaget in Switzerland had informed his training as a clinician and researcher, giving him unusual breadth, and he had continued collaborating with Will Carpenter. They had numerous publications about symptoms, diagnosis, and prognosis, and they had even had the audacity to argue that people with schizophrenia had diverse lives. "Neither diagnosis nor individual symptoms are substantial predictors of outcome," they wrote in 1976.[53] That observation led to an even more provocative question a couple of years later about patients who recover.[54] Strauss would later note that an article he had submitted "showing a wide variation in the outcome of people with schizophrenia" was rejected by a prominent journal. "One of the reviewers stated blankly and without evidence: 'This is not true.'"[55] Strauss and Carpenter suspected otherwise.

In addition to inviting Strauss, Mosher asked Malcolm Bowers, a Yale psychiatrist researching dopamine, and Jack Maser, a NIMH psychologist, to round out the evaluation team going to Vermont. Site visits were common, and this one included a tour of the hospital and grounds, plus a meeting with this young nurse, Harding, to assure themselves she understood the basics and had access to all that she claimed. Perhaps more than others on the team, Strauss wanted to learn more about her topic, "Chronic Mental Patients in the Community for 20 Years."

————————

Harding began the eighteen-month NIMH grant a rookie, as she called herself, piecing together information nobody had thought to assemble the way she would. She was interested in people who struggled each day: How did they do it? Who helped them? What did they need? And what did they want? These were the questions that made sense to her. Having met some patients on the wards during nursing school, and speaking to others later while working for Brooks, she bubbled with insights and information. When she received the award, they became mentors, as did roughly a hundred people who would help her acquire the tools of a social scientist while she learned to stratify samples, match for comparability, and employ protections of research confidentiality. All this would be on display in the next proposal NIMH funded to complete the work. Running from 1979 to 1984, the research would become the mainstay of her dissertation when she made a career change to become a psychologist.

Harding had to answer an essential question in order to establish the legitimacy of her findings: did the patients, once diagnosed with schizophrenia based on the *DSM-II*, meet the diagnostic criteria for the *DSM-III*? Given the buzz, she knew her findings, no matter how compelling, would seem inconsequential if the 269 former patients did not meet the *DSM-III* criteria. "Without the re-diagnosis," she told me, "no one would take the project's findings seriously in the heat of the excitement about the *DSM-III*."[56]

A re-diagnosis was imperative after she moved to Yale University for a fellowship. John Strauss had recently joined the faculty and, with Alan Breier, the chief resident in psychiatry, undertook the project. They worked with redacted files for the 269 people, asking only if their diagnosis was a match for *DSM-III* criteria for schizophrenia. They found that 118 of the original group of 269 patients did meet the *DSM-III* criteria. Better yet, eighty-two of them were still alive.

For her doctoral dissertation, Harding would analyze these eighty-two patients and test whether the *DSM-III*'s presumptions about a persistent decline held up. What she discovered was that roughly two-thirds of the discharged Vermont patients had shown different "degrees of productivity, social involvement, wellness, and competent functioning." Or to answer the question, no, the persistent decline, a holdover from Emil Kraepelin, did not hold up. With this, she planted a flag for recovery.[57]

While still working on her various grants, even before writing her dissertation, Harding hit the lecture trail and conference circuit. Initially she accompanied Brooks and Albee, proud sponsors as early as 1977, when they addressed a group of international psychiatrists in Canada. Soon Strauss joined the troupe, explaining that the *DSM-III* had run afoul because it had compressed nuanced clinical information; diagnosis was compacted over a relatively short time, perhaps the worst of times, and often marked by psychosis; and its negative prognosis was unsustainable. Strauss accused *DSM-III*'s architects of pigeonholing patients with preordained uniformly poor outcomes.

Beliefs that patients could not do well had defined policies and organized services. They influenced clinical assessments, informed what doctors and psychologists told patients and their families, affected insurance policies, and led to vast self-doubts and avoidance behaviors. Stigma led to self-censorship. The *DSM-III*'s campaign to clarify an opaque diagnostic stew had ignored international studies pointing toward recovery. Long-term tracking was more common in Europe than in the United States and already part of the research of Luc Ciompi, Manfred Bleuler, and Gerd Huber. In 1980, the *Schizophrenia Bulletin* devoted an entire issue to research in Austria, Scandinavia, and Switzerland. A review of the studies published up to 1979 led Ciompi to say that "for everyone who does not link the concept of schizophrenia itself to an obligatory bad outcome, the enormous variety of possible evolutions shows that *there is no such thing as a specific course of schizophrenia.*" His optimism came from his own work in Bern, allowing him to boast, "The potential for improvement of schizophrenia has for a long time been grossly underestimated."[58] Despite documented evidence to the contrary, Spitzer and *DSM-III*'s backers accepted only one outcome, the increasing residual impairment, for schizophrenia.

Research psychologists and married colleagues Patricia Cohen and Jacob Cohen introduced a slightly different understanding about the limitations of diagnosis. They asked, quite simply, what was the bias of professionals who saw only people who remained ill? Even the clinical setting where someone met a patient could affect a diagnosis of schizophrenia or opioid/alcohol addictions. Did treatment take place in a public clinic or in a private office? And what of the patients who moved on, who got better? If the physicians saw only those who didn't improve, which was the basis of Kraepelin's initial work with hospitalized patients, it had to inevitably skew their perceptions. And that became the title of their article, "The Clinician's Illusion," appearing in the December 1984 issue of the preeminent *Archives of General Psychiatry*.

Harding's message could be equally provocative, and her keynote of a Community Support Systems conference in 1982 accelerated her visibility. The next year, she lectured at Yale, NIMH, the APA, and more. She was becoming recovery's rock star. She didn't meet her teenage dream of becoming a Pan Am stewardess, but over the years she would rack up 750,000 miles of airline credits.

In October 1984, with a doctorate in hand, she delivered grand rounds at the New York State Psychiatric Research Institute, on the Washington Heights medical campus of Columbia University. It was home to the field's eminent biological researchers, psychiatrists as well as psychopharmacologists. Patient beds for research in a university hospital, a postgraduate center for psychoanalytic study, and a school of public health added to its luster. Her topic, Vermont's outcome study, drew on her dissertation's findings about recovery. With data packaged in statistics about long-term rehabilitation, she spoke to an august gathering. Spitzer was there, as were many of his colleagues. It was also home to Patricia Cohen and her colleagues.

Harding's findings about recovery amplified a counternarrative to the *DSM-III*. She delivered her lecture, answered a few questions, left some in the audience amazed and others protecting the guild. Spitzer would have none of it. "I don't believe it," he told colleagues. A seasoned researcher was heard whispering as he left the auditorium, "Those numbers are as good as we get with medication."[59] Spitzer was revising the diagnostic manual *DSM-IIIR*—R for "revision"—to fill gaps and plug holes in the authoritative guide that was now directing the future of psychiatry, insurance billing, research, and patient care. But Harding's reputation was gathering momentum, and in 1985 she delivered a plenary address at NAMI's annual meeting in New Orleans.

NAMI's conference bracketed an entire day for workshops about rehabilitation. One of the speakers, John Talbott, who had become president of the American Psychiatric Association, proclaimed, "Quick fixes will not work." Good treatment, he said, is "much more than a pill and doctor visit."[60] Bill Anthony, a psychologist who founded Boston University's Center for Psychiatric Rehabilitation, encouraged families to challenge erroneous myths about the intractability of diseases. Use the facts, he said. John Strauss sat with NIMH's Sam Keith, both cheering from the audience.

With a commanding frame and striking red hair curling softly between her ears and shoulders, wearing slacks and a colorful striped blouse, Harding entered the auditorium. Seeing lights, microphones, and chairs set up for fifteen hundred people, "took my breath away," she remembered. She had come to tell these families that the story of recovery in Vermont was real. She would tell them about George Brooks, about the subgroups of thirty-eight patients they studied intensely in 1976, about the 118 patients who lined up with the *DSM-III*'s diagnosis, and about the group of eighty-two she had selected for her doctoral investigation. Here, she thought, parents nursing angry wounds would be happy to learn about recovery. Clinicians had told them to expect little and given them bad news, perhaps unwarranted. These families should have been the ones to cradle hope. But when she looked around the audience, the faces she saw seemed sad. Mothers and fathers had come to hear about recovery. Some confided that recovery hadn't touched their children, and they worried it might never. They were impatient, not heartened to learn that recovery was a journey that could meander for years, even decades.

Rather than bringing these families the good news they wanted, she feared she had unclogged a reservoir of pain. For them a different kind of research, biological research at NIMH, seemed more promising. Already there were discoveries about molecules and neurotransmitters, fluids that traveled the body and could be seen under a microscope. Perhaps they were carrying something magical, something more immediate, with a message of hope just sitting there waiting to be discovered on a slide. No, there was no magic, not in Vermont as Brooks had said, not anywhere.[61]

NAMI would soon confirm that the parents Harding had met had reason to lament. A first-of-its-kind study of the membership revealed just how many of their offspring struggled mightily, and that one in four were in prison.[62]

Harding and Strauss treated the *DSM-III*'s description of a perpetual decline as something akin to humbug. She would tell an audience at the APA annual meeting in Dallas in 1985: "If more than half of the patients improve over the long-term course and get on with their lives, then changes must occur in policy, programs, treatment, education, and training to foster this slow struggle back to wellness."[63]

Some pointed to Vermont's unique rehabilitation programs admiringly but paid little attention to its components. An opportunity to compare them to a similar group of patients in Maine would answer whether Vermont's rehabilitation services, with an emphasis on employment, housing, and eclectic community services, brought additional benefits. She collaborated with Michael DeSisto from Maine's mental health bureau to compare matched subjects, including a re-diagnosis of a sample of patients.

The results of this comparative study became the basis of several talks starting in 1990 and publication in the *British Journal of Psychiatry* in 1995.[64] It showed that 68 percent of Vermont's patients benefited from the emphasis on continuous services, including employment and rehabilitation. They displayed fewer disturbing symptoms, higher levels of sustained employment, and more robust community functioning than the Maine patients. Harding thought the hope and optimism grounding Vermont's program explained some of its better results. Still, nearly half of Maine's patients improved. The results, Harding said, "got us thinking about human resilience."[65]

In the twenty years since Robert Spitzer and Courtenay Harding worked in parallel space, their positions cemented. In 1994, the American Psychiatric Association released the next iteration of its manual to assist in diagnosis, the *DSM-IV*. Like its predecessor, the *DSM-IV* discouraged hope for people with schizophrenia saying, "Complete remission (i.e., a return to full premorbid functioning) is probably not common in this disorder." It gestured toward a softer landing, saying that "numerous studies have indicated a group of factors that are associated with a better prognosis."[66] But it bypassed the ongoing work showing recovery's steady climb.

Harding continued posing questions to learn about the person behind the diagnosis, a stance on full display in an article she coauthored with James Zahniser at the University of Colorado School of Medicine.[67] They challenged seven persistent myths about schizophrenia, starting with "Once a schizophrenic, always a schizophrenic." Evidence about heterogeneity of outcomes had long since challenged that dictum, and still the *DSM-IV* reiterated it. The debate would have seemed but an abstraction, the type of argument in which academics engaged, had it not influenced the expectations of tens of millions of people.

Harding and Zahniser contend that the "long process of recovery implies a revision of what the clinician tells patients." With studies showing that half of the patients significantly improve or recover, "This new message keeps a small spark of hope alive. Hope promotes the self-healing capacity inherent in any recovery process for any illness." They say that reducing that, eliminating hope, promotes "pessimism about outcome for these patients thus significantly reducing their opportunities for improvement and/or recovery." More so, it can also "discourage clinicians, significantly impact the view of the patient, and thus his or her treatment."

For each of the myths about which they write, they detail opportunities "to enhance the possibility of improvement and recovery." It was the place she started when George Brooks asked her to find out what happened to patients nobody expected to blossom.

CHAPTER 11

THE SOUL'S FRAIL DWELLING HOUSE

F IVE YEARS AFTER THEIR LAUNCH IN MADISON, WISCONSIN, IN 1984, and with a membership nearing fifty thousand people, NAMI hired Laurie Flynn to become its second executive director. Flynn was in her forties, mother to eleven children, many of whom she had adopted when she was working her last job at a child welfare agency. And she was fiercely confident. A Washington native, she prided herself on knowing how to use influence, and she intended to build the organization to assure families got the help their mentally disabled relatives needed.

Flynn took command of an organization that was understaffed and overwhelmed. When Flynn walked through the office doors at Fifteenth Street NW on her first day, all she saw were bags stamped "US Postal Office." They had started to arrive the previous July, after television host Phil Donahue showcased mental illness and encouraged viewers to contact NAMI. They did, and now, ten months later, their letters filled unopened bags stuffed in every corner and spilling over desks. Almost immediately she hired two staff who would become key: Ron Honberg, a social worker who subsequently earned a law degree while developing policy initiatives, and Dick Greer, a family member and former staff managing government relations for Democratic senators.

Greer prepared NAMI's 1984 legislative priorities. Confident that NIMH scientists were close to understanding the differences between "diseased" and "normal" brains, NAMI called for tripling NIMH funding to $532 million from $174.3 million.[1] Fortunately, NAMI's membership included the families of politicians. Nancy Domenici, married to New Mexico's Republican senator Pete Domenici, had shown her mettle organizing congressional wives for educational seminars. Her husband would show his by assuring that the Appropriations Committee kept funds flowing to all the health institutes, especially NIMH.

When NAMI's ally Herbert Pardes announced he would leave NIMH by the end of 1984, Flynn wanted his replacement, Shervert Frazier, to meet families before arriving in December. Frazier came from Harvard's McLean Hospital, where, as chief psychiatrist with clinical experience, he had organized research. He had also served on the public relationship committee for the American Psychiatric Association, so he knew the value of shaping impressions.

Science reported that Frazier was expected to "liberate NIMH from its underdog status in the biomedical health establishment."[2] Anxious to speak to him, Flynn called his office three times to schedule an appointment. Each time, his secretary put her off. The fourth time, Flynn asked for his speaking schedule to find out which medical schools, hospitals, or professional conferences Frazier would be attending. She forwarded the schedule to local NAMI affiliates with instructions: sit in the front rows; as soon as Frazier finished speaking, shoot up a hand; identify yourselves as representing NAMI; ask, "What is your agenda for schizophrenia research?" This is how the incoming director of NIMH met NAMI's parents, learned their concerns, and saw their tenacity.[3]

In December 1984, when Frazier was introduced to staff and advisors at NIMH headquarters in Rockville, Maryland, Flynn heard him pledge to "search for new knowledge in neuroscience and behavioral science."[4] With or without NAMI's prodding, his priority would be research, as it had been at Harvard. He would reorganize the institute around disease entities aligned with the *DSM-III*.[5] He would further initiatives already underway and benefit from the recent excitement about the discovery of genetic markers for depression in the Amish community. He organized consensus statements about the pharmacology of mood disorders. He announced a schizophrenia research branch and named Sam Keith its head. He directed additional funding for schizophrenia research and authorized a national plan to rapidly expand knowledge about schizophrenia, fully aware that, as Keith would write, "there are not simple and unequivocal answers to the challenges posed by schizophrenia."[6] Four months into the job, *Science* noted Frazier's "driving purpose." Some, however, worried about whether NIMH should organize its work around disease entities. Was there not more to mental health research than drugs or hospitalization? asked *Science*.[7] Where did education or services belong, two of the three elements of Robert Felix's original three-legged stool? Felix's model, said a psychiatrist familiar with its organizing principles, intended that "basic scientists were not left isolated at the bench." The ideal meant that "clinicians were expected to develop bench projects. The clinical research wards were [situated] on one side of the building and basic labs studying neuropharmacology in rodents and primates were 50 feet away on the other side."[8] These intersecting features no longer seemed pertinent to the culture that had changed so much that, by 1985, a revised mission statement notably omitted the phrase "mental health."[9]

Developing a relationship with NIMH was only one item on Flynn's agenda. Another pertained to NAMI itself. This she knew her first week when a mother called from Seattle to welcome her before she unfurled a manifesto of woes challenging Flynn to redress the indignities visited on her and her son. Where were the services her son needed to resume a life? Why did doctors still accuse her of the baseless charge that she was a schizophrenogenic parent? Flynn felt battered as much by this parent's harangue as she did by the persistent discredited and nonscientific beliefs about schizophrenia's origins. Flynn again felt battered by parents in New York's affiliate who looked to her to remedy the state's failed social services. Two-thirds had adult kids living at home. They suffered tardive dyskinesia's potentially irreversible twitches. They cycled in and out of hospitals and jails and spent time living on the streets. Members' families worried about the federal government's threats to Medicare, Medicaid, Section 8 housing vouchers, and basic food stamps—federal programs the states ran.

Flynn didn't minimize these concerns, but she didn't see how NAMI could build a strategic plan around improved services when states were as different as New York and Washington. She was hardly indifferent to these parents and their day-to-day burdens helping their children resocialize. She considered herself one of them—a "NAMI mommy," as they called themselves in playful moments. She often mentioned her oldest daughter who struggled with serious depression and had spent a turbulent Thanksgiving weekend in an emergency room after a suicide attempt. Yet she didn't see, or believe, that a campaign for better services would accomplish what was needed. Already families had spent "years pounding Medicaid, and still we had crappy public services," she said. No, NAMI would prioritize research to discover a cause and hasten a cure. "Science is telling us these are brain disorders and we have to support that and own that," she said.[10] It would drive NAMI's "highest goal," which would be "to launch a war on mental illness."[11]

Funding basic laboratory research became NAMI's driving priority. At that moment, the trial spectacle of John Hinckley Jr., who had attempted to assassinate Ronald Reagan just two months after his inauguration, had marked psychiatry a soft science with hairsplitting bickering about the significance of brain size or evidence about ventricles for schizophrenia. There was the important matter of how to understand Hinckley's actions. He had carried guns across state lines, mapped out his hopes for future celebrity, and shot the president of the United States in broad daylight—all for the love of an actress, Jodie Foster, whom he had never met. Was he suffering from schizophrenia, as one set of psychiatrists and his defense attorneys claimed? Or was twenty-seven-year-old Hinckley self-absorbed, immature, aimless, irresponsible, yet firmly in control of his behavior, as another set of psychiatrists argued for the prosecution? The jury's decision that he was "not guilty by reason of insanity" rumbled through the public on June 21, 1982. ABC announced a poll saying 76 percent of the public thought jurors had reached the wrong decision.[12] Syndicated columnist George Will attacked "the quicksilver axioms of a 'science'" in which "psychiatry is ideology masquerading as medicine." Calling psychiatrists "itinerant experts-for-hire," he said they were less principled than alchemists.[13]

Lawmakers immediately revisited the federal insanity plea. Who should be responsible for proving that the alleged criminal behavior was caused by a mental defect or illness? The prosecution in Hinckley's trial had to prove he knew what he was doing, that he had capacity to plan, organize, and act purposefully, and that he wasn't psychotic at the time of the shooting. The defense disagreed. They said his deteriorated mental condition, while not uncontrollably psychotic, was sufficiently grave and impaired that his judgment was compromised. Four congressional hearings in July and August assessed federal law and rewrote it to make defendants responsible for proving, beyond a reasonable doubt, that they were mentally ill at the time of a crime.

———————————

Hinckley's trial introduced new ideas for public consumption about the brain's influence on behavior. It became a newsworthy organ, opening a niche for science journalists. No more would the brain exist primarily in a metaphysical sense, or as Shakespeare's construct, the "soul's frail dwelling house." In February 1983, *Newsweek* ran a cover story about the brain, "a human computer," and included cartoons depicting "neurons [as] the brain's relay station." In August, *Psychology Today* profiled Richard Jed Wyatt, chief of NIMH's neuropsychiatry branch, whose work on tissue transplantation described "neurons, regeneration, and the brain as a privileged site."[14] The next month, in a five-part series, the *Washington Post*'s science writer, Philip Hilts, hailed NIMH's biological pursuits researching the brain. "Even some of the subtler things, the supposed personality problems, are also heavily influenced by biology," he wrote.[15] Seizing on public interest and the need to play some role repairing psychiatry's damaged image, NIMH organized a seminar to introduce science journalists to two of its luminaries, Julius Axelrod and Daniel Weinberger.

Hinckley's trial tapped into a curiosity about brain research. In 1984, PBS aired an eight-part special, "The Brain," five years in the making. The series addressed the workings of a mysterious organ, which Richard Restak, author of a stand-alone companion book, called a "gnarled mass of cells." How was the brain structured? How did it cue danger, or calculate where a baseball would land, or direct muscles for a ballerina's pirouette? How did it store memories of poetry, or of love?[16] Questions that had been discussed since Cicero could now be studied scientifically, and even pinpoint where, in a specific part of the cerebellum, memories most likely resided.

The seventh segment of *The Brain*, "Madness," opened the doors to a locked ward for people with schizophrenia at the federal government's St. Elizabeths Hospital. NIMH staffed three wards devoted to schizophrenia, for as many as forty-eight voluntary patients. In exchange, they partici- pated in research, making their blood, urine, central spinal fluid, tears, or saliva available for chemical analysis. Four psychiatrists appeared along- side talking heads from Stanford University and UCLA. But it was the patients, as symptomatic as they were sympathetic, who touched viewers' hearts. Jerry, in his twenties, could have been anybody's son or brother wanting to be understood, asking to be useful, and hoping, unrealistically, to return home to Lexington, Kentucky, where he had once been a police- man. After many hospitalizations, he and his parents believed that NIMH was his last hope. On camera, and in the presence of onlooking research staff, he spoke to his psychiatrist while frantically twirling the dark hair atop his head faster and faster as if he were cranking an engine for takeoff. With his free hand, he pointed to a framed portrait on the opposite wall and said the person had a headache. Gibberish flowed about "dudes with green teeth." Jerry screamed about being electrocuted. He shouted at his mother while trying to strike a bargain. Stay here, move to Washington, he said, or he might leave treatment.

Another patient, Heather, missing most of her teeth, tears streaking her furious pink blotched face, begged her mother to allow her to stay home after a weekend visit. It wasn't clear who was suffering more: Heather, des- perately pleading and visibly heartbroken, or her mother, painfully strug- gling to cajole her daughter to accept a decision she knew was inevitable?

Science called the series a "brilliant, no-nonsense documentary" mak- ing it "abundantly clear that the brain is our badge of humanity." Other reviews were just as favorable, especially in Phoenix, Arizona, where it turned PBS pledge week into an unprecedented success. But Mrs. Anita Cline, from Falls Church, Virginia, was angry. "Absolutely devastating," she called the segment. Why had the producers focused on "two hopeless, incurable individuals"? For her, as the parent of someone with schizophre- nia, it was a hope-killing "horror show."[17]

Producer and science writer Richard Hutton drafted a careful letter saying they had intended to educate the audience: "Thirty-five years ago antipsychotic drugs didn't even exist; thirty years ago, psychiatrists still routinely blamed parents for their children's schizophrenia; twenty-five years ago, nobody knew anything about the possible role of genetics in schizophrenia; fifteen years ago, the mechanism of action of the antipsy- chotic drugs was still a mystery." Of Jerry and Heather? "Personally I don't see them as incurable, except under present levels of knowledge. . . . I sincerely believe that what we offered was the truth, and that it was not without its moments of hope. . . . We hoped that the exposure would help change the way they viewed the disease."[18]

Former patients, organized psychiatric survivors, saw none of the benefits Hutton outlined or of Jerry and Heather's dilemmas as part of their organizing campaigns. With her eyes set on the movement's goal, Judi Chamberlin boomed, "This program will further the stereotype of mental patients as helpless victims, and will ignore our efforts to organize on our own behalf and regain control of our lives."[19]

NAMI had invested their hope in science to solve problems associated with mental illnesses. Research was their priority, and scientific research would be their salvation. Flynn was well versed in theories of fetal brain growth, hunches about in utero brain development, or seasonal variations of childbirth. The announcement NIMH made soon after her arrival, that psychiatric researcher Elliot Gershon had discovered a gene associated with depression, augured hope that more breakthroughs would soon come. Fred Goodwin, then heading NIMH in-house research, appeared on the *MacNeil-Lehrer News Hour* to applaud Gershon. "Every time a biological finding is uncovered in a psychiatric illness," Goodwin said, "it helps take away some of the mystique of the illness. . . . People need not be ashamed of having these problems."[20]

Information about biology helped counter baseless charges of bad parenting or character flaws. To arm parents with information about research then underway, in March 1985 NIMH invited NAMI to meet and greet scientists in their laboratories. When Jim Howe, NAMI's president in 1985, testified at the Senate Appropriations Committee two months later, he could speak passionately about the "mismatch of meager resources against a sick population numbering in the millions." He insisted that "the penny ante approach" must end, and he reminded lawmakers that the brain is "our most important human organ, [and] has become the newest frontier for research."[21]

Despite one breakthrough after another, science hadn't closed the gap between biological research and clinical treatments. NAMI was still disappointed that it wouldn't partner with the newly formed NARSAD to fund scientists. With this venture closed off, NAMI mounted a campaign to secure a scientific agenda through NIMH.

Early in 1987, NAMI's board voted unanimously to endorse returning NIMH to the National Institutes of Health. According to the new board president, Don Richardson, that would put all the health institutes under one roof. It would send "an important signal that mental illness is a disease—like heart and lung and kidney diseases."[22] It would restore the head to the body.

———————————

Could basic laboratory research at NIMH flourish when the mental health institute was not independent but governed by ADAMHA, the Alcohol, Drug Abuse, and Mental Health Administration? Should laboratory and scientific research be separated from the other NIMH activities, such as staffing clinics, educating a professional workforce, or undertaking health services research? These questions struck at the heart of Robert Felix's original concept of a three-legged stool, and they had not been revisited since 1946 when President Harry S. Truman signed the National Mental Health Act. Nor had Congress raised these issues during previous reorganizations of the mental health institute, starting in 1966 when it unfastened NIMH from the NIH. Nor did it come up when Congress again moved NIMH in 1973, this time assigning it to the newer institutes for drugs and alcohol to create ADAMHA.

These questions seemed relevant again, and they came up during a routine reauthorization of ADAMHA. It happened that an interdepartmental study team from the Department of Public Health asked whether NIMH belonged under ADAMHA. Weren't NIMH scientists compatible with and often collaborating with other health institutes with whom they shared standards for reviewing and funding off-site projects? Should services, where people got treated for serious mental illnesses, be separated from laboratory research endeavors? These were heady questions for the forty-year-old institute that had guided the federal government's mental health portfolio despite the fractured community it served. And they would reverberate for the next five years, leaping from the Department of Health and Human Services, to congressional hearings, to the

American Psychiatric Association, and onto the agenda for NIMH advisory council meetings. They would touch NAMI, where Laurie Flynn and parents itched to expand wet bench research. In this, they aligned with Fred Goodwin.

———————————

Nobody's identity was interwoven more with NIMH research accomplishments than Fred Goodwin's. His life had matured inside this institution. In 1965, he bolted a residency at the University of North Carolina in order to accept an unanticipated staff vacancy. In a sense, he was coming home. Goodwin had grown up in Washington, where his father was a New Deal assistant labor secretary, and his summer jobs, starting in high school and continuing through medical school, had all occurred at the NIH, where he absorbed discoveries about physiology and biochemistry. An appointment at NIMH was his dream, and his rise started in the Adult Psychiatry Branch, under William "Biff" Bunney's mentorship, studying how the brain synthesized proteins. Duties for patient care brought him to the Clinical Center's Depression Treatment Unit, where research with two patients informed his groundbreaking and consequential discovery about the clinical properties of lithium.

Goodwin rose rapidly. He became a unit chief three years after he was hired, chief of a laboratory in another five, and chief of an entire branch in four more. Six years later, in 1982, he became director of in-house (intramural) research for NIMH. He had published more than 360 articles in peer-reviewed journals, as well as book chapters, and his résumé noted he was among the most frequently cited scientific authors. Many people would have been satisfied to stop there, savor the taste and the commensurate success of a stellar rise. But there was more to come for Goodwin. In 1988, when ADAMHA housed NIMH, a political appointment made him ADAMHA's administrator with oversight responsibility for three institutes—drug, alcohol, and mental health—whose challenges engaged some of the world's most accomplished scientists.

Despite all he had done that was commendable, Goodwin still yearned for an independent NIMH. It mattered not that the director of NIMH answered to him on a flowchart. He still smarted thinking NIMH had been emasculated in 1966 when Congress broke its ties with the NIH. At the time, Goodwin was a newcomer, but thinking he understood how power flowed, he called on Arkansas representative Wilbur Mills, chair of the House Ways and Means Committee, and implored him to keep NIMH within the nation's health institutes. Years later, and seasoned by experience, Goodwin couldn't imagine how brash and galling he must have seemed as a junior research psychiatrist appealing this congressional decision to one of the most powerful men in Congress.[23]

Goodwin had long suspected shuffling NIMH from institute to bureau and back again had something to do with public attitudes that psychiatry was a weak science, similar to doubts raised during the trial of John Hinckley. NIMH scientists had been sidelined, even though, according to his count, they were the second most frequently cited authors of the NIH's institutes.[24] He had never believed that social science research belonged in the pantheon of NIMH's laboratory science, a position at odds with some of the interdisciplinary staff of the founding generation. Now he said he wanted the "the fundamental defining mission of ADAMHA" to be research.[25]

NAMI had already spoken, and Laurie Flynn urged Goodwin to act. "Either we are a disease or we're not," she said. "The brain belongs in the research institute as a wholly fledged body part, or it doesn't," she said. The dichotomy between mind and body, mental health and physical health had to go. Otherwise, the mental illnesses would remain a second-class priority.

Despite pushback from those who worried about losing ADAMHA as a power base, Flynn remained steadfast. "Goodwin could do this because he knew that NAMI was backing him," she said years later. "There weren't a helluva lot of other folks going up to the Hill and talking about mental illness. There was us . . . and there was us!"[26]

———————

When *Parade* magazine interviewed Lewis Judd as he prepared to take the helm of NIMH in 1988, he was asked whether "just a 'little willpower'" might help a depressed person "become cheerful again."[27]

No, he snapped. "It's a real disease, just as a heart attack is real."

The persistence of the mind-body dichotomy was, as Judd put it, "distinctly counterproductive." That they should be united was every bit as obvious as the fact that the brain was in the body.[28] Like his predecessor, Shervert Frazier, as NIMH director Judd was concerned with the brain's function, its mechanisms, and its "relevance to mental disorders." With a specialty in mood disorders, he proposed collaborating with a European multicenter gene bank working in brain sciences. He renamed the NIMH Basic Science division, making it Basic Brain and Behavioral Science. He used Sam Keith's schizophrenia initiative to persuade Congress to increase funding. Mental illnesses were not the pursuit of mental health, which depended on a balanced diet, alcohol in moderation, adequate sleep, and a happy face.[29]

Modeling himself a doctor-researcher, Judd donned the medical uniform of a white lab coat, an oddity in the administrative halls of NIMH. He regularly met with Flynn, who by now chaired the National Mental Health Leadership Forum, an umbrella organization for twenty mental health constituent groups. Alan Leshner joined them. He had been acting director before Judd arrived, and he would be again when Judd left. A psychologist with a specialty in primates, he added depth to their conversations mapping the institute's strategy. By 1988 it was apparent that the concept of a schizophrenogenic mother was outmoded, even damaging families' clinical concerns. Yet Flynn still heard from tearful moms and wanted an official rejection of this odious suggestion when all arrows pointed to an organ. Obsolete at best, inaccurate in its premise, Judd agreed it was time to retire the schizophrenogenic mother in the service of science.

When President George H. W. Bush signed the proclamation declaring the 1990s the Decade of the Brain, it underscored that this organ was worthy of research attention. But only Congress could authorize funding to enable the work to proceed, and congressional lawmakers had dawdled about the proposal to return NIMH to the NIH in the five years it discussed reauthorizing ADAMHA. At the 169th meeting of the National Mental Health Advisory Committee, on February 10, 1992, NIMH acting director Alan Leshner announced that returning NIMH to NIH was stalled. Thus a meeting started, plain as vanilla, but it ended with a calamitous event making Fred Goodwin fight for his future.

Before launching into his remarks as ADAMHA administrator, Goodwin reminded everybody that NIMH was special to him, and coming to these meetings was the equivalent of "homecoming." Everybody knew he was expected to swap heading ADAMHA for directing NIMH, a lesser spot on a flowchart but where his heart wanted to be. He gave the announcements that were routine at these meetings, and he had an update from the Health Department about the increase in urban violence. Everything from street crimes, to self-destructive behavior, to homicide, to domestic abuse was becoming epidemic. It was worrisome. Then Goodwin veered off course and seemed to lose his bearings. He rambled a bit and talked about urban youth in inner cities. Then he referenced oversexed, antisocial, aggressive male monkeys copulating profusely and killing one another in the wild. Stunned, twenty-six people around the table looked at one another—and him. Goodwin continued talking about monkeys and said about half of them died before becoming adults. Then he connected the dots to social unrest in urban areas. "Maybe it isn't just the careless use of the word," he said, "when people call certain areas of certain cities jungles. . . . We may have gone back to what might be more natural, without all of the social controls. . . . The loss of structure in society is probably why we are dealing with this issue." He wrapped up his comments talking about television violence.[30]

Goodwin's remarks clung like a moist vapor. Sam Keith sucked in his breath. Delores Parron, sitting next to Goodwin, was shocked. Was Goodwin really linking biology and violence? Primates in the wild and urban youth? What is wrong with him? Parron asked herself. She had known him for years, had been on an earlier surgeon general's task force researching violence. That was in 1985, and a lot had changed in seven years, but as an activist and an African American in government's ranks, and someone who had worked with and liked Goodwin, she was dismayed. "This man is smarter than this," she said to herself. But he seemed oblivious, not reading the room, unaware of what he had said or its impact. "Fred is not acting himself," she thought.[31]

Before rushing from the meeting to catch a train at Union Station, Parron whispered something to Goodwin while others sat in silence. Primate specialist Leshner thought Goodwin's remarks were manifestly stupid. He guessed Goodwin didn't get what was wrong with juxtaposing "male monkeys in the wild" with youthful inner-city unrest. How could he ignore poverty, racism, unemployment, and failed gun control? Did Goodwin really intend to stoke images of biological reductionism reminiscent of eugenicists? Nobody had a clue, and all were on edge.

Word spread as soon as the meeting broke up. A couple of folks stopped Goodwin in the hall and asked for an apology. Nope, none needed, he said, seeming tone deaf to America's racially blistered stage. It hadn't even been a year since the brutal beating of Rodney King, a Black motorist the Los Angeles police had stopped for a traffic violation. Or rioting six months before when a Jewish motorist drove through a pedestrian crosswalk in Crown Heights, Brooklyn, killing a Black child in a neighborhood where an ethnic truce was already dubious. But science was also at risk, and neuroscientist Dominick Purpura, dean of the Albert Einstein College of Medicine, was shocked that Goodwin seemed impervious to "five thousand years of evolution."[32]

Secretary of HHS Louis Sullivan, himself African American, thought an apology was needed and insisted that Goodwin make one for "the embarrassment" he had caused the agency.[33] Rumors circulated that Sullivan had kept Goodwin waiting for two hours, as if he were a naughty schoolboy, sitting on a bench outside his office. Some were tickled, some horrified, but nobody was satisfied with Goodwin's apology of "profound regret to anyone I have offended" and for "insensitivity" and "inappropriateness." Some wanted nothing less than a public shaming. Disappointed legislators wanted contrition.

Goodwin dug in his heels, as if that were the best strategy for dousing an explosion. He refused to be interviewed, wouldn't speak to the press, nor would he talk to friends or colleagues, even to clarify his remarks.[34] His silence bred the perfect medium for brewing a controversy. Critics filled in the gaps of what wasn't said, denouncing a racism wrapped in science, with memories of the Tuskegee experiment's heinous disregard for the lives of Black research subjects, and of bogus IQ testing and forced sterilization decades earlier.[35] Defenders parsed what Goodwin did say, cried foul, demanded free speech, not what they considered political correctness. Debate took place on the campuses of colleges and universities, and on the front pages of newspapers and magazines, including the *Chronicle of Higher Education.*

It was an election year with President George H. W. Bush up for reelection, and there was no room for this kind of controversy. Damage control required a resignation, and after two weeks of unyielding criticism, Goodwin told the president he wanted to prevent further distortion of complex issues. He believed the issue was being "exploited politically."[36]

Goodwin's two-week fall from grace seemed as spectacular as had his two-decade rise. Despite trying to put it behind him and resign, nothing quieted after Sullivan announced that Goodwin would, as had been previously arranged, head NIMH. It was a remarkable golden parachute, critics said. Former patients shouted, "Fire Fred."[37] Friends rallied again. Biomedical researchers, chiefs of the NIMH research laboratories, and individuals with long associations from academic health centers wrote to support his lifelong pursuit of science, praising his humanitarian ambitions and his support of patients and families. "He's no David Duke," said one psychiatrist who believed his remarks, though serious, more likely reflected a clumsy turn of phrase. African American psychiatrists were more aggrieved.[38] And twenty-six members of the Congressional Black Caucus protested Goodwin's fitness for NIMH leadership, after which the *Wall Street Journal* charged caucus leader John Conyers with mudslinging and piling on in an editorial headlined "Speech Police."[39]

Meanwhile, where to house NIMH remained unsettled. Should it be pulled out of ADAMHA to return to NIH, severing the services that were part of Felix's original vision? Three psychiatrists met with Senator Edward Kennedy at the end of March, asking him to oppose separating brain and behavior research, something that would disrupt the flow of information from producers of knowledge, researchers, to practitioners, clinicians working with patients. Joseph Coyle, chair of the Department of Psychiatry at Harvard College, and president of the Society of Neuroscience, thought it would be "unfortunate and destructive to separate 'mind from brain.'" Besides, he didn't think NIMH needed to worry about its image. The "research program is viewed as being the highest quality of science," he said, and it needed no further validation.[40]

When Congress passed the ADAMHA Reorganization Plan in the summer of 1992, it kept biological and genetic research at NIMH labs, where they would be governed by NIH. It created the Substance Abuse and Mental Health Services Administration, now called SAMHSA, to focus on services—guiding, expanding, and researching them. Superficially, it seemed an accommodation to benefit all. There would be children's mental health services, renewal of the protection and advocacy for mentally ill or disabled people, and block grant budgets to states for services. It broke what had been central to NIMH's original mission, the flow of conversation between research and practice.

By year's end, Secretary Sullivan announced a blue-ribbon panel to study the NIH's portfolio for violence, aggression, and race. The panel would conclude that violence in America "should be declared a national emergency." A review of more than two hundred research projects found no association between race and violence. Yet the turbulence unleashed by the Goodwin debacle, and the untenable continuation of debate, led Secretary of Health and Human Services Bernadine Healy to cancel a $100,000 contract for a conference at the University of Maryland to discuss "Genetic Factors in Crime." Panelists settled on a recommendation for a public health model with "interdisciplinary research that considers the total human experience."[41]

The five-year campaign to bolster research by unyoking NIMH from ADAMHA began with the expectation that this would better serve people with a mental illness. That was yet to be determined. What was clear with the arrival of a new president, when Bill Clinton defeated Bush, was that in 1993 separate engines would drive research and services, something that would unleash challenges as well as opportunities.

CHAPTER 12

THE CLOZAPINE STORY— RISK-BENEFIT OR RISKY BENEFITS

D OCTORS STARTED CHECKING INTO THE HILTON HOTEL near the Twinbrook Metro Station on Wednesday, February 22, 1984, a day before they were to head over to the Federal Drug Administration's (FDA) meeting of the Psychopharmacologic Drugs Advisory Committee. They had come from Iowa, Texas, New York, Illinois, Michigan, Indiana, Wisconsin, Minnesota, and Pennsylvania. And Lou Gerbino, from Iowa, couldn't sleep. Apparently neither could Gil Honigfeld, for when Gerbino looked out his hotel window at 4:00 a.m., he saw Honigfeld running circles around the parking lot. Calming his nerves, thought Gerbino. The next morning would be a meeting, and the FDA would discuss whether to grant Sandoz Ltd., a Swiss drug company, permission to market clozapine, a new drug. For Honigfeld, who had staked his career on clozapine, it would be the biggest meeting of his life.

Honigfeld's belief in clozapine had led him to accept an offer from Sandoz Ltd. in 1973, when the company was investigating a drug different from others on the market. The other pharmaceuticals were banking on drugs similar to chlorpromazine, trade name Thorazine, in the chemical family of phenothiazines. They were derivatives, or what the trade called "me-too's"—a euphemism for copycats. Clozapine was notably different. It was also the first new drug for schizophrenia coming to market in thirty years, which made it attractive to Honigfeld.

To work for Sandoz, Honigfeld bypassed offers from pharmaceutical companies with better pay, and an easier commute than his hour-plus each way on the New Jersey Turnpike in a gas-guzzling Chevy Suburban. He was a psychologist, and smitten by the same idealism as the friends who said that working for a drug company was selling out. Some had become clinicians treating patients, others were professors stoking learning in the academy. He knew his attention span was incompatible with that of a clinician, but he still hoped to change the world for thousands of people. He had been tutored by psychiatrists Donald Klein and Max Fink at Long Island's Hillside Hospital, where they had pioneered research methods to monitor the links between drugs and behavior. He had also spent a year at Rockland Psychiatric Center, where Nathan Kline was experimenting with clozapine. Kline's work, and a small clinical study underway at Bellevue Hospital with thirty-one patients, had built his hopes for this drug.[1]

When Honigfeld joined Sandoz in 1973 as director of research and development, the animal testing phase was near completion. The next phase, a multisite research project under the direction of James Claghorn, a psychopharmacologist at University of Texas Health Center in Houston, would enroll subjects for the make-it-or-break-it phase of pre-marketing. Recruitment of patients was half completed, with 151 of the 300 patients enrolled in September 1975, when an article published in *Lancet* shocked the research world. Eight of the two thousand people in Finland who were being treated with clozapine had died. Their deaths were sudden, and in quick succession. Nobody expected this.

Of the nineteen countries where clozapine had been studied in clinical trials, Sandoz knew of twelve cases of agranulocytosis. Later it would be known that when undetected, a rapid collapse of white blood cells robbed one person in a hundred of their infection-fighting ability and posed a lethal risk.[2] Agranulocytosis had caused these deaths, but why? Were the tablets impure? What was unique about this cluster? This specific region?

In 1976, Sandoz halted all sales. In Europe this would be temporary. In America, where people settled grievances with lawsuits, the environment was risky and costly. A case in point was what happened surrounding the drug thalidomide, a German-made medicine pregnant women took for morning sickness in the 1950s and 1960s.[3] Two decades later, the pharmaceutical giant Chemie Grünenthal was still mired in the American court system, dealing with class-action lawsuits based on forty babies whose stunted limbs sprouted from their torso or organs grew in the wrong place. Thalidomide had forced Congress to revise laws regulating drug safety, but in the meantime, lawsuits about the onset of tardive dyskinesia were beginning to appear.[4] Word came from corporate headquarters in Basel, Switzerland, telling Honigfeld to close out recruitment for the multisite study. Sandoz considered the United States too risky a place to do business and abandoned the goal of seeking FDA approval. No new patients were to be added.

It was a huge blow to Honigfeld. Halting the enrollment of new subjects was one part of it. A different challenge, one that struck at his moral sensibilities and was even bigger—what should he do about people who were already enrolled? He didn't want to have to cut anybody who was benefiting. Even in the earliest stages of testing, it seemed to abate symptoms and improve the quality of life unlike any other drug. As the research director, he received reports on each and every person enrolled in the trial, and he had evidence that there was new life, new behavior for people with seemingly intractable symptoms. No other drug had relieved anxiety, restlessness, delusions, hallucinations, and negative symptoms—those associated with emotional or social withdrawal, or a blunted and flat affect—in people diagnosed with schizophrenia. It was astounding. At first the gestures were small: lips parted in a smile, the words "good morning," a gesture, a nod acknowledging other people or their surroundings. People who had sat in a corner, some for years, were starting to engage.

It wasn't just Honigfeld who was shaken. So were doctors who had brought patients into this study. Since 1975 there were doctors affiliated with Harvard's McLean or Columbia's College of Physicians and Surgeons whose authority came from a compassionate care protocol. They were among those who begged Honigfeld to find a way to keep this drug available for their patients, and he in turn begged Sandoz. Eventually Sandoz told the doctors they could come to Key Biscayne, where the American College of Neuropsychopharmacology was meeting at the Sonesta Beach Hotel, to plead their case to the company's executives and lawyers. Lou Gerbino was one of the doctors flying to Florida. He had been on Bellevue Hospital's research team of the double-blind study of psychotic patients in 1972 and had subsequently moved back home to Iowa. He also had diagnosed one of two patients in America who developed agranulocytosis. It had been a terrifying case, and the patient needed to spend several weeks in the hospital where a broad-based spectrum of antibiotics, delivered intravenously, saved her life, and she recovered.

In the end, what mattered was the correct medical intervention. But Sandoz's lawyers wouldn't budge. He remembered they gave the impression that they thought "general shrinks don't do medicine." They said, "We own the molecule and we have the right to say who gets it." America was not the right environment.[5]

Flying home, Gerbino imagined having to deliver news to his patients that they couldn't have this drug any longer. Prior to clozapine, they had been in and out of the hospital two, three, four times a year. Now they had jobs, steady employment. They had lost the defining shuffle or the frozen face, and the trembling hands while trying to light a cigarette. When the mother of one man who had resumed work after seven years heard that her son's clozapine might be stopped, she screamed at him, "Is he supposed to go off the medicine and become schizophrenic again?"[6]

For humanitarian purposes, Sandoz allowed people who had started receiving clozapine under compassionate care to continue. Honigfeld monitored lab reports for vital signs, reports about neutrophils and white blood counts, looking for clues about seizures or heart problems. For the next five years he tracked every person receiving clozapine under the umbrella of compassionate care, and he also received reports about their social interactions. Honigfeld learned of people who, for the first time in years, smiled or laughed, played cards, told jokes, or fell in love. A patient who said "Thank you" after years of silence touched him deeply. Dormant relationships were rekindled; a son or daughter who had declined family events had returned. Nearly as enthusiastic as their parents were their doctors, walking testimonials telling colleagues about lives restored. Soon these other doctors started to call Honigfeld, concerned about a patient, perhaps two, who couldn't tolerate Thorazine, Stelazine, Prolixin, or the other commonly prescribed neuroleptic drugs for schizophrenia. Honigfeld couldn't deny them, didn't want to, and as long as he was scrupulously monitoring each and every patient receiving this drug through compassionate care, he agreed. "Even though you're a researcher, when you have skilled clinicians calling you, it's the kind of information that tells you there is something really important," Honigfeld said. He felt he had to persist.

Clozapine's risk for depleting white blood cells in one person out of a hundred was matched by other drugs causing agranulocytosis, or agran. Antipsychotics such as Thorazine, or Mellaril, which was eventually pulled from the market, had a comparable risk. So did chemotherapies for cancer, overactive thyroid, and bacterial infections. For two decades German researchers had been studying agranulocytosis, and they knew treatments could jump-start bone marrow production of neutrophils.

Honigfeld hadn't quite appreciated that the FDA didn't reject new drug applications only because of dangerous side effects until an official whispered this in his ear. Of course, the toxicity of drugs was important, but there were ways to manage them, and Honigfeld urged Sandoz to renew the expired application; recent changes in American laws governing drug marketing now seemed favorable.[7] It might also give Sandoz an opportunity to recoup some of its investment going back five years. Sandoz agreed on the condition that Honigfeld could pull the application together in one year and only use data from the aborted study. There would be no more funding. Honigfeld agreed. With data he had mined from 151 subjects, plus that from the 429 people receiving the medication under the compassionate care standards, he submitted a new drug application to the FDA in April 1983. It was hardly the ideal model, but it was all that he had.

Meeting in Rockville nearly a year later, on February 23, 1984, the FDA discussed bringing clozapine to market in the United States, as twenty other countries already had done.[8] A double conference room was set aside with a podium, wires spooled for microphones, and bleachers for an unusually large number of observers. Paul Leber, head of the FDA staff and a physician board-certified in three subspecialties, opened the proceedings. All of the commissioners, except for one from the Veterans Administration, were affiliated with a university.

Leber started with a reminder that he expected them to focus on the drug's risks. He had worked at Bellevue Hospital during its initial clozapine study, and he certainly knew that clozapine's story was complex. He believed that were it not for what happened in Finland, the drug would have most likely been approved. But the risks warranted singular attention. Leber had become something of an expert on adverse drug reactions and had authored an article about sudden deaths associated with neuroleptics. As recently as 1981, he believed the jury was still out.[9] That Leber had circulated a memo telling witnesses to focus on the risks surprised Honigfeld, who was not on the distribution list. Should agranulocytosis prevent marketing clozapine in the United States? Did the risks outweigh the benefits? With one death per one hundred people, clozapine was ten times riskier than other drugs treating schizophrenia. Was it too risky? Witnesses packaged their remarks in epidemiological models, case-fatality ratios, incident estimates, and how to calculate a denominator.[10]

Lou Gerbino asked to speak in an open public hearing, wanting to make sure the benefits of clozapine were introduced before the experts began with prepared remarks. Now director of the Southwest Iowa Mental Health Center, Gerbino's experience included treating many patients, including forty-five in the three years he was on staff at Bellevue Hospital's Prolixin Clinic between 1976 and 1978. During that time, he testified, he would overhear residents describe the clinic patients by saying, "They are not all schizophrenics." These doctors couldn't imagine people with schizophrenia who behaved with spontaneity, who weren't psychotic— who behaved the way patients did on clozapine.[11]

In Gerbino's estimation, real people were hidden in the thicket of charts and graphs as numerators and denominators—a mother, father, sister, brother, and especially a son or daughter for whom the drug had dramatically altered life. He asked that the panel remember these were actual patients whose stare had become a smile. Some had so few symptoms that their friends, even their treatment team, doubted they had a serious mental illness. He concluded modestly, "These are not things that came out in any of the measurements."[12]

Leber interrupted Gerbino. They had had an agreement to talk about risks.[13] Gerbino said he had received the memo, but he hadn't made an agreement. Risks were not the whole story, and he worried that Leber's memo had biased the committee. Benefits should also be part of the discussion, and among them was resolving TD's "neuroleptic malignant syndrome." A number of patients from state hospitals had TD of such severity that they could no longer stand or feed themselves. After clozapine, half showed a functional improvement.[14] Gerbino said clozapine was "the kindest antipsychotic drug" he had ever seen, even after his experience with a patient who developed agranulocytosis.

Other speakers, including John Kane from Long Island Jewish Hospital, started as skeptics. Kane dated his working knowledge of clozapine to seven patients he'd agreed to treat who were already taking it. When he stepped in, they seemed to be doing pretty well, so well, in fact, that he didn't think they needed it and took them off. They started to deteriorate. Four ended up back in the hospital, one attempted suicide, and a fifth relapsed. He didn't wait to see what would happen to the other two before putting them all back on clozapine.[15]

Herbert Meltzer from the University of Chicago was another champion. He'd been investigating clozapine in the laboratory since the 1970s and could discuss the actions of the drug on a cellular level as well as the clinical picture from heading an inpatient unit at the Illinois State Psychiatric Institute. That's where he met Kane, who had come to consult about TD. In 1982, the DOJ received allegations of patient mistreatment and sent Kane to investigate. He saw the worst case of TD he'd ever seen. The patient was female, thirty-two years old, and had been taking conventional neuroleptics for the eight years she had been hospitalized. She could no longer move her jaws. Still delusional, hallucinating, and kept in restraints, she had lost sixty pounds. Meltzer received permission from Leber and Honigfeld to enroll her for compassionate care use, and within a month of taking clozapine, she could feed herself. Off came the restraints, and symptom scores improved. She had maintained her progress up to and including that very day when Meltzer told the FDA committee about her. She was not the only patient he'd seen react this way. He'd also seen a thirty-six-year-old woman hospitalized in a state facility for ten years where she was delusional, hallucinating, and in restraints despite taking nine antipsychotic drugs (Sparine, Mellaril, Stelazine, Haldol, Navane, Loxitane, Prolixin, Serentil, chlorpromazine). Her functioning scores were near the bottom of the scale until she was given clozapine. Soon the score doubled, and within a short time she was deemed able to go to a less acute hospital setting. There she was removed from clozapine, and her delusions, hallucinations, and thought disturbances returned.

Meltzer apologized for veering from Leber's request to focus on the risks. But he wanted the committee to understand the background to his clinical judgments and what led him to become a fan.

James Claghorn, the principal investigator of the halted multisite Texas study, was another of clozapine's enthusiasts. Pointing to data-filled slides, he couldn't suppress his enthusiasm and said it was "boringly repetitious" to hammer clozapine's "emergence of therapeutic superiority." Everybody knew he was there to describe Study 16, the double-blind study comparing clozapine to chlorpromazine on which that morning's discussion would hinge. Already, however, clozapine's favorable results had become near legendary. With benefits in mind, it was easy to minimize side effects such as a drop in blood pressure, hypotension, or seizures. These could be eliminated by adjusting dosing, making it gradual. Drooling while sleeping might be a nuisance side effect but not a serious risk.

As requested, FDA's consultants dwelt on the risks. Nobody challenged clozapine's clinical superiority. It was the fuzziness of the data from Europe as well as from the scant number of cases Sandoz presented that led to doubts: What was the frequency of side effects? Methodological differences yielded different ways of presenting the data. One person in a thousand or 3.23 cases per thousand? How many ended in death? How much time did clinicians have to treat an abscess? Tissue infections? Other conditions needing infection-fighting white blood cells? Critics challenged Sandoz's methodology. Sandoz defended its results allowing for better lives.

Committee chair Bernard "Barney" Carroll moved the discussion in a different direction. Was superiority really the issue? he asked. Carroll, just forty-four, was esteemed, known for laboratory tests for a hormone associated with melancholia. Since that discovery, at the age of twenty-eight, he had become one of biological psychiatry's stars. Now, as chair of Duke University's Department of Psychiatry, he was an ideal person to chair the FDA's panel on psychopharmacology. With nuanced thinking, he asked whether the more important question was whether clozapine was an "effective alternative for patients who are unresponsive to regular management." Might that suffice? He acknowledged that agranulocytosis could be fatal but said that was also "relatively uncommon."

Carroll's questions foretell why he would later be called the "conscience of psychiatry." What was more common, he said, was the "general demoralization and impaired relationships" suffered by people with schizophrenia. He was struck by the quality of life clozapine enabled and noted how suicide, in the range of 10 percent, seemed more of a threat than agranulocytosis.[16] Even if quality of life weren't on the FDA's list of criteria, it mattered. And it should be the patient's choice whether to take the drug after laying out the alternatives and their risks.[17]

Leber hesitated. He knew that legions of medical do-gooders backed treatments to alleviate suffering, soften horrible lives, even postpone death. That wasn't the FDA's job. Theirs was to assure that treatments didn't impose an additional burden.[18] Otherwise, he feared they might be facing a public health problem.[19]

As the time to adjourn neared, Carroll worried about missing his return to North Carolina. They were stalemated until Dr. Bonnie Camp from the University of Colorado offered a compromise: Change conditions for marketing clozapine. Allow Sandoz a chance for an FDA-approved drug to treat people who had not responded to other drugs. They might be the very patients who would benefit, and they might belong to a subgroup of nonresponders whom some considered mythical and others disparaged as "treatment resistant."

Leber was moved.[20] In quick order, eight of the nine members of the Psychopharmacologic Drugs Advisory Committee agreed that they needed to answer whether clozapine benefited a defined group of patients that other drugs had not.

Sandoz accepted the FDA's challenge and, in collaboration with Leber, Honigfeld formatted a study to be known as Study 30, to answer whether clozapine helped a defined subgroup of patients. If it did, would only those patients be eligible for a drug with clozapine's known risks? The answer could affect the presumption of schizophrenia's progressive decline.

Study 30's selection criteria were rigorous. Candidates needed to have a five-year continuous history of illness and three failed medicines from two different classes of antipsychotic drugs. They also had to do poorly on a test in widespread use measuring symptoms (BPRS) and one assessing functioning (CGI). By definition, they were people for whom treatment had not worked. They were the most ill of all patients at a VA hospital or a state mental health facility.

Once someone was accepted into Study 30, the first two weeks required washing all drugs from their bodies so that all started with a natural base.

For six weeks everybody received haloperidol (Haldol). Then they were retested to see if Haldol brought a change. If it did, by definition they were not considered the "special treatment-resistant population" and would be ineligible. With these restrictions in place, sixteen clinical centers studied 268 patients in a six-week double-blind study starting in 1984.[21] Nobody, especially Leber, thought Study 30 would succeed, because, as he said, it was nearly impossible to work with "chronic, treatment resistant schizophrenic patients." He doubted they could deliver the precision they needed. Honigfeld worried, he told historian John Crilly, that the FDA's bias worked against Sandoz.[22]

In addition to its stringent criteria, Study 30 was unique in another way. The usual drug trial compared a placebo to the study drug. Study 30 compared two drugs, turning this into a competition between clozapine, a new drug, and chlorpromazine, the standard-bearer. In addition, he had firmly believed, he would later concede, that "active control trials invariably fail to find a difference."[23]

Study 30's results came quickly in 1985. Some patients showed improvement on measures of hostility, cooperation, and social interest in one week. Chlorpromazine subjects showed none. By week two, there were statistically significant differences for psychosis, irritability, and suspiciousness (.001 level). Week three showed chlorpromazine subjects leveling off where clozapine patients continued to improve in fourteen of the sixteen study centers. European studies showed similar results in forty days. The earlier Bellevue Hospital study had shown demonstrable results in thirty-five days.[24]

While assembling data, study leaders Kane and Meltzer, with Honigfeld, broadcast clozapine's results about people once considered treatment resistant.[25] The message was clear—they weren't resistant to the right treatment. The results spoke for themselves: Study 30 showed that of those taking chlorpromazine, fewer than 5 percent of the patients showed therapeutic benefits; 38 percent in the clozapine part of the study showed therapeutic benefits.

The results seemed incontrovertible, and Leber had no choice but to concede this point in the next set of hearings in 1989. Opening that meeting, he acknowledged that Study 30 "unequivocally demonstrates a group of patients, prospectively demonstrating its resistance to high doses of haloperidol" did better than those on chlorpromazine. That was an accomplishment in itself given how few studies produce beneficial results. After commenting on the difficulties they had faced in 1984, evidence from controlled clinical trials, the efficacy for a subgroup of patients for whom no other medications had worked, the risks to 1 percent of patients, and the program Sandoz was intending for mitigating risks, the FDA would discuss Study 30's results.[26]

Five years before, the question had been how many deaths Sandoz Ltd. was willing to accept in exchange for bringing clozapine to market. This time it was whether the monitoring system Sandoz proposed would mitigate the risks.

In various forms, that question would wrack the federal government, research and clinical psychiatrists, and patients and their families, and would eventually find its way into the courts.

———————————

By now everybody knew the benefits of not causing TD. They knew clozapine was superior to chlorpromazine, and equal to or better than all other available antipsychotic drugs. Leber wanted more. His background in medicine, radiology, and psychiatry armed him with unique skills.

Leber had originally gone to work for the FDA in 1977.[27] His training coincided with psychiatry's upheavals from psychoanalysis to biological psychiatry, from the *DSM-II*'s vague reliance on psychodynamics to the *DSM-III*'s attempt to standardize communication while building a diagnosis resonant with medical terms. He had witnessed attempts to employ a medical model and suspected it didn't apply to psychiatric illnesses. Many factors seemed to interact to produce psychiatric illness, and teasing out the specificity of who might benefit from which treatments was more complicated. Had agranulocytosis not been a side effect, Leber later said, clozapine would have sailed through the process. This risk, however, made it imperative to show that it was superior to other drugs. The creation of a new diagnostic category of nonresponsive narrowed the range when considering for whom it would justify the FDA's approval.

Leber often modified the word "risk" with adjectives like "terrifying" or "dangerous." More data points were coming. Since 1984, another nine people in the United States had developed agranulocytosis; none had died.

In the decade between 1977 and 1987, a hundred people died in Europe. But European doctors had managed the risk by monitoring. Clozapine didn't cure. The questions, then, were how much improvement justified the risk, and how could that risk be monitored in the United States? Honigfeld thought medical management could avert a catastrophic drop in white blood cells. They could stop the drug, or boost bone marrow production, and reverse a hematological crisis. Could psychiatrists, whose routine clinical care didn't include managing a medical crisis, do this? Regulators were as concerned about this as about the potential collapse of white blood cells.

Data from Sandoz indicated that 80 percent of the cases of agranulocytosis occurred in the first four months. Most others happened within two years.[28] Based on this, Honigfeld designed a staged monitoring system with an independent national registry that didn't depend on an independent doctor. It was designed to avoid duplication and tracking errors, and also retain information when patients moved between systems or doctors. Tests and retests would be pegged to results: if a decline in white blood cells occurred, a mandatory medical intervention could follow. His phrase "No blood—no drug" became the cardinal rule. It was a simple, elegant design that would eventually prove impossible to implement but that in the short term calmed the FDA.

Balancing hope against safety was novel. By the end of the 1989 hearings, the advisory committee was ready to vote. It had addressed clozapine's unparalleled performance, the monitoring system to manage risk, and whether a uniquely defined group of people might be eligible. While clozapine's toxicity remained a concern, the vote was unanimous, nine to zero, to permit two hundred thousand people access to clozapine, trade name Clozaril, starting in 1990.

Sandoz had reason to celebrate. In January 1990, a publicity campaign trumpeted "Hope for a New Beginning." *Psychiatric News* carried a six-page advertising insert for three consecutive months with a glossy insert of Lady Liberty beckoning a future of freedom, along with a story about Honigfeld's role piloting clozapine. It listed the side effects, including the frequency of agranulocytosis. A flowchart specified steps in what was termed the Clozaril Patient Management System for blood tests. An article boasted that clozapine "frees psychiatrists from routine tasks" yet reassured them that "at all times, the physician retains clinical control of the patient."[29]

Sandoz planned a symposium for the upcoming meetings of the American Psychiatric Association. Meltzer, now at Cleveland's Case Western Reserve University, would chair the panel discussing clozapine's potential to promote social integration. It would include John Strauss and John Talbott's ideas discussing social functioning as a factor for helping people with schizophrenia. John Kane, by now well known for his lead in Study 30 and subsequent publications, would join them. A cocktail party uncorked champagne afterward.

Celebrations were short lived. A hailstorm of publicity—outrage, chaos, confusion, and criticism—blitzed Sandoz. Annual patient costs for clozapine amounted to $8,944, a per-person profit of $3,000 a year. Accusations of greed, profiteering, price gouging, and unfair and unjustifiable profit margins embroidered the public narrative. Critics pointed to weekly charges of $172 for Americans compared to $35 a week in Britain; Germany's annual costs of $1,666 were roughly one-fifth of those in the United States.

The patient monitoring system, which Honigfeld designed to minimize patient risk, invited a potpourri of woes. Attorneys general in thirty-four states mounted a federal antitrust lawsuit. Inadequate Medicaid financing led states to develop waiting lists and lotteries. Other institutions involved in the patchwork American healthcare system—insurance companies, state mental health departments, and hospitals—refused to pay for clozapine.

The number of people actually receiving the drug became a scandal. Michigan added six patients. Iowa restricted access to ten hospitalized people. In New York, it was seventy-five. Maine had allocated twenty slots to two hospitals; California let patients start Clozaril only if their home county had already agreed to continue access; Ohio refused outright.[30] Of the 3,600 patients in VA hospitals who qualified, only eight received it. Added to field trial participants, the VA had a total of sixty-one patients.[31]

The VA's associate director for psychiatry, Dr. Laurent Lehmann, asked Sandoz for permission to save costs by using its own laboratory. Sandoz refused. Other states were similarly denied. It seemed, Lehmann said, this was a "rich man's drug for a poor man's disease."[32]

Lawsuits followed. In Pennsylvania, where a class-action lawsuit, *AMI of Pa. et. al., vs. White*, charged a violation of the Fourteenth Amendment, only one-quarter of the eligible population could be entered into a lottery system. In an interview, Honigfeld told Daniel Goleman of the *New York Times* that during the clinical trials, even psychiatrists at very good hospitals had been complacent about blood monitoring. Adverse side effects had put Sandoz at risk,[33] and doctors needed oversight. Consumer activist Joseph Rodgers partnered with NAMI parent Mary Ellen Rehrman to have Honigfeld teach consumers and relatives how to "monitor the monitors."[34] NAMI's Laurie Flynn agreed that doctors had not shown they could track patients successfully.[35]

New York's family activists Vera Hassner and Ethyln Honig were enraged that only 371 of the fourteen thousand eligible people had received the drug. None of the state's clinics, medical centers, or psychiatrists had gotten approval to dispense Clozaril.[36] Public interest lawyers also filed a class-action lawsuit, *Steven G. v. Cuomo*, to place Clozaril on the Medicaid formulary. Hassner and Honig headed the AMI Clozapine Family Information Network to broadcast inequities and spread news about where Clozaril was being prescribed—or not. Their granular analysis revealed differences, hospital by hospital. For most of NAMI's membership, activism was a survival strategy, and they led a well-designed challenge to the restrictive policies.

———————

The pricing controversy laid bare the nation's failures to regulate healthcare while depending on each state to modify its Medicaid policies and separately appeal to Sandoz. It also forced disclosure of differences between local and national strategies for NAMI. When the national office struck a deal with Sandoz to fund five hundred people for one year, critics hollered. It seemed like a sellout to settle for minuscule numbers. "Cruel manipulation," said a parent. Was NAMI being manipulated "as window dressing" for an "outrageously priced sales strategy?" asked a California member. What would happen in a year when the funds ran out?[37] Was the family advocacy organization becoming a service system?

Appeals to the FDA administrator, to HHS secretary Sullivan, and to Sandoz itself cited European prescribing patterns in an effort to bring down the price. Consider invoking federal law placing the drug in public domain, urged Tom Posey, NAMI's chair.[38] Flynn would later tell *Time* magazine that Clozaril was like a mirage: "You can see it. You can read about it. But you can't get it."[39]

Confronting these offenses, Sandoz fought back. Honigfeld was all over the news, as were grateful parents. In January 1991, Sandoz purchased full-page ads defending itself in the *New York Times, Los Angeles Times, Wall Street Journal, USA Today,* and *Washington Post.* In 1992, a federal lawsuit for $21 million was settled in thirty-three states where clozapine blood monitoring was tied to Caremark and Roche, but by then Sandoz had dismantled the system.[40]

With barely two years remaining on its patent, and with other pharmaceutical companies lining up similar drugs for market, Sandoz assessed market share, America's litigious culture, and the new competition. Corporate interest in Clozaril sputtered. Over Honigfeld's objections and profound disappointment, despite the promise, and after its halting start, Sandoz had spent millions of dollars in development and testing. It had advanced a solution for people who had run out of choices. But it could do this no more. Two years later, in 1994, in a company retrenchment, the Swiss-based company called it quits. They offered Honigfeld a buyout, and after twenty years, he left the company.

The pharmaceutical industry calls someone who refuses to let go of an idea a "product champion." For his persistence to a dubious project, Honigfeld's colleagues called him "pigheaded." His confidence never faltered during the monthly meetings when Sandoz reviewed products, even though people thought he was clutching a drug that was, by their estimation, a loser. For several years, clozapine had remained outside the formal review process. Earning nothing, its future was uncertain. But Honigfeld never wavered. "If it hadn't been for Gil championing the drug," said William Reid, the medical director of the Texas Department of Mental Health and Mental Retardation, "we would have lost clozapine."[41] Honigfeld is quick to credit doctors like Meltzer, Kane, and Gerbino, grounded in science, treating patients, pushing the promise. But Reid, among others, has credited Honigfeld with improving the lives of tens of thousands who were facing a dead end with no light and little hope.

Clozapine was heralded as much for its impact on the *negative* symptoms, which had been part of schizophrenia's signature since Kraepelin, as for its abilities to blunt positive symptoms. Yet they had been only vaguely understood. In 1974, John Strauss and Will Carpenter postulated that impaired social functioning should be another of schizophrenia's predictors.[42] This fit into their expansive review incorporating biology and psychology in schizophrenia's social context.[43] When the *Schizophrenia Bulletin* devoted a special issue to discussing negative symptoms in 1985, it paid tribute to Strauss and Carpenter's insights.[44] At the time, no commercially available drug addressed negative symptoms and social functioning. Most doctors were exasperated that there was "little to suggest that current medications have much to offer in the treatment of these symptoms."[45]

It took a few more years for the field to overcome the daunting image of a dangerous drug to appreciate how clozapine worked on the negative symptoms, and how this was another challenge to the orthodoxy of an inevitable and irreversible decline.[46] Meltzer addressed clozapine's benefit reversing negative symptoms at the FDA's second set of hearings in 1989. "We have patients from back-ward state hospitals who are now working in the competitive commercial area, having obtained jobs on their own," he said. "We have patients back in college getting B+s and A-s. We have patients living on their own who formerly could not even make it in the sheltered care setting."[47] He was then investigating thirty-eight hospitalized treatment-resistant patients to determine whether a six-month trial of clozapine altered their quality of life.[48] According to standard scales assessing symptoms and quality of life, they had shown notable improvement. More than half (55 percent) could volunteer, continue school, or work for pay. And the benefits were not just to them and their families. These had accrued over time, showing fewer hospital days and less public spending.[49]

Clozapine forced doctors to ask whether psychiatry had been too conservative by accepting the abatement of some symptoms. Meltzer asked whether they ought to accept anything less than a person's return to his or her prepsychotic level of functioning. That meant rethinking psychiatry's expectations for treatment outcomes, quality of life, and reducing suicide.[50]

Clozapine wasn't for everybody. But Sam Todd in Louisville, Kentucky, was among the lucky 99 percent for whom clozapine worked. He had been living at Wellspring House since its founding in 1982, and he had stayed out of hospitals. There were no more car crashes. But he didn't thrive until starting clozapine in the early 1990s. That's when he perked up and his life expanded. He went fishing with his dad, Bos. He returned to music, slinging his guitar over his shoulder wherever he went. He became part of the family, joining his two brothers and parents in shared events. Social workers at Wellspring said he seemed like a different person. He was still a heavy smoker, but the last ten years of his life included a sociability once made dormant by his illness. When he was stopped, at the age of forty-six, it was not by schizophrenia but by lung cancer.

Sam's doctors' early optimism about new medical treatments had been based on the dopamine hypothesis—they had told Bos how dopamine flooded Sam's brain and then prescribed the first generation of antipsychotic medicines to block it. That didn't work for Sam. His hope came from something that didn't bind to the dopamine receptors. That would be clozapine.[51]

As Honigfeld had hoped, this drug was different. And it had the potential to reach and help thousands in America as it had worldwide. The challenge would be not whether the psychopharmacology worked but whether psychiatrists would or could adopt it. Once fear became a factor, it was another of the hurdles to overcome.

PART 3

SOLUTIONS

CHAPTER 13

BUILDING A VILLAGE

NOTHING UPENDED THE NEAR-PERFECT EXISTENCE DAN AND ELAINE WEISBURD had built for their family like the phone call from Harvard College in 1978 telling them to retrieve their son, David. The dean explained to them that David had fought demons and angry voices, and a short hospitalization had confirmed that he should withdraw from school. Immediately Dan flew east to bring David back to Toulaca Lake, a Los Angeles suburb and the storied home to movie and television artists like him and Elaine. For the next forty years they would turn somersaults fighting for David's future. The oldest of their three children, David was musical like his mother, handsome like his father, had at one time excelled at tennis and piano, and had had near perfect SAT scores. To his parents, the creative force for the children's television show *Captain Kangaroo*, and to his teachers and camp counselors, he was a marvel.

Frustration chased Dan and Elaine while they struggled mightily to help David and protect others from his outbursts. He would bang his head against doors and walls, rip phones from the socket, and once, wielding a knife, had scared the hell out of his younger brother. Wanting the best psychiatrist that money could buy, Dan called his friend Herb Pardes at NIMH. "Save your money," Pardes said. "There is no best, but I'll give you the names of the 'least worst' psychiatrists in Los Angeles. We know almost nothing about the brain," he added.[1]

Dan and Elaine wouldn't relax their search, and at a meeting sponsored by the Los Angeles branch of the Mental Health Association (MHA), they met Richard Van Horn, an Episcopal minister who was becoming the go-to guy for mental health services throughout the county. Van Horn, who'd studied with renowned theologian Paul Tillich at Harvard, embodied liberal theology's social activism. Before the diocese assigned him to the MHA, he'd worked with Hispanic teens whom he'd tried to divert from drugs and gangs. He'd learned to remain focused on solutions despite broken systems.

Van Horn directed the Weisburds to a consumer-run, peer-support program, Project Return, which opened in Santa Monica in 1980. For the next four years, David floated in and out of their daytime activities while his parents tangled with board-and-care operators. Dan called them shills, unaccountable to patients' needs, collecting money for providing a roof, a bed, and often little else. David did his own tangling with the police, jails, courts, and judges. He was on the way to his eighth psychiatrist—there would be more—and had had more hospitalizations than he had fingers. Nothing had worked.

Dan and Elaine's vigilance brought them to the California Alliance for Mental Illness, CAMI. Irrepressible, Dan soon became its president, and lobbying took him to Sacramento. When Assemblyman Bruce Bronzan held hearings about the need for services, he testified with a fierce dedication about the son he intended to rescue from a consuming illness. Gray speckled his goatee, his clothes fit with elegance, and he carried himself with confidence and a stealth-like anger. That, and tenacity, led Bronzan to nickname Dan "torpedo."

Throwing himself into avenues of influence, Weisburd joined a project at UCLA discussing standards for delivering services. He and Elaine, along with Van Horn, produced a documentary, *Interrupted Lives* (1984), which was narrated by their friend Burt Lancaster, whose son also battled schizophrenia. That Jackie Parrish had green-lighted funding from the Community Support Program led to an unexpected quarrel with consumers. Families applauded its depiction of bleak services and research. Survivors and ex-patient consumers attacked its portrayal of mentally ill people as hopeless.

On a trip to CAMI's headquarters in Sacramento, Dan met Rose King, who also had a son in his twenties who had been diagnosed with schizophrenia. Untreated mental illness had already claimed her husband, who, in her presence, took his own life two weeks after being denied mental health services, and now she worried about her oldest child. King was regarded as a fierce and feisty political strategist who'd originally entered the arena as the Sacramento County coordinator for the "Recall [Governor Ronald] Reagan" campaign in the 1970s.[2] It was rumored that she'd leaked the governor's tax returns, showing that he'd paid no income tax in California at the same time he was slashing social services. Since then, she'd served as the executive director of the California Democratic Party and, having worked for different legislators, knew her way around politics. When she and Dan met, she was chief of staff to the lieutenant governor, Leo McCarthy, a liberal Democrat who'd established himself protecting the environment and vulnerable children and was fiercely supportive of services for the elderly. She scheduled a meeting to see how McCarthy could help Weisburd.

Interspersing anger with grief, Weisburd unburdened himself to McCarthy and King. Nothing had worked for David. Not the therapies, not the drugs, not any of the programs falling short of David's needs. He worried about Elaine, who had gone from a svelte size nine dress to a malnourished size zero. He worried about his two younger children, who had seen things no parent wants their kids to see. He had come to Sacramento that day intending to announce a lawsuit against Los Angeles County on David's behalf.

King and McCarthy were sympathetic but thought a lawsuit was a weak tool given Weisburd's goal. Courts were expensive. They took a long time. Remedies, even based on good legal decisions, could take even longer. They might create newspaper headlines and bring attention, McCarthy said, but he preferred something more lasting.

McCarthy and King believed they might have a secret weapon: public opinion. It came from a survey King had commissioned from Berman and Associates in 1985 to learn how the public wanted to spend a windfall budget surplus of $700 million. The unpublished survey had revealed the public's willingness to spend it on people struggling with mental health problems. This was as much of a surprise as it was a gift. The survey had asked respondents to choose from a list of items such as fighting crime, cleaning up toxic chemicals, pairing roads and highways, supporting the frail elderly or children, and even a cash refund. The list was exhaustive, and 63 percent of the voters opted to help people with mental illness, close to the 64 percent favoring improvements to public education, and slightly less than the 66 percent voting for better nutrition and care services for the frail elderly. As King later said, "It took a lot of people by surprise."[3]

This ranking seemed almost astounding, and it informed McCarthy's thinking that morning while he paced his office and tossed out ideas in a stream of consciousness. Public hearings were probably not the answer. Everybody knew that funding tipped toward hospitals starving counties of community services. It might be informative for the public to learn that the $1.2 billion California budgeted for mental illness was misspent on services that were flawed, fragmented, and stuck. But it would point fingers, not build a coalition. What works? McCarthy asked, shrugging and not really expecting an answer.

"Nothing works," Weisburd shouted. "My son goes from one crisis to another." It was ridiculous that California put people on waiting lists, and when their name was called, providers got reimbursed even if the patient got no help. "The concept's missing," Weisburd answered.

It had been six years since David had returned home, and Dan feared time was running out for his beloved son. Program directors said his needs were incompatible with their services. He was too interested in the world around him to be satisfied watching afternoon television, too restless to tolerate group therapies, too intelligent to be satisfied with sheltered workshops. And he was irascible. He disregarded rules that made no sense, disrupted routines, and was ejected. None of it made sense to Dan or Elaine.

Dan despised programs treating David like a faceless case, a so-called schizophrenic, known only by a diagnostic label. One of his and Elaine's earliest artistic achievements in the 1970s had been a series of three-and-a-half-minute musical cartoons animating the "Most Important Person in the World." *Captain Kangaroo* embodied this segment, giving primacy to kids' emotions.[4] Only in retrospect did it seem a preamble to positioning David's needs as the focus of the services he deserved for a life of good quality. A decade later, their storytelling had grown to include documentaries about mental illness, including *A System in Shambles*.[5]

In an NPR interview in 1986, Dan and Elaine described David's infrequent demonstration of his warmth, intelligence, and talents. Even the smallest particle—a hug for Dan or a piano improvisation—softened the hurt of abusive, obnoxious, even threatening behaviors. They couldn't abide hearing that nobody knew what to do. If herculean efforts were required to keep the essence of David alive, that's what they would do. They vowed not to allow their son to expire with an illness.[6]

Love couldn't heal David, but it certainly fueled Dan's mission for his firstborn. He told McCarthy that services should put the patient's needs before agency or staff comfort. McCarthy understood. He too was a father; he too believed government should be there for frail citizens, whether children or the elderly. To "figure out an alternative to this mess," as he called it, McCarthy suggested a task force. As lieutenant general, he could authorize it under the sweeping authority of the Economic Development Commission. Although its major focus was intended to promote international trade, he could use it to provide a workable home for this work. Would Weisburd chair it?

Without blinking, Dan agreed, saying, "It was the opportunity I had been waiting for to roll up my sleeves and attempt to do something with the mess I had experienced and observed."[7]

"Let's get cracking," McCarthy said.

With help from King, Van Horn, and Assemblyman Bruce Bronzan, Weisburd recruited professionals, politicians, a couple of high-profile executives, and an experienced consumer activist. Of all the people he wanted, none was more important than Art Bolton, still a legend for LPS and a pillar in Sacramento. King had enthusiastically endorsed him, knowing he could shape ideas into laws.[8] Bolton, in his mid-fifties, still harbored hopes of completing the package of services LPS had intended. Although he might have nursed a grudge or a fantasy of revenge toward the politicians who had crushed this in 1967, he was just happy to be back in the fight. He believed mentally ill people had been wronged by politicians stripping LPS of community support. He shelved his consulting work to join Weisburd and spearhead a statewide reform under the banner of "The Lieutenant Governor's Task Force for the Seriously Mentally Ill."

The task force spent eighteen months evaluating successful programs to understand what made them so. Studies about community services now filled libraries. Research was beginning to identify how quality of life was an objectively measured criterion, how it should be part of the assessment of services.

Like tourists in cathedral cities, task force members visited the arche-types. The team consisted of Art Bolton, Dan Weisburd, and Jay Mahler, a first-generation consumer activist from Northern California. They went to Wisconsin to speak with Mary Ann Test and Leonard Stein, whose fifteen-year-old ACT model of providing on-site assistance to people in their communities had been adopted widely. Bolton and Weisburd went to New York City to visit Fountain House, the flagship of the clubhouse movement offering safe haven and helping discharged patients live in the community. Their unique job-training program enabling clients, called members, to enter the competitive workforce was worthy of study. The team stopped in St. Louis to learn about Independence Center, a rehabilitation-oriented clubhouse that was expanding a housing program for its clients. They went to Chicago, where the National Council of Jewish Women had founded Thresholds as a social service agency in 1959, and where a decade later Jerry Dincin developed employment programs taking members into the paid workforce. In Ohio they consulted with leaders Pam Hyde and Mar-tha "Marti" Knisley, whom everybody knew had had remarkable commu-nity support successes. And they stopped in Rochester, New York, to learn how a novel county financing program had innovated paying for medical services. Called capitation, it attempted to rationalize services, to allow a fixed budget for each person and give independence to service providers to spend flexibly and creatively.

With their knowledge of the most promising programs, many of them helped by CSP grants, they proposed "An Integrated Service System for People with Serious Mental Illness." It was a synthesis of ideas to synchro-nize services around the individual receiving them, not the systems offer-ing them. It was bold, it was idealistic, and it threatened the foundations of political patronage dispensing authority to agencies in a crowded field.

———————

Dan Weisburd thought services should address a person's specific goals. But since everybody's needs were unique, the challenge would be how to help someone meet his or her goal. McCarthy agreed, seeing this through his eyes as a father of four, a grandparent of two when he spoke at CAMI's spring conference in San Mateo in April 1987. "We must create a system, driven by love, that will serve the whole person and the family," he said. It shall come with the "sense of duty and responsibility—out of love—that we have for our own children."[9] Melding his family life, social values, and political ambition for higher office, he criticized the current system, which he described as "driven by bureaucratic and economic considerations to be fragmented, unresponsive and wasteful." In this way he foreshadowed the task panel's priorities. It would focus on people like David, to find out what he needed, not what service providers wanted or what limited them.

"So sweeping are these reforms," Weisburd said, that they required "full public participation and debate." Citizens needed to hear how taxpayer money would be spent, how pilot projects exploring integrated services would actually work. The lieutenant governor's task force held fourteen town hall meetings across the state, each of which Bolton and Weisburd attended. Van Horn's Mental Health Association underwrote the costs. In San Francisco, Times Mirror newspapers hosted a town hall, as did Levi Strauss, the textile company. In Sacramento, McCarthy sponsored a task force in his garden office. Some county supervisors sponsored meetings. But others feared losing fiscal control over local clinics.[10] During the buildup, Weisburd and McCarthy received intimidating calls from people fearing their jobs would end. To give McCarthy cover, Dan offered to resign. No, said McCarthy. Meanwhile, the crosshairs of politics left Weisburd breathless, literally, as he was racing back and forth, in his early fifties, ignoring his health, and near collapse.

The task force recommendations became the blueprint for the next phase, an Assembly bill officially called the Wright-Bronzan-McCorquodale Act of 1988 but known as AB3777. It boldly articulated that "mental health care is a basic human service." It conveyed "all the rights, privileges, opportunities and responsibilities [to people with a mental illness] accorded other citizens." This became the foundation for service integration. It was a model linking food and shelter, medical and dental care, education, money management, vocational training, and protective services.

AB3777 uniquely promoted integrated services to replace piecing together disconnected programs. Bundling everything under a single mental health director cut into California's county leadership with local offices, all open at different hours, or with staffs unfamiliar with one another. The new model called for a multidisciplinary team for each patient—social workers, nurses, psychiatrists, and personal service representatives, elsewhere called case managers, working together.[11] AB3777 incorporated the federal law for protection and advocacy, PAIMI, requiring families and consumers on advisory panels.

The legislature was mindful, all of California was aware, of the social and political reasons people lived on the streets. People leaving jails, hospitals, or nursing homes qualified if they met the *DSM-III*'s diagnosis of schizophrenia or bipolar disorder. The same applied to people who were homeless, of whom 40 percent were estimated to have a mental health condition. The program also had to reverse skyrocketing costs for mental health. It had to show that California could save enough from inpatient hospitals or jails to offset these new comprehensive services.

Rotated through a kaleidoscope, AB3777's priorities reflected the bill's authors. Assemblyperson Cathie Wright wanted Ventura County's successful model of children's services to guide integration. Turn the dial one notch to see elements of Van Horn's existing outreach program in Long Beach, which was already finding accommodations for people who were homeless. Turn it another notch to bring into view Art Bolton's recommendations for emergency services, an idea dating from his days of LPS reform. Turn it once again and there was the focus on individual needs, what the Weisburds feared for David's future. When it came time to vote, only a single person in both chambers opposed passing AB3777.

Before a statewide adoption, the bold changes in AB3777 needed testing to show they worked. For this reason, the law funded demonstration projects that would iron out the wrinkles. Seventeen submissions, including two of the winning projects, came from county health departments to pilot an experimental integrated system; one came from Assemblywoman Wright's Ventura County, the other from Modesto, in Northern California's Stanislaus County. Van Horn's proposal turned out to be the third. It would be located in Long Beach, where the MHA already had a foothold with an outreach program for a drop-in day center and a job-training program for homeless people. MHA's proposal endorsed a "no-fail" provision. This meant that idiosyncrasies and symptoms, such as those troubling David, would not jeopardize eligibility or receiving services. Van Horn also insisted on "one-stop shopping," which meant access to services with a single enrollment.

Despite Van Horn's role in bringing AB3777 to this level, the decision was not a shoe-in. Weisburd had to recuse himself. A discrepancy in the competitor's application tilted the decision to Van Horn, pleasing those who considered the MHA's application best of all.[12]

In 1990, the MHA opened in a three-story brick building at 456 Elm Street, in Long Beach. Inland from the coastal harbor where the US Navy had once dry-docked its ships, the neighborhood had become thick with people using drugs and street dwellers, and the empty buildings and warehouses where they found refuge. AT&T International had once occupied this space, but it had been vacant for years by the time the MHA bought it for $2 million. From the outside, 456 Elm Street looked tired. It was hard to imagine it could be anything as quaint as what was implied by its new name: Village.

If Dan and Elaine Weisburd personified parents wanting better services, Mark Ragins epitomized those psychiatrists who were also frustrated with a failed system. Then ensconced at Harbor General Hospital, a UCLA affiliate, he was baby-faced, on the cusp of thirty, with rumpled bangs and a Fu Manchu mustache. And he feared California was careening toward disaster. Governor George Deukmejian had already vetoed adding a $25 million expansion of mental health services. People in psychiatric crisis were sleeping on the floors of the local emergency rooms. Police officers in Northern California reportedly let vulnerable people sleep in the back of their cars. They called it "squad therapy."[13] Meanwhile, the lame duck governor Deukmejian announced another $100 million in cuts for the 1990 budget.

From his days as a medical student at Washington University in St. Louis, Ragins had gravitated toward nontraditional services. This led him to seek postgraduate residency training at the University of Southern California, which had an unusual community-based program, USC Alternatives. It was being run by Richard Lamb, whose work with families in PAS in San Mateo had exposed him to a family-friendly viewpoint ten years before; now, at USC, Lamb was documenting mentally ill people who were ending up in jails. USC was also a ten-minute drive from downtown LA's skid row, which was on the verge of becoming an iconic image of homeless encampments. It fit Ragins's sense of mission with purpose.

The challenge of "connect[ing] to somebody that nobody else could" compelled Ragins. He was drawn to people who "had serious things wrong," people who had soaring fantasies, nattering voices, odd fears, and vivid suspicions, or were actively psychotic.[14] But did it make him right for the Village? Or the Village for him?

Martha Long, whom Van Horn had hired, interviewed Ragins and let him know that the Village was not hiring doctors embedded in a hierarchical medical model with a preordained formula. She shared Van Horn's and Weisburd's goals of putting a client's voice at the heart of services. Her success building a clubhouse in Virginia had exposed her to this vision of integrated services. She wanted everybody she hired, especially a psychiatrist, to share that excitement of innovative multidisciplinary teams.

On paper, Ragins didn't appear to be her guy. He had attended one of the country's premier medical schools but one steeped in biological psychiatry focused on diagnosing and treating symptoms. In that world, *good* patients followed instructions. Client empowerment and the person-centered approaches were atypical, as were personal service coordinators. The Village enrolled "clients" who were considered "members," similar to the clubhouse model. They received a lifetime entitlement to services and worked with personal service coordinators (PSCs). All this was a new frontier.

Ragins liked the idea of working with a team providing services. Patients he knew in downtown LA were similar to those the Village served. Long Beach was also close to his home in Torrance—an added plus. That the job required only a four-year commitment meant he had time to figure out next steps while California's economy improved. Mostly, however, he could bail from the disagreeableness of working at Harbor General Hospital. He wanted this job. And he stayed for twenty-seven years.

––––––––––––

Martha Long expected finding a psychiatrist to be the biggest personnel challenge. Ragins turned out to be the easiest. The next candidate revealed her inadequacies when she told Long she wouldn't eat in the same dining room as the Village members and wouldn't use the same toilet facilities. Interview over.

Strategically, the Village had to hire people who could grow into the roles required for a still-evolving integrated rehabilitation model for seriously ill people. That meant balancing a start-up staff while renovating space at 456 Elm Street, and simultaneously enrolling new members, engaging the external community of merchants and landlords, and understanding local transportation networks. Village members would be using it all. Staff needed to know how the system could support a member or intervene to divert a crisis. For someone needing to get to a hospital, Village doctors obtained local admitting privileges. Meanwhile, plans were laid for an on-site eatery, the 456 Café, where members could get on-the-job training in food services. The staff also wanted an on-site bank so members could cash checks and obtain small loans. The bank could become a payee for Village members while they developed financial management skills, and it could introduce people to the essentials of financial health.

To promote a patient-centered culture, the Village eliminated organizing around the typical hierarchy of hospitals and public clinics. There were no private staff lounges, and everybody used the same lavatory. A single line formed for lunch at the 456 Café and at the on-site bank. Members had access to their own treatment records. They could add to the commentary and notes. Long usually kept her office door open, surprising members as much as staff who had worked elsewhere.

Clinical integration required on-the-job relearning for everybody, including Ragins. He would later say the unique service needs of individuals couldn't be predicted from "a clinical or historical analysis of our members. The solution was to have the members' needs generate a highly individualized and forever changing list of services."[15] New roles emerged, and Long knew that she too had to get out from behind the desk and spend time in the field where the members actually were.

Village members also presented challenges the team found familiar. They relapsed by using street drugs or stopping their medication. They destroyed their belongings, got evicted from apartments, or became malnourished. They also disappeared to the streets, moved back with a relative, or isolated themselves under a bridge, in an alley, or a locked room. Elsewhere, they would have been terminated for poor attendance or lack of initiative.

One member, Libertad, had come from the streets. She spoke only Spanish, was highly suspicious, and was devoted to her church and priest. Through the Village, she landed a place to live. But after a good start she deteriorated, and in that phase she demolished her furniture and hoarded garbage in the shower. Intending to permit the devil to escape from a wall, she pushed her refrigerator to the outside balcony, and she cooked the pages of her Bible. She was evicted and hospitalized for six days, but she refused medication and was discharged. Ragins attended, and the multidisciplinary team saw her throughout her stay. The team had worked with her priest, urging him to bless her medicine in the hope that it would keep her engaged. The Village maintained access to emergency beds at the local board-and-care housing service, but she declined one. She declined further treatment with the Village. Unwilling to force her, Ragins and her coach, Clara Alvarez, emptied their pockets to give her forty dollars before she walked away. A former landlord gave her shelter. A year later, she returned to the Village seeking a job so she could donate money to her church. It just so happened that there was an opening for a dishwasher at the 456 Café and she was hired. When she noticed that her suspicions were interfering with her earning capacity, she asked Ragins to prescribe the medication he had wanted her to take all along. It was her choice. He believed their collaboration, rather than his insisting on compliance, became the foundation for the ongoing rehabilitation relationship.[16] Not everybody's situation resolved so well, of course.

Ragins had been working at the Village for four years when he described what he learned from another member, Gail. She had progressed "from years in a state hospital to self-sufficiency and a full life."[17] Gail had heard about clozapine and wanted Ragins to prescribe it despite what she had learned about its potentially dangerous side effects. Her history of seizures worried him, and he tried to discourage her. But she insisted, and together they mined the research literature. They also consulted with experts, and he reluctantly agreed. In an open letter to Gail when she left the Village, he wrote: "I supported your choice to take the medication even though I wouldn't have chosen to take it. . . . The lesson for me [was] that you turned out to be right and I was wrong."

How the Village managed risk became an ever-present concern. Psychiatrists worried about reducing stress for people with a psychiatric condition. But choice often brought risks, as did competition, and even having dreams involved an element of risk. At the Village, where they used shared decision-making, managing the stress of making choices became part of the culture of therapy and required a team effort. The core team was watchful when Gail started clozapine, knowing that the consequences of failure could be devastating. This vigilance was repeated dozens of times for members whose ambitions other programs would have discouraged or prevented.

Learning how to manage risky situations resembled Mary Ann Test and Leonard Stein's earliest challenges in Madison, when they had moved patients from the classroom to the community, where they had to navigate crowded supermarkets or laundromats with broken coin machines. The Village adopted similar real-time problem-solving, while helping clients accumulate confidence. When Test visited the Village during the pilot phase, she was delighted to see how they were implementing these practices promoting empowerment.[18]

Ragins accepted that he couldn't cure schizophrenia, bipolar disorder, or major depression. But he could help people develop a resilience to meet their goals despite their symptoms. Hope, he believed, was a powerful motivator.[19] And while some goals were grand and others prosaic—budgeting until the next check arrived, learning to drive, managing a stutter, and not breaking into a sweat trying to court a romantic interest—he saw his role as helping people have a better life despite their having a mental illness.

———————

In the early phases, the Village invited experts to train staff in rehabilitation principles. Rehabilitation introduced a conceptual framework for dealing with psychiatric conditions rather than focusing on what clients didn't have, what their illness had robbed them of, or what deficits needed repairing. Weisburd invited Bill Anthony, whose name was becoming synonymous with the idea. Perhaps because he was a psychologist, or perhaps because he once worked on a ward showing how rehabilitation practices helped Vietnam vets resume a civilian life, Anthony disdained the status-quo practice of just maintaining patients.[20] He intended to foster building skills and self-determination.[21] He shared Weisburd's dislike over "unappealing, inappropriate, or demeaning" services. But rehabilitation was nowhere near mainstream in mental health, despite his twenty-year effort honing a conceptual framework at the Center for Psychiatric Rehabilitation, which he had founded at Boston University in 1979.

Anthony had watched the Village craft its program. He and Long had worked together in an international association for rehabilitation service, and Weisburd had invited him to speak to CAMI families before visiting Long Beach in 1991. By the time Anthony arrived, he was considered a soft-spoken guru with avuncular kindness and patience. Ragins asked him what was next on the agenda.

"Recovery," he said.

"I nearly fell off my chair," Ragins told me.

Bill Anthony believed the conventional treatment system had gotten in the way of helping people recover. What was missing was a vision of recovery as strong as the vision of cure, or of prevention. He argued that the prevailing system, which assumed indefinite dependencies, shorted hope. With an aversion to risk, it promoted chronicity.[22]

Anthony credited consumers with promoting recovery's vision, which he thought would blaze in the 1990s. It was significant that scientific research, as he put it, sought "better treatments and, eventually, cures for mental illness." But it wasn't the full story for treatment services. Those hinged on enabling someone to put in motion their own goals and ambitions, to structure choices about how to get there, and to be supported for the duration. These self-determinative steps were ingredients of recovery that would shade the "guiding vision that pulls the field of services into the future . . . of what we hope for and dream of achieving."[23] For that, Anthony predicted the 1990s would be known as the Decade of Recovery. It was parallel to the Decade of the Brain's pursuit of science.

Rehabilitation, unlike cure, focused on "the consequences of the illness rather than the illness per se." Consequences might start with stigma and discrimination but also include lost opportunities or skills, self-doubts associated with stereotypes, or a depleted social world. Calling the 1990s a decade of recovery was bold, but no more bold than his endorsement of consumers taking charge of their lives, "even if one cannot take complete charge of one's symptoms."[24]

However preposterous the idea of recovery seemed to some, to those like Ragins, who was becoming familiar with Anthony's work along with that of Courtenay Harding, it was beginning to fit. Over the next couple of years, he too would write about the differences between the medical model in which he had been schooled to prescribe and decide what was best for patients, and rehabilitation and recovery in which a relationship tied to patient preferences prevailed. While psychiatry still struggled to understand what schizophrenia was and had no exact model for recovery, its practitioners had a lot of hunches. What Strauss and Carpenter had earlier proposed about dissimilar outcomes for people diagnosed with schizophrenia resembled what Ragins himself had seen in Gail or Libertad. It seemed to be "clear evidence of the growing efficacy of our treatments and more benign outcomes than traditionally thought." He wrote, "The problem may be as much in our conceptual model of treatment and recovery as the inherent nature of the conditions."[25] By 1995 he considered the differences between a medical model and a psychosocial rehabilitation model. The medical model, he wrote, characterized recovery in negative terms. Doctors worked to eliminate symptoms, or worrisome signs of an illness. The rehab model focuses on a life, and how the restoration of a function, not the eradication of a pathology, can enhance that life.

Ragins was coming to grips with the fact that people expressed mental illnesses differently, and some for an indefinite period. He said that in medical school, he had been "taught to be a strong, helping professional, ordering medication for weak, helpless, dependent, sick patients, and then to assess their 'compliance' with my regimen." At the Village, where he focused on health instead of weaknesses, he said he had to "discard my white coat, my coat and tie, and even my professional distance."[26]

Reflecting on his work, he said that, after the first year, what he liked most was the opportunity to innovate. "We didn't have to do anything a certain way because 'that's the way it's always been done.'" That freedom paid off. "We were all newly hired staff, who wanted to create a better way, and were willing to try new ideas and learn from our mistakes."

Ragins and the Village team believed the program was working well. Gradually members had shorter hospital stays, and the team learned what mattered. "This highly experimental approach made us keep our focus on what worked and what didn't," Ragins wrote. "We didn't have regulation driven, or payment driven, or even philosophy driven. We could figure out 'whatever it takes' and do it. We learned very fast that way."[27]

All this happened while the Village was enrolling new members coming from various referrals. Dan Weisburd suffered a considerable heart attack but remained involved after recovering. And despite many of the component parts having been tailored to David's challenges, it would take David more than a year to feel comfortable availing himself of the services.

California lawmakers needed answers to two questions: Did clients at the Village get the services they needed to help them get better? Did this model save taxpayers money?

AB3777 required an evaluation of the $9 million demonstration projects. That evaluation interviewed service recipients and available families. It established comparable sample sizes of roughly one hundred people in each of the three demonstration programs and compared these groups to an equal number of clients who received traditional services from local county clinics. They began in 1991.[28]

When it came to the Village, the evaluators, Lewin-VHI, needed to answer whether it "improved [a] system of care which would be beneficial for the most seriously mentally ill clients." Had the rehabilitation model offset costly hospitalizations? Were costs for courts or homeless shelters reduced? Had members found employment? On each of these measures, recipients of services at the Village performed better than the recipients of nonintegrated conventional programs to which it was compared. They had spent fewer days in the hospital. They also engaged in activities where they acquired skills, including self-care in the community. Symptoms had decreased, but that was secondary. As Weisburd had wanted, there were no failures at the Village—nobody was kicked out or summarily discharged. And nobody was forced into anything.

Lewin's analysis favored the integrated services model. It concluded, "The client outcomes at the Village represent the best achieved to date—in California or elsewhere." An integrated system, they said, solved many problems of "inflexibility due to categorical funding restrictions" and represented an "improved system of care which would be beneficial for the most seriously mentally ill clients." The costs for staff were higher than for the public clinics, however.[29] Case management, socialization, and employment services absorbed three-quarters of the Village's resources. The mental health director of Los Angeles County, Areta Crowell, testified at the Senate Labor and Human Resources Committee about mental health benefits in the fall of 1993. She told Senator Paul Wellstone, whose brother suffered with schizophrenia, that the Village cost about $17,000 a year per person, compared to $100,000 a year for someone in a state hospital. It was also more favorable than the $60,000 it would cost for someone in twenty-four-hour residential care. Crowell credited the integrated services model with flexibility, without which people would drift into the public sector, or end up in hospitals or prisons, and nobody would benefit. The structure of programs like the Village allowed for what she called an "intimate knowledge of the person over time to engage them in appropriate treatment and rehabilitation." These are not, she advised senators, traditional health organizations. But they were successful, and ignoring elements of their success would be a mistake.[30]

Despite the success of the Village, David Weisburd never got the breaks his father wanted him to have. For a while he seemed to benefit, but he drifted in and out, had makeshift jobs including work at the Village, and pocketed change from occasional piano gigs. But he never found a pathway to a future. For six weeks, clozapine changed his life. Ecstatic, he told his father, "I'm back . . . I'm not my illness . . . I'm David." A life-threatening drop in his white blood cell count ended that all-too-brief interlude.[31] He knew schizophrenia had robbed him of relationships and achievements he once assumed were his birthright: family, children, a measure of satisfaction with self and others. The inability to tame schizophrenia had cost him the good qualities of life. It was not what his parents had wanted, and certainly not what the Village had wanted when they designed what would become state-of-the-art integrated services.

CHAPTER 14

LEADERSHIP IN THE SERVICE OF PEERS

IN THE DECADE AFTER JUDI CHAMBERLIN AND HOWIE THE HARP first marched on the streets of New York, a robust core of activist consumers challenged laws and lawmakers from California to Vermont while they were developing programs through which clients could help one another. Remembering their own experiences in the mental health system, they sought change. Howie's experience was deeply rooted in Creedmoor Hospital, from which he had eloped at the age of sixteen to land on the streets of New York City. With his wit, his vivid memories, and his network of other crazy folk, in 1986 he moved to California. While the state closed hospitals and gutted community mental health services, he opened the Oakland Independent Service Center (OISC) in a hardscrabble neighborhood. He envisioned turning an empty storefront into a welcoming place where anybody could drop in for food, coffee, a bathroom, or a place to shower; obtain a mailing address; or get practical help to answer questions such as how to enroll in Social Security or locate a food pantry. There were tips about real jobs and tips for managing money. In his mecca, nobody should feel alone, nobody should be "isolated, outnumbered, defeated, and powerless." With this base, Howie wanted to build a "client force in the mental health politics of California."[1]

For the next six years he worked round the clock turning OISC into a safe space. People came from jails, from hospitals, and from the streets. Trust was a big part of the welcome. "Often people like us, who are never trusted, will go out of our way and work ten times harder," he said, "to come through when we are trusted."[2] He showed clients how to navigate government bureaucracies, how to advocate for others as well as themselves, and how to work with neighborhood resources. To him, this was the peer experience. Offer hope. Solve problems. Listen more than you talk. Learn what someone needs.

Howie's north star, self-help, required choice because no single program exclusively held "the answer." He worried that the medical model's emphasis on sickness and disease was oppressive. Medicines were not a substitute for solving a person's social and political problems. Medication may have helped some, he said, even people who loathed the side effects. But validation of oneself meant remembering that as human beings they were more than a diagnosis.[3]

Writing grants, mentoring volunteers, filling the coffee pot at OISC—these only partially filled his time. He worked with Sally Zinman expanding the California Network of Mental Health Clients in Alameda County. He stayed involved with Project Release, a pioneering self-help collective he had organized in New York City. He collaborated with Judi Chamberlin who was then building the Ruby Rogers drop-in center in Boston. Each person, each activity furthered his soul-defining mission: "mental health client controlled/self-help groups."[4] After securing another grant for the OISC in 1992, he realized he was tired. A long-term relationship had ended, and sleep apnea, a condition in which a breathing irregularity interrupts sleep, left him depleted. He considered leaving Oakland. "OISC will get along without me," he told his friend Peter Stastny, a psychiatrist with whom he had once worked delivering food to homeless New Yorkers. He told Stastny how he missed "the dirty, gritty, intense, and real people and streets I knew, and loved, and hated."[5] Stastny contacted Steve Coe, executive director of a New York–based mental housing program, Community Access.[6]

———————

Community Access had been around since 1974, when thousands of homeless people wandered New York City streets. It would take a class-action lawsuit, Callahan v. Carey, to begin to address the situation, but that wouldn't happen for another seven years. Meanwhile, 185,000 disabled people needed services citywide.[7] One Manhattan neighborhood, the Upper West Side, had become an epicenter for tens of thousands of discharged patients who lived in run-down dwellings with grease-lined halls, sheets of peeling paint, broken windows, wobbly bannisters, missing floorboards, broken hallway toilets, and few creature comforts to mitigate heat, cold, cockroaches, or rats. Here Howie developed grassroots organizing skill with Project Release, working with people who were victimized by the breathless pace of gentrification and turning these dilapidated buildings into expensive market-rate apartments, and leaving poor and powerless tenants one step from being out on the streets. This was the environment giving rise to Community Access. It was born from one man's efforts to buy an apartment building so his sister wouldn't become homeless after she left Manhattan State Psychiatric Institute. Manhattan's problems mirrored the national crisis in which housing was disconnected from comprehensive services.

In the 1970s, while studying at the New School, Coe interned at Community Access. It was a largely volunteer-run organization that was managing two poorly maintained tenement buildings on the Lower East Side. On his first visit to one of the buildings with a student team in January 1979, the outside temperature was barely three degrees and residents were using ovens going full blast to heat their apartments. He thought to himself, "These were the people who got left behind, and we could have been doing a lot better job than we were."[8]

By July, Coe was hired as an intern and he rolled up his sleeves, literally. The son and grandson of carpenters, he knew how to hang doors, fix toilets, and repair electrical outlets. He could type, so he could help people fill out forms. Tall, skinny, and bearded with relaxed red hair and a vision, he was a transplant from a West Coast farming town who was willing to wield a hammer.

Coe stepped into a leadership role after the founder had a fight with city hall and left the next year. By this time, the New York State Office of Mental Health had launched a program for not-for-profit agencies to lease apartments and provide support services. Community Access was a good candidate, but Coe knew it needed a lot of shaping. It had a board of directors and two apartment buildings but only one staff person responsible for the whole operation, which by then included forty-four rent-paying residents. And many more wanted housing. Over the following year Coe was able to find two landlords willing—and many who were not—to rent apartments to former patients. For the next forty years, he built and expanded Community Access, his vessel for community service and activism.

Change was in the air in the 1980s, and regulations about case managers, service plans, medication regimens, reimbursement, and housing codes and restrictions demanded attention. Each legal or bureaucratic modification changed the relationship Coe had built to address tenants' needs. Knowing he needed to reshape the organization, he began meeting leaders in the patient rights movement. From community activists such as Laura Ziegler with Project Release, he learned more about what clients needed. He viewed a documentary film, *Hurry Tomorrow*, and even though it came from one of California's state-run hospitals in 1975, the themes about dehumanized treatments were applicable and relevant. Film critic Vincent Canby wrote in the *New York Times* that any single three-minute sequence was filled with "more bitterness and outrage" than all of *One Flew Over the Cuckoo's Nest*.[9]

Coe intended to avoid the problems blighting treatment programs, including forced treatments or malicious disregard, and with this in mind he wooed staff who wanted human rights values to infuse clinical practice. Some people wanting nonprofit work came from city government. He hired a consultant who helped develop strategic plans. Since visiting Fountain House during his student days, he had nursed the idea of building a clubhouse on the Lower East Side. In 1988, with a $400,000 grant from the city, Coe turned a six-thousand square-foot empty supermarket on Avenue C into Club Access. In 1990, Community Access upgraded apartment buildings, the first of which opened on Avenue D.

Howie's interest in returning to New York corresponded to housing issues spilling into the city's hot-button politics. The question of what to do about the homeless population stirred passions in the mayoral election with federal prosecutor Rudolph "Rudy" Giuliani challenging the incumbent mayor, David Dinkins. With his typical bombast, Giuliani promised to end encampments under the city's bridges. He would get rid of the city's squeegee men who would surround cars at traffic lights and perfunctorily wipe their windshields before demanding money from the drivers. In the meantime, homeless people crowded shelters, some as big as Civil War–era armories. Some had fled a catastrophic fire leveling their homes; others were jobless, penniless, or among the fragile and vulnerable with a mental illness. After being elected as mayor, Giuliani basically starved the support system when he halved public funding and capped the service in Manhattan's city shelters at ninety days. Residents were effectively exiled, and many ended up northwest of the city, in Orange County,[10] a cosmetic solution that hardly repaired the social catastrophe.

Headlines about housing shortages fed Coe's desire to expand Community Access. That's when he learned about Howie's work training homeless ex-patients to become advocates. He had gotten a copy of the Alameda County evaluation of the Oakland Center that was linked to a CSP grant. In six years the OISC had helped nineteen hundred people remain in the community. It had employed fifteen ex-patients, and another twenty were training to become advocates to learn the ABCs of coaching. Evaluators praised the center's governance. It was fiscally sound and kept good records.[11] This aligned with Coe's goals of expanding Community Access's housing anchor program. He would later say, "Howie's 'genius' was carefully documenting everything he was doing, including evaluation studies like this one. He made sure he had a seat at the table, such as the boards and oversight committees that determined how research funds got spent."[12] Coe told Howie, "We have a vision for Community Access that requires people of your skill and stature . . . to transform a fairly traditional, licensed, community residence into a cooperative model."[13]

In New York, Community Access was a beacon amid a scandal-ridden and unregulated industry of adult group homes in which former patients were routinely scammed. Even legitimate operators imposed arbitrary rules about bedtime, roommates, phone calls, medicine, or access to public spaces. With more need than availability, it was easy to eject someone for infractions. Others left because they didn't want a roommate forced on them. Howie wisecracked about what it would look like, what the challenge would be for any twelve mental health professionals to live together. He once lived in a house that required residents to prove they were ready for independence by preparing a meal for a dozen people on a fifteen-dollar budget.[14]

Howie welcomed Coe's invitation to come for a visit. He met staff and members. He gave a talk at Club Access about human rights and social justice, and he dazzled everybody, including state officials who came from Albany. Howie too was impressed with what he saw. Opportunities danced in his imagination. "With more consumer involvement and empowerment, you could be doing an even greater job," he told Coe. "Even now, you are decades ahead of most other states, even California!" Coe wanted to expand. "Advocacy is a key part of the mission of our agency," he told Howie when he offered him the job. "I believe you would be an ideal person for that position."[15]

Howie and Coe spent fourteen months negotiating before he took the job. He wanted to know whether consumer employees had a status equal to staff doing similar work. After the American Disability Act passed in 1990, requiring accommodations for people with disabilities, he asked Coe, what had Community Access done? The truth was Community Access had done nothing yet, and this spurred Coe to act.[16] Wary of tokenism, Howie demanded independence to create the program he imagined.

Both knew what was at stake by offering Howie a position. The rest of the Community Access staff consisted of college-educated, professionally trained people, and Howie's formal education had ended at the eighth grade. But he had experience, and he had developed skills and insights different from and often more nuanced than a textbook's printed page. Neither an education nor a diagnosis defined him. His three-year hospital stint "does not describe who I am," he once said, "but it identifies a profound aspect of my life." He had worked as an offset press operator and a personal care attendant, and he liked to describe himself as a "musician, a lover of nature, and a frustrated comedian."[17]

Coe rewrote job descriptions for Community Access crediting a candidate's unique background in the mental health system. It would be important for hiring future staff, a prerequisite for anybody doing consumer advocacy.

As director of advocacy, Howie would "promote initiatives that will enable consumers to achieve independent lifestyles in the community." Part of his role also required applying these values "both within Community Access and the broader community." Howie saw the danger to this—it might be double-edged. What happened if this role required "advocating on behalf of a client against the employer, namely CA?"

To create parity, Coe set a new goal for Community Access: going forward, people with a psychiatric history would comprise 51 percent of the payroll. Some on the board of directors and the staff found this unacceptable. Over time, preferring a more traditional work environment, they left Community Access.[18]

Howie returned to New York in 1993. He moved into an apartment in the East Village, and on Sunday nights, with borrowed chairs, he set up for potluck and music with friends. He was a large man, barrel-chested, overweight, sporting wild blond curls and huge aviator glasses. Using a cane, he was unmistakable in a crowd or on a subway platform. But it was when he was seated at a table at Club Access, talking with members, enlisting them to develop their skills for advocacy, that he seemed larger than life.

To outfit a clubhouse environment at Club Access, Coe renovated the former grocery store and added small offices. Movies, workshops, or structured activities such as lectures about entitlements drew some members. Others came to play pool, or watch those who did. Club Access was becoming common ground for companionship, and all other activities that didn't emphasize fixing someone's deficits.

Howie's goal to expand housing mirrored Coe's. "Where a person lives," Howie said, "affects every aspect of that person's life."[19] He told an audience of psychiatrists that the "lack of housing, [plus] housing discrimination," sent people back to hospitals.[20] He didn't think there was a conflict between living independently and receiving help. "Only a hermit on a mountain top is truly independent. We are all interdependent," he wrote.[21]

As he had in Oakland, he wrote grants, and New York State responded favorably with $150,000 for a curriculum to train peer specialists. It was one of the nation's earliest, if not the first project of its type.[22] He knew the touch and feel of safe harbor, the warmth of a welcome at a drop-in center, and he also knew the challenge of staying upbeat when a thousand leaflets attracted only thirty people to a meeting he had planned. He repeated a lesson he learned in the early days of organizing Project Release: "Don't get discouraged."[23] With that upbeat confidence, he cajoled power brokers while remaining true to his values.

He was both tactful and strategic, and when providing feedback about New York State's 1994 plan for comprehensive mental health services, he adroitly complimented state commissioners for wisely knowing "the value of recipients as service providers and of consumer-run programs." But don't be stingy, he said, especially when financing something that was "absolutely necessary" like shifting the emphasis from institutions to the community. It was incomprehensible that even though everybody knew the CSP programs were "the service model of choice for most recipients," these initiatives had been budgeted for "the lowest level of funding."[24]

With a peer specialist curriculum nearly developed by the winter of 1995, Community Access announced a date to begin training the first class of advocates. Excitement grew as applications came from members of Club Access. Until Howie's program could become self-supporting at some future date, Community Access agreed to provide the infrastructure and sponsorship. Meanwhile, a board of directors consisting entirely of consumers (with the exception of Peter Stastny) took shape.

But tragically, two weeks before their big event, Howie had a heart attack. He was forty-two years old and died instantly. Bereaved, Steve Coe announced the program would be delayed for three months. When it opened in June, it was called the Howie the Harp Advocacy Center.

Both of the cities Howie called home, New York and Oakland, held memorial services. New York commemorated his political activism with a march. Each stop on the march was purposeful. The first was Community Access whose application for a group home had just been rejected. The second stop was at the home of the Assembly speaker, Steven Sanders, who'd led the fight for the denial. The third stop was to rally across the street from Bellevue Hospital, where a pilot project was underway to study involuntary patient commitment.[25]

In Oakland, Howie's memorial service at the First Unitarian Church comforted mourners with a song of simple protest, written by the popular Holly Near: "We Are a Gentle Angry People." Next was a poem by William Matchett, "Quaker Funeral," and the service closed with a selection from Walt Whitman's "Song of Myself."[26] They captured the way Howie the Harp lived in his community with humor, friends, and music. It paid tribute to one of his favorite adages, something attributed to Popeye, whom Howie had quipped had been "one of the greatest philosophers of our time." He quoted him often: "I am what I am."

Howie the Harp had been a builder, and Judi Chamberlin remembered him as "single-minded with one goal, perpetual energy, a commitment to unity." When the movement burst into two after the Alternatives '85 breakdown, he joined the competing factions and urged others to do the same. But it took until his funeral, writes Sally Zinman, after a decade's animosity, for warriors to reconcile and put down their swords. "Howie would have been happy," Zinman wrote.[27]

About the time Howie the Harp was building programs for Community Access, Larry Fricks was organizing the grass roots for recovery in Georgia. He'd come far since his life had careened out of control a few years earlier. Bouts of mania interspersed with depression, along with drugs and alcohol, had driven brawls, a failed marriage, financial catastrophe, and hospitalizations. If he hadn't been white and affluent, surely he would have spent time in jail instead of getting bailed out and sent to a hospital.[28]

During his third hospitalization, which included seclusion with four-point restraints, he was convinced he was being persecuted. Raised a Southern Baptist, he knew scripture. He knew that Psalm 31 called them to God's hands for protection from persecutors. Didn't Peter 5:8 warn about the likelihood of the devil devouring adversaries? Medicine was Satan's instrument. Of this he was certain.

"Absolutely not," said his doctors. "This is not God. This is an illness."

A fellow patient on the same floor shared Fricks's faith. And he told Fricks that he, too, had a special relationship with God and that since taking lithium, their conversations had gotten better. Give it a try, he suggested.

"My trusted peer had walked in my shoes," Fricks would later write, explaining why he started lithium.

Before this other patient, his peer, spoke up, nobody else had understood that Fricks's spiritual yearnings extended beyond something to check on his symptom profile.[29] Although he hated gaining sixty pounds, lithium turned out to be okay. When he left the hospital, staff solemnly dispensed their advice. Avoid stress, they said. He would never remarry, they warned. He would never work productively. He already knew what he had lost—a wife, considerable sources of income, property, family relationships, self-respect, dignity. Psychosis takes away your soul, he would later say. The prediction of a doleful future didn't help. Later, he attended a meeting of the Depression and Bipolar Support Association (DBSA) and was heartened seeing people who weren't woeful or hopeless. They had lives, careers, partners, and plans for a future. They also had bipolar disorder. There was hope in that room. For him, it was a new beginning.

Fricks's move toward advocacy was unplanned. He got a job as a journalist covering local events in northeastern Georgia, for twenty-five dollars a story. In 1989, he covered a meeting of the Habersham County Commission where a day program for people with a mental illness was under consideration. Should the commissioners approve this? Scribbling notes, it was clear to him that fear and misunderstanding framed the debate and bracketed their worries. "I was upset and did something very unprofessional," he later told his biographer, Richard Cohen. He spoke up and shared his personal story, crossing a boundary that journalists hold dear: to remain impartial. "I told people that I was in recovery from a mental illness. . . . We have to give these people a chance," he said. Fricks hadn't intended to self-disclose. But he saw an immediate impact. "They gulped, and then they passed the proposal."[30]

After he disclosed his battles with bipolar disorder, Fricks met other people who had also been hospitalized. They too had heard it said that they would have no future. They too had become discouraged. No longer bound by stigma, like a piñata broken, Fricks's secrets fell. He was invited to join a conversation about building a consumer network in Georgia. About thirty people came, and they began the Georgia Mental Health Consumer Network (GMHCN). Fricks says he became president immediately because he had a big mouth. More likely, it was because his talents were evident. He quit his job at the newspaper. When the GMHCN pressured Georgia's mental health director to hire a consumer advocate, Fricks got the job. He stayed for the next thirteen years.

From its earliest days, the GMHCN was action oriented. Wearing two hats—one leading the GMHCN, the other as the director of consumer relations—Fricks organized a conference for Georgia's consumers. In 1992, 650 people packed Mercer College in Macon, Georgia, and voted to incorporate. They vowed to end every meeting with a strategic plan guiding the next year's activism. "From day one it was the vision that we would bring together the people experiencing what it's like to live in recovery from mental illness and addiction," Fricks said. "And we would let them speak."[31]

That first year, and most years thereafter, the GMHCN voted to make employment of consumers their top priority. "People wanted something meaningful to do. They wanted purpose," he still tells his audiences. Then comes the planned ad-lib: "They never said 'give me more doctors, give me more medicine, give me more therapy.'" They wanted to become integrated, as contributors, and wear the dignity employment affords.[32] He told his boss, Commissioner Eddie Roland, "Consumers want to work!"

Fricks set out to make that happen. If they couldn't locate jobs in the regular workforce, as had he, they could become peer service providers, offering assistance, support, and guidance. A movement was taking shape state by state, leader by leader, and in Georgia, Larry Fricks was leading the way.

———————

Fresh out of library science school, Darby Penney stumbled into the leadership role she would play in New York. She hadn't seen herself as a leader or even an activist when she took a job at the New York State Department of Mental Health. She just needed to support herself, and even though she had no training in mental health, she got hired for an entry-level position for a study about the mental health needs of refugees. When the study ended, she moved over to the department's Health Planning Advisory Committee. That was about the same time the PAIMI law went into effect, requiring the inclusion of former patients and family activists on policy or planning committees. Her job required recruiting ex-patients, for which she tapped into the membership of the local patient liberation movement.

Penney had never actually considered her own mental health issues more than what she called "personal junk." Coordinating meetings for ex-patient consumers, and hearing men and women describe their stories, led to an awakening. "I'm one of them," she realized. "I'm not those bureaucrats in suits over there."[33]

Around that time, New York's ex-patient activists were petitioning the mental health commissioner, Richard Surles, to create a bureau of recipient affairs. People had been talking about Joel Slack in Alabama and Larry Fricks in Georgia, who had become consumer affairs advisors to their respective health departments. The job could be daunting, and at a workshop at Alternatives '91, Slack outlined the work of consumer bureaus and the practical challenges they faced. Penney was there, and the next year, when Commissioner Surles was ready to announce one, he asked her to become the commissioner of recipient affairs.

She wasn't sure she wanted the job. She hated speaking in public. She suspected some bureaucrats would consider her part of the "lunatic fringe" asking for "ridiculous things." What about boundaries? Who would she be serving? The Department of Mental Health or former patients who were often its critics? When she accepted, she reminded herself, "Even though I was working inside the system and paid by the system, . . . my ethical and moral responsibilities were to people with psychiatric disabilities."

Soon she displayed the talents Surles suspected would shine. After about a year, a task force report crossed her desk recommending hiring aides to work in state hospitals, men who were big enough "to take people down." She was stunned that this recommendation had been made without consulting her or others about the experience of seclusion. The task force was made up of people whose knowledge came from secondary literature, not experience. Based on their reading, they recommended hiring "bigger people to throw people down on the floor."

Penney complained up the chain to Surles. So did the head of the task force, but about Penney. "I can't believe Darby had the nerve to question me about this," he barked.

"She's right," Surles replied. "You should have had the right people on there and you've got to deal with this now."[34]

As commissioner of recipient affairs, Penney wanted staff who understood the coping skills required to manage psychiatric symptoms. It had to be someone who understood the rights of recipients, someone familiar with federal entitlements. Candidates had to be good listeners who could model strategies for overcoming the social challenges associated with their illness. They would carry the voice of consumers in all matters when the department evaluated its policies or organized its services. To do this, she needed a new job classification to hire consumers for peer services. She drafted a job description that included personal experience. It read: "By virtue of their own experiences in the mental health system, Peer Specialists model competence and the possibility of recovery, and assist recipients in developing the perspectives and skills that facilitate recovery."[35]

With a job description in hand, she sought approval from the civil service commissioners. Two colleagues accompanied her for the interview. One was also a consumer, the other a psychiatrist. The commissioners' reputation for rejecting new positions made her dread this meeting. To her surprise, they bubbled with enthusiasm, said it was great idea, and instantly approved the position. She was ecstatic and thought to herself, "Two months from now we'll have a hundred peer specialists."

Next she needed approval from the budget division. After her recent success, she hadn't anticipated objections. But one commissioner, a former social worker, was mortified that Penney expected people with a history of mental illness to hold a job. She accepted the civil service pay grade, the lowest for paraprofessionals, but couldn't accept that Penney would hire consumers. Unaware that two of the three people before her were themselves consumers, she strutted her ignorance. "I used to be a social worker and I know that nobody with a mental illness could ever hold a job." Penney and her colleagues were dumbstruck while this commissioner killed the proposal and continued her ridicule: "This is the stupidest thing I've ever heard. I'm telling you as a mental health professional, it's impossible."

Penney said it took another six years to officially arrive at a new pay grade and hire consumers to staff New York's regional offices, and all "because this dimwit woman decided to expose her prejudice."

That same year, 1993, eight people who had recently taken jobs staffing state offices of recipient affairs met in New England, where they formed the National Association of Consumer/Survivor Mental Health Administrators. Joel Slack became the president.[36] The next year, six more states filled similar cabinet-level jobs. In this way, writes Laura Van Tosh, they opened "an avenue for consumer participation in the formation of policy and development of consumer-operated programs and services."[37] According to Van Tosh, Georgia, Connecticut, and Florida owed their positions to activists. Other states such as Maryland undertook a formal needs assessment that called for a similar position.

Paradoxically, the emergence of consumer leadership grew while local, state, and federal governments were under a microscope for spending patterns that failed to develop adequate outpatient services. Every state had fewer hospitalized patients, but most of the resources still went into bricks-and-mortar maintenance. In 1987, after four years of planning, Ohio's mental health commissioner, Pam Hyde, expected to integrate the state's services for outpatients, who accounted for 95 percent of the patients and a staggering 48 percent of the budget.[38] Governor Richard Celeste endorsed the work but neglected to provide the requisite leadership on which its legislative success depended.[39]

Pennsylvania's decision to close Byberry Hospital in 1989 exemplified the difficulties of closing even the most primitive institutions. It still resembled *Life* magazine's shocking photo essay after World War II. Governor Bob Casey agreed with a blue-ribbon committee that this five-hundred-bed hospital should fire the abusive predatory guards, who were actually inmates borrowed from the local prison, that made up the staff. He recruited two of Ohio's seasoned professionals to develop community alternatives for which the state initially offered $16 million for case management and housing. Furious, families screamed; Joseph Rogers demanded $50 million.[40] When former patients with nowhere to go were found dead in the Schuylkill River, it was apparent that the cost of Casey's humanitarian impulse to close this state hospital was inadequate. Nor did the outcome affect the state's remaining fifteen facilities.

New York's 1993 campaign for reinvestment lays bare how one governor, Mario Cuomo, responded to the opportunity to redirect money saved from downsizing hospitals into housing, social programs, and the creation of peer services. The legislature's allocation of $200 million for local mental health services was waiting for his signature at the same time he was deciding between a reelection bid or a campaign for president, and mindful that union as well as nonunion hospital employees would be affected. New York's hospital costs, the nation's highest, amounted to about $70,000 a year for a bed, times twenty-two hospitals, potentially amounting to a billion dollars a year.

While Cuomo hesitated to sign the bill. In the meantime, NAMI families felt whipsawed and demonstrated across the state. Six hundred people marched in New York City. In Suffolk County it was 150 people outside state offices.[41] Outside the Sheraton Hotel in Manhattan, where the governor was addressing the New York Bar Association, the crowd chanted, "Off the streets and into care, Governor Cuomo show you care!"[42]

Activists also met in Albany that fall. Among them was a research psychologist, Ed Knight, who had a deep, booming voice that could actually be scary when he was angry. Knight headed the Mental Health Association's Recipient Empowerment Project. New to politics at that meeting was Harvey Rosenthal, who was emerging as one of the East Coast's premier consumer activists.

Knight and Rosenthal had constituents and could get out the vote, and they were tired of the governor's delays and his pushing blame onto the legislature. "We're in a meeting," Rosenthal recalled, "in the Red Room of the Capitol. The governor gets up and says, 'This bill is being brought forth by the legislature. The legislature is not your friend. I'm your friend.'"[43]

They were dumbstruck. With reelection fever in the air, the governor was cranky. But so was Knight hearing Cuomo disavow his responsibility and blame the legislature. To him, politics was not a game. With his loud voice reverberating, Knight got to his feet. He told Cuomo, "Well I've been homeless. And I have a diagnosis of schizophrenia. And people like me belong in the community. And we need the housing. And we need the support."

Cuomo grew still, suddenly realizing how his offhanded comment actually affected people sitting at the table. He gestured to Knight respectfully and called him "doctor."[44]

Cuomo agreed to sign a revised version of the nettlesome reinvestment bill, and activists were elated. But they were also guarded, and they vowed to demonstrate at the Capitol until Cuomo affixed his signature to the Community Reinvestment Act. He did so in December 1993, in New York City at the flagship community clubhouse, Fountain House. Cuomo might have sounded off the cuff at the signing ceremony when he credited those "who refused to leave," but he could have said nothing more serious to mark his respect for their impact.

The sweet taste of victory soured when the newly elected governor, George Pataki, did an about-face. Despite having been a coauthor of the Community Reinvestment Act, as a governor facing a $4 billion deficit he was about to starve that law. He proposed cuts to mental health that were four times larger than elsewhere. Already New York spent less on community programs than the national average (21 percent versus 38 percent);

already it spent more of its budget on hospitals. In a front-page story, the *New York Times* headline read, "Pataki in Switch Seeks Cuts in Programs for Mentally Ill." Kevin Sack wrote, "The state hospital system, which cared for 93,000 patients on 19 campuses 40 years ago, now uses 22 campuses to care for 9,000 patients." Pataki's own Republican colleagues tarnished him. "Somebody said, 'Find me savings,'" said Binghamton's Republican senator, Thomas W. Libous, "and that's where they found it," while keeping local jobs in Republican districts.[45]

Pataki reminded activists that politics was fickle.[46] They knew they had been duped and could not leave reform of an obsolete system to politicians.

CHAPTER 15

STAND ON CUE

CONVERSATIONS LEADING UP TO THE RETURN OF NIMH TO THE NIH IN 1992 emphasized the benefits to scientific research, but how this would benefit mental health services was less clear. For Robert Felix, who died in 1990, it would have seemed a wrecking ball to his dream, far from his vision linking science and services under one roof. On the eve of his retirement from NIMH in 1964, Felix allowed his imagination to soar beyond the dreams he carried after World War II when hospitals were lamentably the only service option. Drafting the bill for NIMH, he was confident that the changes he expected would be revolutionary. Hospitals might even become museums twenty years hence, testimony to a bygone era, he mused. His optimism came from scientific achievements and from people like Seymour Kety, the first scientific director of NIMH, who helped build a foundation for studying biological processes. Felix would have been troubled that NIMH had been dismembered, and with it the synergy driving discovery and clinical treatments, that hospitals still absorbed most of the funding for public services, and that scientific disputes, even the basics of a diagnosis, were far from settled.

Although discussions about returning NIMH to the NIH had percolated since 1985, it took place rather suddenly. It had barely been a year since Alan Leshner, NIMH acting director, oversaw an optimistic report to improve services as a companion to Sam Keith's plan for schizophrenia research. After services were sectioned off from NIMH in 1992, new agendas evolved, occasioned by a new president, Bill Clinton, and an entirely new structure, the Center for Mental Health Services (CMHS), which would live in a new bureaucracy called the Substance Abuse and Mental Health Services Administration (SAMHSA).

Before Clinton arrived in 1993, the Bush administration had asked the Department of Health and Human Services to review the Community Support Program. At NIMH, community resources for reintegration of former patients had existed on the margins of biological research, a margin that the CSP filled with robust ideas about programs and services, a godfather to innovation. The resulting HHS report, *Revitalizing the Community Support Program*, which rolled out in the new Clinton administration, equivocated with both praise and criticism. The report hailed the CSP's pragmatic "conceptual framework for serving adults with severe mental illnesses." It saluted collaborations with states. But it worried about the manifest influence of consumers, wondering if this tipped preferences away from what it considered the legitimate "treatment community, professionals such as psychiatrists, and providers such as CMHCs and hospitals."[1]

These questions skirted the psychiatric establishment's failure to meet the palpable service needs wrought by deinstitutionalization's discharge of tens of thousands of patients. And David Stockman's insistence proved consequential now. It had been a dozen years since he had said government wasn't going to fund services nor would it study them. The reach of that dictum was apparent in the paucity of data about social supports, self-help initiatives, and rehabilitation programs conceived with CSP guidance. Now consumers worried about how a new leadership would view their priorities, and whether the new office, CMHS, would slight them and reinvest in "more traditional research-oriented projects."[2]

While the reorganization was underway, the Community Support Program continued to hold brainstorming meetings for grant holders. For the October 1993 meeting called CHANGE, two hundred people checked into a Hilton Hotel in Rockville, Maryland, in roughly equal numbers of family members, government employees, nonprofit service organization staff, and former patients, consumers, and survivors. The agenda featured NAMI's Laurie Flynn as keynote speaker. Two ex-patient consumer leaders—New York's Darby Penney and Maryland's John Allen—had been asked to facilitate breakout sessions. A ten-minute introductory slot went to Joseph Rogers, representing Project SHARE from Philadelphia's National Mental Health Consumers' Self-Help Clearinghouse. Other than that, ex-patient consumers had no visible role. Still smarting from NAMI's insistence on prioritizing biological research, former patients thought they had been slighted. And they were angry.

Ex-patients agreed to protest with a walkout the next day. Later Penney chuckled that they had easily settled on a walkout, as she recalled earlier fights over strategies and tactics, or what to call themselves, and how they had parsed who was trustworthy. The issue of whether they could accept government funding had almost broken them. Could they really synchronize a protest? It would be unprecedented, but on this they agreed: they would wait for a cue, and then they would stand to leave when Laurie Flynn spoke from the podium.[3]

Former patients found it easy to indulge their anger toward Flynn and NAMI. Tensions had only grown since consumers perceived an insult as long ago as NAMI's launch meeting in 1979. Despite CSP's efforts to build bridges by bringing families and ex-patients together, sniping had continued. At the first Alternatives conference in 1985 they bickered, and they still hadn't resolved who among them could be considered a "consumer." By default it had fallen to former patients, who settled for being called consumers/survivors. Personality and style may have driven some of the tension, but conspicuous differences about policy, as well as language, put them on a collision course. NAMI's focus on "persistent brain disorders" or insisting on calling mental illnesses "chronic" were among the flashpoints. West Coast ex-patient activist David Oaks portrayed NAMI as the equivalent of an Antichrist in the journal he edited, *Dendron*.

At the 1993 CSP meeting, consumers/survivors believed NAMI leaders had usurped the agenda. Flynn had recently attacked the Protection and Advocacy program for being "out of step with NAMI." This seemed extreme even to other parents, one of whom reminded them that P&As were established for clients, not for what NAMI believes is best for clients. Flynn angered partisans in the legal community, including one lawyer, a parent whose daughter's abuse at a New York public hospital, Pilgrim State, sparked his activism.[4] Consumers/survivors were on the lookout for these kinds of internal differences, and this seemed to be a moment to show their displeasure.

On that second morning of the CSP conference, Laurie Flynn spoke from the lectern with an abundance of confidence. But she seemed to have a tin ear when it came to understanding the gulf separating the former patients from families, or how their priorities differed. Allen was waiting for the right time, and when she implied there was "a consensus of clients and consumers," he stood up. As planned, ex-patients followed. With one-quarter of the audience on their feet, Cindy Hopkins, from Texas, read a 122-word statement reminding the others that it was because of consumers that they were there that day. "You could take out the families, the providers, and even the bureaucrats," Hopkins read from the prepared statement, "and we would still be here with the same issues. . . . If you take out the consumers/survivors, there is no reason for you to be here."[5]

When she finished, Allen and Penney led the protesters out of the auditorium, through the lobby, across the parking lot of Rockville's Twinbrook Metro Station, and up the road for ten minutes to SAMHSA's home in the Parklawn Building. Bypassing the receptionist's desk, they took the elevator to the fifteenth floor, where psychiatrist Bernard "Bernie" Arons, still awaiting congressional confirmation as the director of the Center for Mental Health Services, was in his shirtsleeves unpacking boxes on this, his first day.

Arons was a twenty-year veteran, new to the job but not to Washington. Over the course of his long career, he had provided clinical services and professional education at St. Elizabeths Hospital. Later, as the court-appointed director for the hospital's discharge plan (known as Dixon), he oversaw the return of patients to community housing and services. He had once worked for California's health champion, Rep. Pete Stark, and he understood politics. He also knew financing as a current member of President Clinton's Task Force on Mental Health Reform, which had been weighing costs and models of insurance reform. Mental health and substance use disorders were elements of that reform, and it was essential to ensure that services were available in the least restrictive environment. That he was an advisor to Tipper Gore meant former patients knew him.

When the demonstrators arrived, unexpected and unannounced, he gave them his undivided attention. About fifty stayed all day explaining what they wanted, who they were, and how they ultimately saw a different role for themselves than that of protesters. He understood they wanted a voice in policies affecting them.

Do something bold, they challenged him. Hire an ex-patient, a consumer/survivor. Make it someone whose vision included personal history and was willing to use their mental health experience to inform policy and action, someone who wasn't beholden to families or to professionals. Arons rushed nobody; he took copious notes. The next day, he attended the CSP conference and took questions from the audience, and in this way he began his work as director of CMHS. It would be apparent the next month, when giving testimony at a congressional committee headed by Senator Paul Wellstone, that he was sympathetic to the extra-hospital priorities of former patients.[6]

The walkout burnished another chapter in the ex-patient consumer movement. Arons already knew that some states had hired consumers and created offices of recipient affairs. The HHS inspector general's report about the future of the Community Support Program had encouraged adding an office of consumer affairs, although it hadn't specified whether that entity would be led by someone from the family or ex-patient constituency.

A search for qualified candidates found Paolo del Vecchio, who was both family and a former patient. A Philadelphia native, del Vecchio battled depression as a child and had flirted with suicide; later he acknowledged that services for him would have been useful. His mother too had struggled with serious depression. That she had also raised four children, finished her education, and gotten a doctorate inspired him. He found a mentor in Joseph Rogers and an internship at the Consumer Self-Help Clearing House, which was offering technical support for consumers calling about self-help services. His leadership skills had grown since organizing the World Federation of Psychiatric Users meeting in Mexico City in 1991. Two years later, he spoke at the United Nations. With a master's degree in social work from Temple University and immediate experience working in Philadelphia's city government, his qualifications were unimpeachable.

Laurie Flynn thought Arons had "caved," she said, hiring del Vecchio in 1995 as the consumer affairs specialist.[7] Although Flynn wanted a prominent role for NAMI, she had to settle for an advisory capacity where their concerns intersected.

NAMI found self-help insufficient compared to professional help; NAMI parents didn't think their children flourished in drop-in centers.

It was hard to champion self-help when so many of their children still lived at home, abandoned by a failed public mental health system. By now, there was no mistaking that the lack of services had swelled jails, including with some of their children. It had become another scandal in places like Los Angeles County, where more people with mental illnesses could be found incarcerated than hospitalized.[8] Never had parents been retired from the job of de facto caregivers, thus again pressuring Flynn to make services one of NAMI's priorities. Hiring del Vecchio seemed an insult to their problems and an end run around science and medicine, the bedrock of the services and therapies they wanted.

Starting his new job in January 1995, del Vecchio was nervous. As a former patient, he was mindful that prejudice and stigma ran through workplace environments, and he also knew that some people in his own community, his friends, even peers considered him a trinket, a plaything of the status quo. He had been branded "King Token Consumer." Others discounted his legitimacy saying he didn't have significant or enough hospitalizations. There was no end to the criticisms.

He learned later that one of Arons's assistants had agreed to unofficially keep an eye on him. She half expected him to personify the offensive caricature of a drooling, shuffling, disheveled person. He now delights when describing how, three years later, they got married. One of the standard lines in his public presentations became, "Now we take care of each other."

Hiring del Vecchio was strategic as well as symbolic. Conflicts between families and former patients had turned from simmer to boil. None was more immediate than addressing what had become a recurring disagreement about forced treatments.[9] Arons addressed this in a memo to the larger community: "Recently, there has been a great deal of discussion about electroconvulsive therapy (ECT)," he wrote, "and, in particular, the involuntary administration of ECT to mental health services consumers/survivors." Opposing viewpoints had led to misunderstanding, even rancor, and he stressed the importance of maintaining "ECT for those who desire it." Forced treatments led to psychological damage, and the difference, he said, was between offering treatment and behavior control. The center would work toward "solutions that will promote alternatives and respect consumer/survivor choice." In this, psychologists, social workers, and consumers agreed.

By using the phrase "consumer/survivor," Arons reflected what activists had said about the importance of language. This infuriated Flynn, and she believed he would embolden die-hards, even encourage Scientologists in their anti-psychiatry campaigns. She implored him to "focus on medical aspects of ECT and avoid the 'politics' of ECT."

Arons held ground. ECT was available for people who wanted it. But he maintained that choice, not force, should determine its use. Flynn also dug in and rather oddly insisted that involuntary treatment and ECT had little to do with each other. Ironically, not all consumers appreciated Arons's studied argument. *Dendron* questioned CMHC's authority and could only hope that del Vecchio offered a "ray of hope."[10]

Arons wasn't posturing about wanting to work with consumers, and he knew hiring del Vecchio might be a gamble.[11] "Consumers Play a Key Role" headlined the Winter 1997–98 CMHS online publication, KEN (Knowledge Exchange Network). This was a new, one-stop resource about "prevention, treatment, and rehabilitation services for mental illness," and tech-savvy Sylvia Caras, a consumer with a three-hundred-person listserv, MADNESS, had helped start this internet program.[12]

Arons intended to dig into every resource. "Collaboration isn't just a matter of reducing duplication," he said. "It also means tapping into gold mines of existing expertise."[13] An early project proposed building technical assistance centers "for developing successful consumer-based enterprises." Philadelphia and Boston, each with robust consumer/survivor leadership, respectively got a nod to open two of the offices. In Philadelphia, Joseph Rogers already had the self-help clearinghouse, and he saw this opportunity to develop "valuable human resources that otherwise might be overlooked."

Boston's technical assistance program, the National Empowerment Center, was cofounded by consumer activists who were also professionals: Pat Deegan, a psychologist, and Dan Fischer, a psychiatrist. Their recovery experiences informed their campaigns challenging myths that people don't recover. So important was it to document the process that, in 1997,

CMHS funded a one-year project collecting interviews with people in various stages of recovery.

———————

Could organized consumers and guild-defined psychiatrists get beyond polemics? Was there common ground? The question led del Vecchio and Melvin Haas, a physician and colleague at CMHS, to plan a meeting in July 1997 to promote dialogue between consumers and psychiatrists for "better mutual understanding and respect" with recommendations for a "more therapeutic partnership."[14] For their part, the invited psychiatrists said they were burdened by the expectation that they should be omniscient, that they should *treat* someone rather than support their recovery. Consumers expressed frustration that everything they did or said was perceived as part of an illness, robbing them of dignity and turning professionals into enemies. They talked about choice, respect, hope, peer support, and voluntary engagement as ingredients for a collaborative relationship, and the center followed up with materials for training psychiatry residents. That success led to conversations for consumers and psychologists. For this, trauma and stigma provided a focus. The successful conversation with psychologists, as was the case with psychiatrists, warranted an encore.

After about a year on the job, Arons introduced del Vecchio to the CMHS advisory board where he described this work, plus plans for developing a veterans' advisory group and teleconferencing with people of color, all of which expanded the audience and the CMHS vision. On the workload for 1997 was "a CMHS survey of self-help groups nationwide."[15]

Research indicated that no fewer than twelve million people—some thought this an undercount—participated in self-help programs. From the University of Michigan's Institute for Social Research, psychologist Ron Kessler reported that self-help programs might account for as many as 40 percent of all mental health visits. In California the Department of Mental Health funded a project to learn what enabled well-being, what helped a client get better. Two consumers, Ron Schraiber, a psychologist, and Jean Campbell, a sociologist, wrote the winning proposal to document what would later be called the "Well-Being Study," and they worked with Sally Zinman and the California Network of Mental Health Clients.

They interviewed 331 clients, 160 professionals, and 50 family members. Each group showed different priorities when it came to questions about what worked, what was important. Schraiber was surprised that as many as half the clients considered medication helpful, and not surprised that all of the psychiatrists did. There was also cleavage on questions about the importance of sexuality and intimacy. More than two-thirds of the clients saw this as important to their well-being compared to mental health professionals and families, none of whom considered it significant. In addition to differences on specific questions, the larger concerns about resiliency differed depending whether one was providing or receiving services.[16]

The CMHS could look to one of their own staff, Ron Manderscheid, to explain consumer-operated services. He was among the field's most prolific and respected researchers, and he had already teed up to measure and evaluate the outcomes of service systems for recipients. Manderscheid understood, earlier than most, the potential of a recovery movement. He was a clear-speaking midwesterner, with a humble confidence and hundreds of professional appearances and publications. With a doctorate in sociology, graduate study in anthropology, and the skills of a statistician, he discerned patterns that could inform policy. Data girded his thinking that managed care, which had limited service options, conflicted with integrated community care. What was needed, he said, was understanding people "in the community who are in need of a service delivery system designed to meet their needs." He urged developing "outcome and performance measures." In 1994, he organized the Mental Health Statistics Improvement Program to design a report card giving weight to consumers.[17] Every provider, every funder, every professional group sought standards, and data, and each intended to establish their own best practices. CMHS ought to provide leadership in the development of a research process, he said, because "the consumer's perception must be primary."[18]

In 1997, the CMHS announced an eight-state study to evaluate patient outcomes. For nearly twenty years, activists had insisted that self-help programs brought success. Did the reality match the rhetoric? Turf wars had too often obscured studying benefits to patients, and political posturing limited resources.

With straightforward questions—who was served, what were the results, and what were the costs—CMHS would answer how consumer-operated treatment programs compared to traditional services. Campbell, at the Missouri Institute of Mental Health, was gaining a national reputation after California's well-being study, and she was chosen to coordinate the Consumer Operated Service Programs (COSP). The COSP spearheaded research employing a random research design in which patients were assigned to self-help organizations or to more traditional services. It would take four years, cost $20 million, and track 1,827 people across eight sites.

A lot was riding on this unique project. Howie the Harp, Judi Chamberlin, Joseph Rogers, Sally Zinman, and a generation of activists had lobbied for self-help. Rigorously constructed research would test whether eleven hundred consumer-operated services, plus six thousand mutual support groups for consumers and families, actually delivered results. They would be measured in categories such as individual empowerment, social inclusion, employment, housing, service satisfaction, and cost.[19]

University-based medical centers partnered with consumer programs to "evaluate the effectiveness and costs associated with consumer-operated services."[20] Although the results would not come in for years, when they did, Campbell summarized the "significant gains in hope, self-efficacy, empowerment, goal attainment and meaning of life in comparison to those who were offered traditional mental health services *only.*" When all was done, it seemed that the people "who actually used the peer services the most" were actually benefiting the most.[21]

On a trip to the 1996 Summer Olympics in Atlanta, Second Lady Tipper Gore asked HHS secretary Donna Shalala, "Who authorizes a surgeon general's report?" Gore was a respected, serious, influential, and reliable activist working behind the scenes, and her question led to what would become a defining moment. For the next three years, dozens of expert consultants met, read, and studied the nation's mental health system for a report that would be hailed a landmark achievement when it was released in 1999, *Mental Health: A Report of the Surgeon General.*

After it was clear that a surgeon general's study was on the agenda, Paolo del Vecchio encouraged anyone he met on his travels to share their points of view with health planners, university researchers, senior government officials, doctors, lawyers, economists, service providers, and just about every health advocacy organization imaginable. For this, he wanted to make sure consumers were included. Of the eight consumers on the planning board, in addition to himself, del Vecchio invited Larry Fricks, who by now had become Georgia's most outspoken consumer.

In the 1990s, Georgia was on the brink of fiscal disaster threatening all service programs: primary care services, rape crisis centers, homeless shelters. There was talk of privatizing prisons, hospitals, and schools. Governor Zell Miller's 1997 budget proposed saving money by cutting 250 hospital beds. Making matters worse, Medicaid had issued a withering criticism of Georgia's publicly funded mental health centers. Day treatment programs were a dead end for twenty-three thousand people. With no services, no staff, and no hope, they were basically holding pens called treatment. Desperate, Georgia engaged a consultant, Colette Croze, to help them rescue Medicaid funding. She encouraged Georgia to amend their Medicaid contract and ask for peer supports. She had seen something akin to peer supports in Washington, but it hadn't yet been implemented or standardized. In New York the program Darby Penney had tried to start was still on hold. In Georgia adopting peer support to provide services would amount to employing a new tool to rescue poorly functioning clinics. This would require reimagining the framework of licensed professionals on which clinics had been built.

When Croze first floated the idea that peers could be employed, the Center for Medicare and Medicaid Services had no idea what she was talking about. How could peer services be useful? they asked. What did peers do? Croze explained that peers promoted therapeutic outcomes, something that fit into Medicaid's standard for medical assistance. It was a bold idea, and fiscal urgency made Georgia frantic. The health department asked Larry Fricks to weigh in.

Fricks had a vague and imprecise understanding, based on limited knowledge of New York's attempt. What he did know was that consumers wanted to work. Paid employment would lead to social and economic independence and make social integration possible. As talks became more specific, as the department drafted proposals to introduce peers to clinics, Fricks brought the proposals to the Georgia Mental Health Consumer Network to hear their opinion.

Initially nobody in Medicaid thought that employing people in recovery might be the linchpin for reorganizing services. Wendy Tiegreen, who worked in Georgia's Division of Mental Health, spoke to Croze and Fricks and fielded the federal government's questions about how peers met Medicaid's medical assistance criterion. Was their "lived experience" sufficient? "There's no rule prohibiting it," Croze replied. What about their knowledge base? A college degree? Not necessary for paraprofessionals, Croze said.

When someone from the Center for Medicare and Medicaid Services had questions about self-help and the evidence about peer support, Fricks could answer. He knew that Paolo del Vecchio and Laura Van Tosh were working on a study about the outcomes of consumer-operated services, and he knew about the favorable outcomes Carol Mowbray was reporting from Michigan. He told Medicaid that the surgeon general's task force was working on a report based on this evidence. Peevishly he said, "You don't want to go against David Satcher and Donna Shalala, do you?"[22] Medicaid reimbursement for peer services in Georgia started on July 1, 1999. Qualifications for peers included those with "lived experience"; they could be in recovery or still receiving service.

Consumers who attended the GMHCN conference were already doing the work of peers without being compensated. They would go to the client who couldn't tolerate intensity, or needed something specific and for a short time. Day after day, they helped people leaving hospitals, searching for sustenance in the community, getting settled on parole, or fighting the bureaucracy. They added flexibility that the larger systems and smaller clinics lacked, and they could be paid for this.

Fricks and Tiegreen knew that implementation would be painstaking: a one-by-one conversation with the directors of mental health programs to explain how peer services could benefit their clients at the same time their agencies increased their workforce. Peers added value. In the meantime, Fricks partnered with Ike Powell, a transplanted New Yorker, to develop a curriculum for a peer training program similar to Penney's model—the one a New York social worker had rejected because she'd been absolutely certain that people with a diagnosed mental illness could not work.

CHAPTER 16

THE IMPRACTICALITIES
OF THE SITUATION

G RASSROOTS ACTIVISTS STEADILY GAINED CREDIBILITY and influence by focusing on specific goals. For some it was building self-
help services, for others it was challenging psychiatry's model, and for still
others it was securing a place to live. As Howie the Harp told a group of
psychiatrists in 1986, "The best therapy in the world wouldn't help when
a person has nowhere to live."[1] These elements were related, and the lode-
star was choice.

Choice was core to Judi Chamberlin's demand of "nothing about us
without us" and intrinsic to Howie the Harp's Project Release for New
York City's tenants. Choice guided Su Budd's ambitions for Project Accep-
tance in Kansas and informed Marcia Lovejoy's decision to fight stigma
with Project Overcome in Minnesota.[2] For Sally Zinman, choice was vital
to defining client-run programs. Choice, she said, meant they were not
"part of the continuum of mental health services that involuntarily com-
mit people."[3]

Choice also defined the battleground for a psychiatrist named E. Fuller
Torrey. He and his widowed mother longed for a silver bullet for his sister,
Rhoda, who suffered from schizophrenia. When he spoke about needing
research, about wanting treatments, it was deeply personal. It wasn't just
because of Rhoda that he felt this. As a staff psychiatrist at St. Elizabeths
Hospital, every day he saw people with schizophrenia and bipolar disorder. Like other families, he often sparred with psychiatry.

In 1982, Torrey attended NAMI's fourth national convention in Arlington, Virginia, still deflecting criticism from the two books he'd authored that criticized his own field. His upcoming book, *Surviving Schizophrenia*, would repair his reputation and anoint him as a family warrior. In the bosom of NAMI, he would shape a new image, rebuild his reputation, and guide the nascent organization. While his peers considered him a rogue, an upstart, and a maverick, families thought him courageous, well traveled, and especially bold.

Earlier in his career, Torrey had mixed idealism with erudition and arrogance. He'd joined the Public Health Service while finishing medical school in Montreal at McGill University, then he spent two years in the Peace Corps in Ethiopia and another year working in the Bronx, where he developed nonprofessional mental health workers. In 1970, he became special assistant to NIMH. Four years later, he published *The Death of Psychiatry*.[4]

Torrey's book foreshadowed a growing belief that mental illnesses were diseases of the brain, not of the mind. At NIMH, he approached the brain as an organ, similar to other organs that could suffer structural or functional deficits, be weakened by a virus, or become diseased. While his colleagues debated the environmental or parental causes of mental illness, he doubted bad parenting was a culprit. And when psychiatry debated the boundaries of diagnosis or fine-tuned therapeutic principles, Torrey paid little attention. Instead, he opined, "Psychiatry is an emperor standing naked in his new clothes." Should there be any doubts about what he said, he insisted, "Psychiatry is dying." He called it "a platypus," designated psychotherapy as "toothpaste," and thought education should help people develop "crap detectors." People who struggled with brain diseases, he claimed, differed from people struggling with problems of living. Did problems of living need doctors? No. Did they need hospitals? No. Did they warrant being called mentally ill? Definitely not.

Torrey denounced claims that hospitals helped "large numbers of 'dangerous mental patients.'" The numbers who have committed crimes were "infinitesimal," he said.[5] Actually, he said, hospitals were places where people get sicker. Judi Chamberlin or Leonard Frank or any reader of *Madness Network News* might have found these ideas more compatible with their views than did his colleagues.[6] Writing in the *American Journal of Psychiatry*, Dr. Jules Masserman considered *The Death of Psychiatry* misguided, with "bias, misrepresentation, illogic, and sophistry."[7]

NIMH director Bert Brown reserved remarks at the advisory panel's regular meeting, saying he would respond to *The Death of Psychiatry* at an upcoming APA convention. He also made it clear that Torrey would be departing, going to the Bering Sea's Pribilof Islands, between the United States and Russia, where he would provide medical, obstetrical, and dental care for the 450 native Aleut residents. Even those who thought him combative, however, considered him a skillful clinician, and after two years he returned to Washington to run two of the schizophrenia wards at St. Elizabeths Hospital.

From this platform, Torrey again predicted psychiatry's demise. He compared psychiatry to a gramophone. "Both were good ideas at the time they began," he said, "yet both have been superseded by technological developments and more advanced design."[8]

Then came thunder with the 1983 publication of *The Roots of Treason*, a biography of the poet Ezra Pound. Pound was a maniacally anti-Semitic fascist who moved to Italy during World War II, and on return he became St. Elizabeths' most famous patient between 1945 and 1958. Torrey blasted Superintendent Winfred Overholser, who'd overseen Pound's care and had overruled his staff's recommendations about a diagnosis. Weighing Pound's putative madness against his apparent treason, Overholser wanted to spare the profession the spectacle of an insanity trial. "Impracticalities of the situation" were at stake, he said. But Torrey believed Overholser deprived the public of a conversation about the differences between delusions and hate. For the dozen years before he was discharged, Pound lived in luxurious incarceration on the hospital's grounds.

Critics were again harsh. *Kirkus Reviews* said Torrey's single-minded focus on Overholser's flaws was a "skewed, one-note exposé." Writing for the liberal Jewish periodical *Commentary*, historian Kenneth Lynn called Torrey "an obscure psychiatrist," with "dim-to-invisible" scientific achievements. This book, he said, became "another stick with which to beat his profession."[9]

It was *Surviving Schizophrenia: A Family Manual*, Torrey's tenth book, that secured his place in the family movement. He hoped he would become the movement's Dr. Spock and believed that he presented "a scientific framework for understanding [schizophrenia's] symptoms and causes."[10] He credited help from Leslie Scallet, an attorney with the Bazelon Law Center, and Paolo del Vecchio, still in Philadelphia becoming a grassroots activist. This collaboration would be hard to imagine when, years later, they occupied opposing trenches.

Surviving Schizophrenia earned praise. In a review for a professional journal, Columbia's eminent biological psychiatrist Donald Klein said he appreciated Torrey's call for "a schizophrenia lobby." Klein agreed there was a "pitiful amount of research funding for schizophrenia despite its enormous public health importance."[11]

Surviving Schizophrenia, unlike Torrey's signature attacks, comforted hurting and confused families in ways nobody else had. He explained theoretical propositions and where evidence was scientifically based. Vitamin therapies lacked proof. Stay away. Medicine worked, he said, but all medications were not equally effective. One chapter addressed what a family needs, another the legal landscape. Surviving Schizophrenia was practical, comprehensive, compassionate, and hugely successful. Five years later, a second edition appeared.

Torrey's star was shining in NAMI's galaxy. Their story was his story. He became their professional envoy in a profession still clinging to shibboleths about family conflicts or parental ill will. In this way he became a cherished, if controversial, ally on behalf of families that other doctors had shamed and wounded.

When Torrey first joined NAMI, there were about a hundred local affiliates. By the second edition of Surviving Schizophrenia in 1988, it had grown eightfold. Part of Laurie Flynn's skill lay in enlisting him to speak for the membership. On behalf of NAMI families, he could charge NIMH with inertia, or say that schizophrenia hadn't received proper investigation, or that this cruel brain disease deserved more research. When NIMH's portfolio included pigeon studies, he erupted, pointing out that there were as many studies of bipolar disorders as pigeons. He led NAMI's campaign to grade the states about its services to answer, "If I or a family member had a serious mental illness, in what state would that person be most likely to receive good public services?" Thus began what would become a NAMI trademark publication, Grading the States.

Seeing former patients from St. Elizabeths Hospital barely subsist in shelters or on the streets saddened Torrey.[12] Many had stopped taking their medicine. They didn't attend clinics. Some had drifted back to drugs. Women suffered rapes. What had their freedom brought, he asked? Had they traded the brutality of the hospital for the brutality of the streets?[13] Turning his pen into a sword again, in 1988 he published *Nowhere to Go: The Tragic Odyssey of the Homeless Mentally Ill*. Now a best-selling author, Torrey sharpened his focus, arguing that the medical model had been abandoned where it wasn't broken.

Unlike the Fuller Torrey of 1974, who'd questioned the medical model's use of force, he now accepted force to get people into treatment. Having once discounted excessive hospitalization, a decade later he viewed this more favorably. Having once brushed aside myths about people with mental illness and danger, he now crafted arguments about dangerous patients: they were a threat to themselves and a threat to others, so forcing them to take medication could be justified.[14]

Torrey's evolution paralleled psychiatry's, from psychoanalysis to psychopharmacology, with drugs at its core. But as Susan Stefan, an attorney at the Bazelon Center, told him, "injections of Prolixin won't cure homelessness." They won't "create housing nor dissipate discrimination against the mentally ill in existing housing." She reproached him for making the wrong diagnosis, leading to "the wrong treatment."[15]

———————————

Curing homelessness was a passion Torrey shared with NAMI families. Problems of homelessness also backlit the Senate committee hearings about renewing SAMHSA in 1995. Added to routine considerations about renewals, the Senate Committee on Labor and Human Resources considered a $25 million amendment funding states to write laws forcing outpatient treatments. This would apply primarily to homeless people, and Kansas Republican senator Nancy Kassebaum chaired the meeting where Torrey urged the amendment's adoption.

Torrey positioned himself pretty much as a lone warrior. He had dropped out of the Washington Psychiatric Society and the American Psychiatric Association, but he kept his hand in treatment by volunteering twice a month at a clinic for local homeless women. He maintained guest status at St. Elizabeths Hospital's neuroscience center, and he chaired NAMI's Stanley Foundation Research Center. That day he spoke with NA-MI's backing.

He argued that people with brain diseases, notably those with schizophrenia or bipolar disorder, didn't believe they were sick. If they did, they would do what sick people do: they would take their medicine. By not taking medicine, given that the public mental health system was broken, involuntarily treatment was needed. Those with proper insight, meaning they accepted medicine's powers, wouldn't need force. But others could be court-ordered into treatment. He estimated this could benefit as many as two-thirds of those who were homeless.[16]

Howard Goldman, a psychiatrist at the University of Maryland, disagreed. Based on his research funded by the Robert Wood Johnson Foundation in nine different cities about delivering services to people with a persistent mental illness, he said the evidence was indisputable—forcing people into treatment didn't work.[17] Voluntary alternatives had been proven effective. He urged the committee to sidestep an "unproven approach." Consumer activist Joseph Rogers also spoke against this amendment's intention to fund involuntary force. Opponents carried the day, and Kassebaum eventually withdrew her amendment.

Six months later, NAMI's board of directors endorsed a policy similar to Torrey's recommendations for court-ordered treatments. Their recommendations changed criteria from the conventional "danger to self or others" to people they now called "gravely disabled," meaning they were "likely to substantially deteriorate." NAMI asked judges to fast-track an outline for treatment during commitment hearings and allow doctors and families to drive the treatment plan.

The levers of power—who controlled treatments—was the issue. Turning this over to families and using vague criteria infuriated former patients. NAMI opposed the choice and self-determination ex-patients cherished. NAMI's official statement, "Past history is often a reliable way to anticipate the future course of illness," subverted ideals of recovery and wellness. Since meeting in Madison, former patients and NAMI had bickered. Now discussions about involuntary outpatient commitment cemented their differences.[18]

Involuntary outpatient commitment seemed close enough to science fiction that activist and ex-patient leader David Oaks called it Orwellian. Oaks was based in Oregon, heading an organization of forty grassroots groups, Support Coalition, and publishing the nationally distributed journal *Dendron*. "The general public will not believe us about the threats," he wrote. Who could imagine such proposals for "deadly chemical crusades . . . needles on wheels . . . mind control"?

Ex-patient activists who'd cut their teeth protesting forced drugs had campaigned about disabling side effects for nearly two decades. The publication of Peter Breggin and Ginger Ross Breggin's book *Talking Back to Prozac* in 1994 seemed a welcome cautionary tome. The Breggins promised to reveal "what doctors aren't telling you about Prozac and the newer antidepressants." The first page contained a black-box warning: "When trying to withdraw from many psychiatric drugs, patients can develop serious and even life threatening emotional and physical reactions. In short, it is dangerous not only to start taking psychiatric drugs but also can be hazardous to *stop* taking them." This came from trusted friends who also opposed forced medication. That outpatient commitment depended on medication furthered activists' worries about NAMI's relationship with the drug industry.

In 1995, D. J. Jaffe, an emerging NAMI leader, angered former patients when he told *Psychiatric News* that "families and consumers agree that the status-quo is unworkable and the new policy marks the first time they have agreed to a better policy approach."[19] Who was NAMI to be speaking for ex-patients? When he said outpatient commitment and court-ordered treatment could apply to one million people, activists saw a "million needle march."[20]

Dendron reported about Prozac survivor groups organizing in the shadows of the blockbuster antidepressant. There were prisoners in California and New York forcibly getting drugs. Didn't that turn patients into prisoners? *Dendron* referenced a story from *Psychiatric Services* describing African Americans being treated with antipsychotic drugs at higher rates than whites.[21] Thirty years after racial stereotypes redefined the diagnosis of schizophrenia, people of color were still overrepresented in state hospitals. Disproportionately large numbers had been involuntarily committed.[22]

"Forced outpatient drugging kills," shouted the Support Coalition, suspicious of drug companies. In 1994, Public Citizen revealed that pharma had spent nearly $2 million underwriting APA activities, nearly a 40 percent increase over 1990 spending. In 1995, the industry spent more than $1.25 million for twenty-six symposia, exhibits, and parties at the San Francisco meeting.[23] It was said this money supported education, and activists thought the lesson plan was clear.

Of the medical specialties, none was more tarnished by its relationship to drug companies and the array of benefits that afforded than psychiatry: Junkets. Tickets and trinkets. Stock options. Speaking fees. Kickbacks. Ghostwritten books and articles. And this was separate from the way pharma seduced psychiatrists to perform at symposia, luncheons, industry dinners, and weekend meetings. In Stanford University's Department of Psychiatry, chairman Alan Shatzberg earned at least $6 million this way. Emory University's Charles Nemeroff was censured, then fired, before his professional violations came out. Shatzberg and Nemeroff were only two of the many who became textbook definitions of conflicts of interest.

Whistleblowing doctors and indefatigable journalists exposed them. One of Sen. Charles Grassley's staff, Paul Thacker, used their tips to launch investigations about astonishing tunnels of impropriety, deceit, and greed, calling out doctors who lent their names to articles or books they hadn't written, research they hadn't conducted, data they hadn't crunched, or speeches others had written for them.[24] This hit a high point with new drugs coming to market. Risperdal, Paxil, Zyprexa, and Seroquel filled the commercial void left when patents expired.

Beyond the conflicts of interest, beyond the misrepresentation of science, beyond the compromised ethics of joining pharma boards while conducting research into its product, what really mattered were lives. Patients were affected by fraudulent studies. Health, wellness, recovery, a future—all hung in the balance. Lawsuits would later identify manipulation of data to obscure life-threatening and dangerous consequences. Plain misery, shorter lives, compromised metabolic systems leading to diabetes and heart problems, plus medicine-related suicide would belie drug companies' claims and the health industry's mission to do no harm.

Former patients understood that, separate from pharma, psychiatrists and pharmacologists had been probing the long-term effects of psychoactive drugs. Their questions had been minimized in this environment where a drug could be advertised as a miracle worker. When NAMI started accepting pharma's gifts, the image of heartland moms and dads fighting with incorruptible independence suffered.

Ex-patient survivors sounded a five-alarm worry. Forced treatments that made medicine the core requirement for community living seemed more and more outrageous.

Pharmaceutical companies lavishly rewarded state and national politicians at the time second-generation drugs were coming to market. This included Texas governor George W. Bush, with long-standing connections to Eli Lilly and Company, where his father, former president George H. W. Bush, had once been on the board of directors. As governor, the younger Bush promoted an algorithm-based model for prescribing psychiatric medications the drug companies sought. In 1995, he enlisted psychiatry's leadership, pharma giants, and politicians for the Texas Medication Algorithmic Project (TMAP).[25] A whistleblower would later observe how this opened "the doors of the Texas prison system, juvenile justice system and Texas state mental health hospitals to the unlimited influence of major pharmaceutical companies in expanding the usage and marketing of their most expensive drugs."[26]

Former patients deplored drug companies' heavy hand. When reporters caught up to David Oaks on a protest line outside an APA convention, he confirmed, "Quite a number of members choose to take neuroleptic drugs." But that wasn't force, and the Support Coalition condemned NAMI's push for national expansion of commitment criteria.[27]

Oaks blamed NAMI leaders, whom he called "crusaders in this traveling medicine show," and accused them of unleashing a "chemical crusade." He pointed to Laurie Flynn, executive director; E. Fuller Torrey, "widely considered one of the most extreme proponents of forcing psychiatric drugs, and excluding other alternatives"; and NAMI board member D. J. Jaffe.

What Torrey and Jaffe had in common was a disappointment that their own relatives—Torrey's sister, Jaffe's sister-in-law—hadn't benefited from billions of research dollars and a belief that current laws were a barrier to treatments. With Torrey's credentials as a psychiatrist and Jaffe's know-how as a marketing executive, they redesigned the public image of mental illness. Their work moved beyond the theater of professional events or psychological theories. The public was their sandbox, and they used fears about violence to achieve goals by unorthodox means.

In the 1990s, when patients were also eloping from New York's psychiatric hospitals, crime and random violence seemed endemic. Talk of violence was multifaceted, Black and white, male and female, in big cities and small towns, in families, on the streets, and in the schools. And it was being packaged, almost prefabricated to mingle with negative cultural stereotypes that maligned people with serious mental illness.

Jaffe absorbed Torrey's ideas characterizing untreated people as violent and came up with a strategy. "From a marketing perspective," he said, "it may be necessary to capitalize on the fear of violence." He explained this to NAMI's families in Staten Island, spinning that it would reduce stigma and reframe services because the public would find it comforting to read messages about "Making Mentally Ill Take Medicines" instead of "Psychotic Killers on Rampage." He argued this would deflate NIMBY—not in my backyard—energies. Forcing people to take medication would be the key, he said, "if they want to live in the community."[28]

Jaffe and Torrey had been promoting involuntary outpatient commitment when Jaffe suggested swapping *involuntary* for *assisted* outpatient commitment. Patting himself on the back, he said it was "a brilliant phrase." Whatever it was called, it needed backing with a change in the law.

Jaffe recommended naming opportunities for the laws he expected to pass. Like the people whose images were indelibly stamped onto buildings or auditoriums at universities or hospitals, he imagined the names of people associated with violence would become part of the public's consciousness. His first choice was Larry Hogue, a homeless man in New York City who'd left Manhattan's Upper West Side terrorized in the early 1990s.[29] But invoking the image of a disturbed man never caught on. The names of victims seemed better, and he let the idea germinate until, a few years later in 1999, a mentally ill man named Andrew Goldstein pushed thirty-two-year-old Kendra Webdale off a New York City subway platform. Her death became the centerpiece of campaigns for involuntary commitment called Kendra's Law.

Torrey, by his own admission, was single-minded and tenacious. A colleague once called him combative. All this was on display when he attacked consumers for describing themselves as "survivors."

Torrey didn't remember how, but he got a recording of a meeting of the California Network of Mental Health Consumers. And it angered him to hear Jay Mahler, who was by now advising the Village and other integrated programs AB3777 had funded. He was a soft-spoken, first-generation activist calling himself a psychiatric survivor who couldn't support involuntary treatment. Torrey thought this was outrageous. He believed survivors were people who beat cancer. They were victims of the Holocaust. They were the ones who had been "unjustly imprisoned and even tortured." Survivors weren't the people who had what he called "neurobiological brain diseases," more commonly called mental illnesses.

His furious back-of-the-envelope calculation projected that half a million people with serious psychiatric disorders "are now prematurely deceased."[30] He slammed "survivors like Mr. Mahler," saying they, and their lawyers, were to blame. "Civil liberties lawyers have made it virtually impossible to treat such patients when they have no insight into their illness or their need for treatment," he said. Psychiatric survivors, and their allies such as Dr. Peter Breggin, were culpable.

He argued this in "Taking Issue," an op-ed column in the February 1997 issue of *Psychiatric Services*, to which seventy people responded—a record number for a single article in that publication. Editor John Talbott excerpted twenty of the letters for a column he playfully titled "taking issue with taking issue."[31] Among them was NIMH's acting director, Rex Cowdry, who distanced himself from Torrey, who had identified himself at the NIMH Neuroscience Center. Cowdry said he was "a part-time guest researcher . . . [whose] opinions do not represent the views of the National Institute of Mental Health."

But it was Torrey's claims that psychiatric survivors had caused half a million deaths that provoked a clash. "A big lie," thundered Judi Chamberlin. Sociologist Robert Emerick said he was "closed minded to true scientific debate and available evidence." Anthropologist Sue Estroff asked him to learn from those who "speak eloquently of surviving both their symptoms *and* their treatment." Consumer leader Paolo del Vecchio challenged him to move beyond a semantic debate to "focus on a shared mission of improving quality of life." Professor Steven Segal explained how a dearth of acceptable services meant that "people are often forced to trade their liberty for care." Joseph Rogers said bluntly, "It's the system of care, not force, that will fix the problem."[32]

Torrey construed their responses as evidence that his "message had been heard, that consumers were ignoring the needs of their sickest colleagues."[33] He failed to acknowledge that, for years, consumers had been developing programs using Community Support Program grants in Maine, Indiana, and Colorado.[34] A study had recently affirmed how Michigan, recipient of three demonstration projects with drop-in centers serving fourteen-hundred people with serious mental illness, had created "an environment promoting social support and shared problem solving."[35] The California Network of Mental Health Clients was then lobbying state authorities for an additional $20 million for addressing problems of homelessness, and David Oaks had spearheaded a forty-member organization helping Oregon's homeless people. Torrey dismissed the existing programs run by his critics, people he dismissed as a "small but noisy subset, misplaced liberals" who postured as "psychiatric radical chic."

Jaffe relished Torrey's attacks on former patients, whom he disdained "a new ruling class: professional survivors" or a "consumertocracy." He was regularly accusing the Center for Mental Health Services of ignoring people with what he termed neurobiological disorders, firmly believing that nobody cared for "those with the most serious brain disorders" more than he and Torrey. They would guide NAMI's leadership.

———

Under Flynn, NAMI had become the families' flagship mental health advocacy organization. She made sure politicians knew about insurance reimbursement plans that discriminated, and throughout the 1990s she vigorously campaigned for insurance parity. She also made sure constituents had talking points to use when Congress considered rolling back services or protections of supplemental security insurance, or amendments to weaken housing, as was the case in 1998. When the Schizophrenia Patient Outcomes Research Team (PORT) published its long-awaited study with specific recommendations, NAMI distilled the drug-related component for each of the 1,140 affiliates into "an easy-to-understand guide." NAMI was one of ten nonprofits the American Institute of Philanthropy celebrated in 1997 for its fundraising practices and cost-effective strategies.[36] That NAMI claimed to be the "voice of mental illness" infuriated former patients.

Keeping the operation afloat, providing member services with timely bulletins, organizing conferences, and preparing testimony were costly. For all of this, drug companies were happy to provide support. With fine-tuned marketing plans, just as they had ensnared psychiatry, drug companies courted NARSAD, the Mental Health Association, the Depression and Bipolar Support Association, and NAMI.[37] A whistleblower named Allen Jones would later describe how pharmaceutical houses became the engine corrupting "the soul of the American university, the ethics of medicine, the integrity of the scientific record, and the safety of patients who serve as human subjects in pre- and post-marketing clinical trials."[38] But for now, it was just business as usual.

At the same time patents were expiring on an older generation of drugs, pharma needed a strategy to influence doctors. Influencing families through the organization to which 145,000 belonged was among the strategies. Of the eighteen companies vying for the attention of NAMI's growing membership, four got there early: Janssen, maker of Risperdal; Eli Lilly, maker of Prozac; Pfizer, marketing Geodon; and Novartis, with Seroquel. They cloaked their marketing efforts as campaigns for educational or anti-stigma benefits. Pfizer's was the NAMI Anti-Stigma Foundation. Janssen's program, Person to Person, was billed as information for people seeking guidance.[39] Lilly's funding was multipronged. It included the Campaign to End Discrimination, and for state affiliates, In Our Own Voice: Living with Mental Illness. Meanwhile, Eli Lilly loaned Gerry Radke, its marketing director, to the national NAMI office.[40]

Through these campaigns, drug companies scripted NAMI's support. When costs or side effects of the new drugs became public, NAMI issued a press release about the "right of individuals with brain disorders to receive treatment with 'new generation' medications." This included "atypical antipsychotics and selective serotonin reuptake inhibitors."[41] Another press release, with the same message, boasted, "A new generation of breakthrough medications—such as atypical antipsychotics and advanced antidepressants—are [sic] allowing people with severe mental illness to reclaim full lives without the devastating side effects produced by the older drugs."[42] This was the pattern, time and again.

NAMI launched Janssen's curated campaign for Risperdal users, Person to Person, in 1997. Among the features touted was a phone service Janssen provided answering questions from families or patients about the drug. Another service was follow-up calls reminding patients specifically about appointments, or when to pick up their prescriptions, or even offering coupons for discounts. Janssen, meanwhile, collected information the industry could later use to enlist citizens to lobby for a specific piece of legislation. The expansion of direct advertising models warranted a front-page story in the *New York Times* by 1998.[43]

D. J. Jaffe, now a member of NAMI's board of directors, suspected Janssen's motives for the free services.[44] "Let's face it," he said, "the reason Janssen is starting this program is to keep more folks on their medicine. . . . The 'person to person counselors' will abandon you if respiridol [sic] does not work for you and you switch." Displeased that NAMI's name was associated with the ploy, he urged his following not to be fooled.[45]

But NAMI had already been bagged. "We applaud Janssen for providing another important key that will help pave the road to recovery," beamed Flynn's April 1977 press release.[46] The next month, she rebuked a California health maintenance organization, citing costs, for cutting Risperdal and Zoloft from its formulary. These drugs should be "reinstated immediately. . . . Lives are at stake."[47] When Governor Bush adopted TMAP's stage-managed recommendations for medication, NAMI applauded the Texas legislature for "Ending Insurance Discrimination in Coverage for Severe Mental Illness."[48]

Whether Risperdal, or any of the other drugs, warranted TMAP's ratings as superior would be addressed later. Only PORT said that, except for clozapine, these drugs didn't merit the rating of "superior efficacy."[49] In the meantime, Texans paid the price when Risperdal went from $250 a year to $3,000 a year.[50] Eventually, everybody would pay the price as the effects of such increases spread throughout the healthcare system.

Torrey wanted NAMI to distance themselves from drug companies. While he remained confident in the therapeutic effects of drugs, he was outspoken about not wanting pharma's incursions threatening his independence, and he was dubious about the whole picture. Could researchers, he asked, "who are paid by drug companies," find themselves "influenced by the source of payment?"[51]

Mother Jones would expose, and lawsuits would eventually reveal, that between 1996 and 1999, NAMI accepted more than $11 million from pharmaceuticals.[52] Some years, these monies amounted to more than half of its operating budget.

Critics considered NAMI a Trojan horse, and looking at Janssen's marketing strategy, it seemed well founded. The company urged using advocates such as NAMI's to deliver a "constant flow of information on Risperdal benefits." This would "minimize exposure" of Janssen because advocates could "educate payers."[53] Using NAMI this way showed benefits. Risperdal sales reached $589 million in 1997, up from $172 million three years earlier. To meet Janssen's target of $1.059 billion for the United States, the strategy included off-label prescribing to children and nursing homes, a deliberate violation of FDA rules.

Other drug companies asked NAMI for testimonials with the FDA. When Pfizer's new antipsychotic drug Geodon came up for review, NAMI's board chair and medical director both testified for Pfizer. By then Torrey had departed NAMI, Flynn was preparing to do so, and Jim McNulty of Rhode Island, who had joined NAMI's board in 1997, was on Pfizer's payroll. The 2001 announcement that he would chair the board noted he was a leader in Rhode Island, a consumer with bipolar disorder, and NAMI's representative to the NIMH Advisory Committee. It omitted his relationship to Pfizer. Laundering Pfizer's payments through affiliates brought his downfall. In the interim, Lilly's Radke became interim director after Flynn's departure.

Pharma's influence spread like an oil slick. The American Association of the Advancement of Science sponsored a discussion about the influence of drugs in January 1999, leading the *Wall Street Journal* to lament the "creeping commercialization of science" the next month. The *New Eng-*

land Journal of Medicine took aim when its editor, Marcia Angell, wrote an outraged editorial.

None of this surprised ex-patient activists. If anything, it seemed old news. But it confirmed their resolve to fight back.

———————

Torrey's easy relationship with NAMI was fraying by the time the third edition of his brainchild, *Grading the States*, was underway. NAMI's demand for transparency and accountability had become a signature, and local affiliates forwarded information for evaluations about services, funding streams, and oversight. Learning that three of their affiliates had received office space or stipends from their state mental health departments disturbed Torrey. Had this already compromised their independence? Asking states for help answering the survey was unforgivable, and he withdrew support from the project Flynn had once called "Torrey's Report on the States."

Other irritants chafed. Consumers on NAMI's client council, which was formed in 1985, wanted more influence in the organization. Torrey thought this too confining. "It was becoming politically correct not to argue with consumers," he said, reflecting on his discomfort. It seemed to him that NAMI was pandering. He worried that NAMI was veering from its founding mission to cure mental illness, lobby for research, and identify service shortages.

In 1996, Torrey issued a tripartite plan for NAMI's future, with ideological, economic, and legal components, to clean up the "current mental illness mess." Mental health, he believed, was now closely associated with social reform, "strongly associated with liberal political causes," and laden with "heavy political baggage."[54]

A case in point was "Woody Allen Syndrome," the comedian's punch line about his psychotherapy lasting thirty-three years. NAMI didn't want to lump together the so-called problems of living with people who suffered from serious brain diseases. Torrey renewed attacks on doctors caring for the so-called worried well of the middle class. He also fed the dubious narrative that reform was mostly driven by an anti-psychiatry vanguard. He excoriated LPS and Art Bolton, erroneously linking Bolton to the anti-psychiatry icon Thomas Szasz. Three decades after evidence accumulated about desirability of community treatments, Torrey still grieved the disappointed ambitions of the 1960s and heaped scorn on Kennedy-era community mental health centers. More than useless, he said, they had "usurped" funds and resources.[55]

Torrey was a hero to some, a villain to others, and he wanted NAMI families to join his campaign for forcing people into treatment, involuntarily if necessary. The governing board had announced support for involuntary commitment as a last resort. This came on the heels of Senator Kassebaum's withdrawal of her proposal for federal funding of laws. Torrey urged his flock to continue to "challenge outmoded laws in the courts. . . . Use the media to publicly confront mental health lawyers with the frequently tragic consequences of their legal action." Don't be naive, he said. "Hope and patience alone are not going to change the system."

———————

Shortly after the publication of *Surviving Schizophrenia*, a wealthy couple from Connecticut, Ted and Vada Stanley, approached Torrey with a million-dollar offer to fund NAMI's research agenda. They had a son with bipolar disorder. This began the Stanley Medical Research Institute (SMRI) and a thirty-year commitment. With Torrey's guidance, SMRI financed a brain bank the next year, a research director working out of NAMI headquarters, and a competitive program awarding stipends to research scientists worldwide. Eventually the Stanleys would underwrite research with more than $600 million.

A decade later, the Stanley family funded a second platform for Torrey, the Treatment Advocacy Center (TAC), devoted to changing laws to make treatments mandatory for people presumed to have untreated mental illness. NAMI considered itself a "supporting organization" to TAC. An advisory board included Flynn, Jaffe, NAMI counsel Ron Honberg, and board members Carla Jacobs and Annie Saylor. "If NAMI doesn't stand up for those who are the most ill and most vulnerable, who will?" asked Flynn when announcing its launch.[56] Both projects left NAMI headquarters in 1998.

TAC would not duck controversy or tolerate political correctness, and it absolutely wouldn't take money from drug companies. What TAC did was announce stories about so-called preventable tragedies. All-cap headlines were typical, such as this in 2000: "VIOLENCE: UNFORTUNATE AND ALL TOO OFTEN TRAGIC SIDE-EFFECT OF UNTREATED SEVERE MENTAL ILLNESS."[57] There were grisly tales of children who killed parents, husbands who killed wives, men and women who took their own lives. The backstory always alleged it was someone with an "untreated neurobiological brain disorder." TAC's database built a searchable library of "preventable tragedies."

As TAC gathered articles to build an online archive of preventable tragedies, it also filled newspapers with editorials about people with mental illness. It drafted "A Model Law for Assisted Treatment," which Torrey unveiled at NAMI's 2000 annual convention. Jonathan Stanley, his benefactor's son, was a lawyer. He explained some of the unconventional recommendations. To end the "inherently cruel delays" between a commitment hearing and the start of treatment, TAC's model law recommended that treatment decisions come during the initial hearing. Their model would replace judicial approval, used infrequently, with a panel that included a close relative of the person in question.

TAC called its critics a small group "who believe that nobody, no matter how psychotic, should be involuntarily treated." Torrey said they came from "anti-medication professionals." These were TAC's enemies, people whom Torrey and Jaffe considered "largely responsible for the anti-treatment bias in state treatment laws." To the standard enemies' list of lawyers at the Bazelon Center, and the federally funded Protection and Advocacy staff, he accused the federal Center for Mental Health Services of funding transportation to "the 'consumer-survivor' conferences," scheming to instruct them how to stop taking medication.[58]

Torrey said he wanted to pull the pendulum back "toward a more reasonable center" using examples of people who were untreated.[59] The problem with his approach was that it fed fear, promoted stigma, and didn't resolve the service shortage. There was no evidence that the people Torrey identified were in fact untreated. It might have been a convenient assumption, but it remained unverified, definitely a supposition, and in part a fiction. Still, the idea that untreated people were dangerous propelled his work, including the headline that they were responsible for "1,000 homicides a year."

Twenty years earlier, Torrey's passion had predicted psychiatry's death. Now he was focused on using a dangerously false narrative about violence. Torrey explained that he estimated a thousand homicides per year based on a Department of Justice study of family violence. Data from 1988 showed that people with a mental illness displayed aggression toward family members seven times more often than against strangers.[60] Family aggression, and that toward strangers, accounted for 4.2 percent of the murders. He labeled people in that category "untreated."

Torrey had calculated this number from the thirteen homicides attributed to people with mental illness reported by the *Washington Post* in 1992, which he multiplied by eighty-five, the number of metropolitan areas of similar size: "My estimate was based on all cases in a metropolitan area of 3 million people for 1 year, then [I] extrapolated to the whole country."[61] He assumed the metropolitan Washington was representative of the entire United States, and relied on anecdotal evidence to further extrapolate beyond urban areas. "I think such extrapolation is reasonable," he said, pointing to that population growth, poor services, and seriously mentally ill people wandering the streets. Hence, he concluded "there are now approximately 1000 homicides a year committed by individuals with schizophrenia and bipolar disorder, almost all of whom were not taking medication at the time of the homicide."[62] Torrey's kitchen-table methodology—estimating, extrapolating, approximating, and anecdotal padding—departed from social science methodology. Yet he would assert that "to date, nobody has challenged this 1000/year estimate."

Actually quite a few people had challenged his work. Dr. Wilson M. Compton, president of the Eastern Missouri Psychiatric Association, was among them. Compton complained immediately after his local television station KSDK broadcast that misinformation: "The promotion I saw this morning spoke about the '1,000 murders committed each year by persons with mental illness.' No reputable scientific data supports the assertion about 1,000 murders, and this inflammatory language does a disservice to a vulnerable population who are much more likely to be the victims than the perpetrators of crime and violence."[63]

NAMI affiliate members in New York, Jean Arnold and Nora Weinreth, founders of the National Stigma Clearinghouse, also challenged Torrey's numbers and methodology. The baseline numbers from 1988 came during a peak in violence, and the numbers had fallen consistently since

1990. He had also exaggerated DOJ's findings by rounding upward. They alleged TAC had employed an "inventive manipulation of research data." Using a different hypothesis, they said they could prove the opposite.[64]

Torrey's misattribution of data trailed him and TAC. When asked to confirm Torrey's exaggerated claims, the public affairs officer of NIMH said, "NIMH did not make the statement that the absence of treatment leads to homelessness, incarceration, or violence."[65] D. J. Jaffe and Sally Satel, a psychiatrist in Washington, misrepresented findings of a large study assessing violence (MacArthur Violence Risk Assessment Study), leading the study's seven authors to presume their words were politically motivated. "Anything that suggests that some segment of the mentally disordered population is unlikely to be violent is seen as taking the pressure off politicians to maintain or expand mental health services, particularly involuntary ones," they wrote. It was "the desperate hope that the public will fund what it fears."[66]

With its campaign for "1,000 homicides a year" shelf-ready, after the death of Kendra Webdale in 1999, TAC used it to crusade for involuntary commitment in New York, which they called Kendra's Law. That Goldstein, her attacker, had sought and been denied help eleven times didn't figure in the campaign.

"People care about public safety," Jaffe told a workshop at the 1999 NAMI meetings. "Once you understand that, it means that you have to take the debate out of the mental health arena and put it in the criminal/public safety arena." He repeated this in a mailing to NAMI affiliates in New York: "From a marketing perspective, it may be necessary to capitalize on the fear of violence to get the law passed," he wrote. "Some have suggested calling the enabling legislation, 'The Hoag Law.' It may be a bitter pill to swallow, but if it benefitted people . . . we should be for it."[67] These were war words, and Jaffe was getting ready for a skirmish.

TAC used Webdale's death to drive fear. Torrey, Jaffe, and TAC's executive director, Mary T. Zdanowicz, placed editorials in the nation's newspapers demanding that state legislatures pass outpatient treatment laws. They added the phrase "mindless and deadly" to their template. In Florida, the *Orlando Sentinel* asked legislators when they will realize that "being psychotic is mindless and deadly." In Utah, the *Salt Lake City Tribune*'s op-ed asked "how many more preventable tragedies" before lawmakers realize that "being psychotic is mindless and deadly." And in California, involuntary treatment roiled debate until a delusional woman killed a passerby, Laura Wilcox, bringing about Laura's Law. Twin slogans, "Mindless and deadly" and "1,000 homicides a year," fueled TAC's campaign.[68]

Despite evidence challenging these claims and studies questioning whether involuntary commitment was beneficial, Torrey and TAC were on a roll.

———————

In California, Dan Weisburd also questioned Torrey's numbers: "It's just not true. It doesn't happen!"[69]

Weisburd had founded *The Journal* in 1989 and relied on guest editors to put the quarterly together. *The Journal* had the air of a high-brow coffee-table literary magazine juxtaposing classical images with stunning photography. With short essays, poetry, autobiographical riffs from parents, patients, and people with a unique perspective, it was unique. Each issue opened with an editor's introduction.

Weisburd liked to provoke conversation and warned his readers that not all "will sympathize with all the sentiments and ideas that they find here, for some writers will flatly disagree with others." For the issue about mental health and the law, a photo inset of the Constitution and Bill of Rights gilded his two-page introduction. Topics for that theme included mental health courts, incarceration, and the perspectives of families and those who'd survived jails. Three articles pertained to involuntary outpatient commitment.

Weisburd, like Torrey, worried about the "uncared for" people on the streets. But he reasoned a thousand murders a year, roughly twenty murders a week for the nation, would produce three a week just in California. It was false, Weisburd said, false on its face, and he came down hard on national news outlets—*60 Minutes, Washington Post, New York Times*—for failing to fact-check the claim. Meanwhile, Torrey "expertly drums home a single point that he presents as fact."

Involuntary commitment, Weisburd said, would brand "unmedicated people with mental illness [as] violent." It couldn't be, and Torrey was peddling "fallacious and unsubstantiated statistics." How would laws allowing for involuntary outpatient treatment serve patients? Would "coercive treatment laws stand the constitutional test?" he asked.

The California Alliance on Mental Illness (CAMI) technically owned *The Journal*, and in a poorly thought-out move, leadership ordered the pages of Weisburd's introduction to be glued closed before its distribution. Brian Jacobs, board president, was married to Carla Jacobs, who'd led the crusade for the involuntary treatment law that California just vetoed. She also served on NAMI's board as well as TAC's.

If Weisburd was rattled by CAMI's glue fiasco the first time it happened, he was unspeakably mad that it occurred a second time. The journal's topic was wellness, and Weisburd had written about his son, David, who had dangerously high cholesterol levels. With a family history of heart attacks and surgery, including his own, Dan was disappointed that David's medical team hadn't seen this threatening side effect of his drugs. But why was CAMI attempting to silence him? He wasn't attacking anybody, yet he wondered if it had something to do with CAMI not wanting to offend pharmaceutical companies that helped underwrite the expenses, all of which were disclosed at the back of the book. Was this self-censorship to keep the dollars flowing?

David Oaks had fun saying NAMI was "unglued" and "is this what 'normal' looks like?" More seriously, he asked, "What does the National Alliance for the Mentally Ill (NAMI) have to hide?" Oaks posted links to the original articles, plus Weisburd's complaints that the leadership went from "mediocre to being a malicious absurdity."[70]

Weisburd felt betrayed by CAMI. He saw himself as godfather to the Village. He had once been a lifeline for CAMI's struggling leadership. And now he had become a target for people who would rather silence differences than discuss them. He could only assume it was because, as he said, "I am pro-consumer and pro-patient's rights."

Weisburd knew that labeling people "violent" perpetuated stigma. He told Oaks that Torrey "has found that dangerousness sells." CAMI responded by halting *The Journal*. A financial drain, they said. Nobody believed it, least of all Weisburd, who sued to publicly air the differences. *Mental Health Weekly* did a story on the controversy. Stigma Clearinghouse lamented the loss. Testimonials to Weisburd's integrity and work came in.

Weisburd thought his introduction showed respect for Torrey whom he regarded as "a good person." But Torrey accused him of deliberately misrepresenting his statistics. Looking back at it, Torrey believed Weisburd simply disliked him.[71]

The prevailing sadness at the dissolution of *The Journal* had as much to do with the frayed family movement as it did with involuntary commitment. It was more than messaging—it was fallen leaders, a painful realization for Weisburd. "What sorry times our family movement has fallen upon," he mused to Oaks, no friend of the family movement. "And what a sad excuse for leadership we have now holding power."[72]

During the heated debate about involuntary treatment roiling California over Laura's Law, the state's premier oversight commission, the Little Hoover Commission, heard from Sally Zinman. She reminded them that tightened restrictions around commitment had influenced the founding of the California Network of Mental Health Clients fifteen years prior. Now, in 1999, it was being revisited. This time, she said, two contradictory trends were at odds: "On the one hand, the California mental health system has grown immensely in supporting client empowerment, [and] more recently, endorsing the concept of recovery as a goal of the system." But recent events were making that insecure because choice, the backbone of their movement, was under attack. Threats came packaged "in the guise of LPS reform" and included "expanding forced treatment, including involuntary outpatient commitment." If California accepted this charade, despite all that had been accomplished, Zinman feared it "would set back the client movement, and by extension, the emerging client friendly mental health system, thirty (30) years."

CHAPTER 17

A VINTAGE YEAR

THE YEAR 1999 MIGHT HAVE BEEN THE CENTURY'S LAST, BUT IT WAS ALSO A YEAR OF MANY FIRSTS. In June, there was a White House Conference on Mental Health. It was designed and promoted by Tipper Gore, with help from Bernie Arons, and hosted by Washington's historic Black college, Howard University. Real-time video streaming linked six thousand sites filled by consumers, service providers, and government offices from Portland, Oregon, to Portland, Maine.

Weeks later, the Supreme Court affirmed the Americans for Disability Act in *Olmstead v. LC*. The ACLU had charged Georgia's mental health commissioner with pointlessly confining two women with disabilities, restricting them against the recommendations of their doctors, lawyers, families, and the wishes of the women themselves. Justice Ruth Bader Ginsberg delivered the Supreme Court's 6–3 majority opinion, writing that the state had consistently underestimated the women's abilities to live in the community with supports. She decried their "unjustified isolation" and opened the legal doors to the aspiration of "community integration for everyone."

Again in Georgia, the next month, peer services received Medicaid funding approval. It was twenty years since Howie the Harp had introduced the idea of a workforce composed of former patients. Now, with Larry Fricks's leadership in Georgia, consumers would be paid for the services they, as peers, provided. This funding mechanism required rethinking providing services to incorporate people whose personal journey could be instrumental to another person's recovery.

To cap the year, and the century, on December 13, 1999, Surgeon General David Satcher released *Mental Health: A Report of the Surgeon General*. Of the fifty-one previous reports surgeons general had released since 1964, twenty-seven addressed smoking hazards. Others focused on cancer, suicide, or HIV/AIDs. These reports had drawn attention to matters warranting a public health priority, and this was the first to address mental health. That alone was a milestone, but so was its message: Mental illnesses are treatable. Recovery is possible. Services mattered.

To prepare a campaign for this declaration, and to challenge myths handed down from generation to generation, the Department of Health and Human Services enlisted the Ad Council, MTV, and the American Psychological Association. Secretary of Health and Human Services Donna Shalala would proclaim, "This report is as important as it is timely."[1]

————————

When Satcher strolled to the podium, the audience filling room 450 of the Eisenhower Executive Office Building stood to applaud. With homespun humor for this friendly crowd, Satcher quipped that standing up probably amounted to that day's exercise. These colleagues were familiar with his soft-spoken clarity and his moral authority. Satcher believed that neither politics, nor religion, nor personal preferences belonged in science. He often mentioned an earlier surgeon general, Dr. Luther Terry, who, along with eight members of his task force studying smoking, was a smoker. Yet they all subordinated their personal behavior to professional duties in 1964 when they warned Americans that smoking was a scientifically confirmed health hazard.

For this public event, Satcher wore his black-and-gold Public Health Service uniform with four stars on the cuffs. A white beard wrapped his boyish face, and he spoke about the "hope and restoration of a meaningful life [that is] possible, despite serious mental illness." Unlike typical medical outcomes, there is no "single agreed-upon definition of recovery nor a single way to measure it." In the field of mental health, recovery "is variously called a process, an outlook, a vision, a guiding principle." His gravitas came from having been faculty at three medical schools, past president of Meharry Medical College, head of the Centers for Disease Control, assistant secretary for health and simultaneously surgeon general—only the second person to do both at the same time, and the first African American to ever do so.

As a specialist in family medicine, not as a psychiatrist, he asked the public to reimagine assumptions, rethink dogma, replace myth, and honor the evidence saying mental illnesses are treatable.[2] Activists had fueled a national debate, he said. Now it was time to acknowledge recovery.

A dress rehearsal for this day had taken place in November at the Fifteenth Annual Rosalynn Carter Symposium on Mental Health Policy in Atlanta. Leaving the White House hadn't dimmed Rosalynn Carter's interest or her leadership. People in recovery, leaders like Larry Fricks and Joel Slack, had influenced her greatly.[3] Since 1985, the annual Carter Center symposium was among the field's most coveted events. Now she applauded the surgeon general's message, saying she hoped it would "close a huge gap between what the experts know and what the general public understands."[4]

Many flying into Atlanta that November had participated in one or more of the research panels contributing to this opus. There were psychiatrists, such as Howard Goldman, who provided editorial leadership while conducting research and editing the journal *Psychiatric Services*. Lisa Dixon, also from Maryland, spoke candidly about her experiences as the sister of someone with a mental illness. She was one of the co-investigators of an important study about patient outcomes with the acronym PORT. Activist Bill Emmet, who had worked at NAMI and NASMHPD, hoped to break the "blame and shame" pattern still afflicting families. Among the consumer leaders, Laura Van Tosh had consulted with several states about peer leadership and collaborated with Paolo del Vecchio about consumer-run self-help programs. Another consumer, Susan Rogers, came on behalf of Philadelphia's National Mental Health Self-Help Clearing House, intending to protest the section allowing continued use of ECT. Of course, there was Georgia's own Larry Fricks, in the throes of building a model for expanding peer services.

To prepare for the public reception of the surgeon general's report, the Carter Center partnered with the MacArthur Foundation for a study. Consultant Celinda Lake foretold their challenge when she reported that two-thirds of the respondents had voiced skepticism, uncertain that mental health treatments were effective.[5] Lake cautioned they shouldn't overestimate public enthusiasm for *Mental Health: A Report of the Surgeon General.*

———————

A month later, standing at the podium, Satcher seemed upbeat and confident when he declared that "a scientific revolution has taken place over the last 25 years in our understanding of mental health and mental illness." Now "people [could] return to productive lives and positive relationships." He reminded listeners that a "pervasive silence" once quashed discussing mental illnesses. None could have said a half century earlier, when Congress established the National Institute of Mental Health, "The brain is the integrator of thought, emotion, behavior, and health." Now they could, he said, because a "revolution has resulted in a vast array of safe and effective options to treat mental disorders." On the eve of a new century, science had proven that "brain chemistry affects behavior and behavior affects brain chemistry." All of this meant that it made no sense to separate the head from the body. "Mental illnesses are physical illnesses," he said.[6]

Treatments for mental illness, Satcher boasted, were "the great news of this report." The challenge would be access to services. Roughly two-thirds of the people needing them neither sought nor had access. Mental illnesses were the second leading cause of disability and the second leading cause of premature death. In 1997, the nation spent $71 billion treating mental disorders. It was nothing less than a public health crisis.

———————

That day, Tipper Gore was one of four people on the stage. A standing ovation revealed that nobody needed to be reminded why she was there. With an avuncular glow, Satcher called her "a bold change agent" and placed a shiny copy of the five-hundred-page report in her hands. She had set the process in motion four years earlier with a question for Secretary Shalala. To organize a working staff, Shalala turned to Arons, and to engage consumers, he turned to Paolo del Vecchio.

Gore was a well-known advocate before her husband, Al Gore, became vice president in the Clinton administration. The public and the press had underrated her then, turned her into a caricature for slamming musical lyrics about drugs, sex, or violence. But she'd lectured at colleges, medical schools, and professional meetings, not only as a figurehead—although she had cut her share of ribbons and delivered luncheon speeches—but with respect for her work on behalf of children needing services. Washington knew her, and activists did as well through her work with Unity Health, dressing incognito and covering her shoulder-length hair with a baseball cap while helping homeless people move from wooded parks into housing. She'd curated dinner parties where politicians could meet Nobel laureates and cutting-edge NIMH research psychiatrists. She was the energy driving the White House Conference on Mental Health that June, which became the backdrop for President Clinton's challenge to Congress to enact insurance parity.

Among Gore's most important accomplishments as second lady, revising a State Department policy stands out. On the books was an automatic rejection of a security clearance for anybody who'd ever received mental health services. She knew her friend and White House advisor Vince Foster hadn't sought help for depression because his would be retracted. On the one-year anniversary of his suicide, in July 1994, at the National Press Club, she announced President Clinton would issue an executive order (no. 12968) overturning this policy. Counseling for nondelusional issues such as children's problems, eating disorders, or grief counseling would no longer automatically trigger an FBI investigation. "What is being corrected," she said, "is this blanket assumption that if you have had a bout of depression, you're a security risk."[7]

Nobody in that room needed an explanation about why Tipper Gore was on that stage, or why she received the first copy of *Mental Health: A Report of the Surgeon General.*

———————

Larry Fricks, the fourth person on that day's stage, personified recovery.[8] His day had started inauspiciously when White House guards stopped him. Dressed in a blue shirt, brown suit, and tie, he identified himself as the person who was going to introduce Tipper Gore at a breakfast meeting at the White House. He was told, Sorry, Mrs. Gore wasn't hosting a breakfast event at the White House, and his name wasn't on the preapproved clearance list. Could he have gotten the date wrong? No, he replied, it was correct. But he started to sweat, worried about whether he had heard the instructions incorrectly.

Was he a psychiatrist? they asked.

No! Not a psychiatrist, he said.

He was beginning "to feel like a hick from Georgia" and didn't want to identify himself as a mental health patient. He remembered feeling foolish: "If you say you're supposed to introduce Tipper Gore at a breakfast and if there's no breakfast here, it sounds a little bit delusional."

A phone call sorted it out, and a taxi rushed him to the National Press Club, where Gore, Shalala, and Satcher were waiting for him. Later they continued together to the White House. Television crews—CNN, NBC, ABC, and a platoon of reporters—startled him. They had come to cover a presidential press conference, but that had been canceled. So the press moved on to the surgeon general's announcement. Sensing his nervousness, Tipper Gore got him a drink of water. Unaware that he had worked as a journalist, as had she as a photojournalist, she whispered, "They are all friends."

When it was his turn, Fricks quickly won over the audience. His southern drawl and slow musical vowels carried warmth. He described a grandmother whom he adored, her impish smile, her deep infectious laugh, and how, as a child, he'd watched her stare and rock in the living room chair. The family never discussed her many psychiatric hospitalizations. He recalled shameful feelings when, as a high school student, he visited Georgia's public hospital in Milledgeville. The touring students paused at the door of a seclusion room where they'd peered through the small window to gawk at a patient lying naked on a table, face down, splayed limbs, wrists and ankles secured tightly. Never did he imagine that he would be similarly bound with a four-point restraint during a hospitalization.

Fricks spoke about his own bipolar disorder. He described the friend who had said taking medicine might help him, the one person who'd reached him when nobody else could. Since then, whenever he describes his recovery, Fricks credits hearing from people with similar experiences. They understand and don't judge. They are peers.

Fricks might have been chary about identifying himself as "the mental patient" to the White House guards, but national news had no such reservation. This he learned when an excited cousin called from California to say he was on the news, identified as a "former mental patient."

Barely six months after the release of the report, presidential candidate George W. Bush pledged that, if elected, he would expand the services covered under the Americans for Disability Act. It was partly as an homage to his father, President George H. W. Bush, who in July 1990 had signed the ADA. The surgeon general's report had provided the scientific legitimacy for recovery, and the President's New Freedom Commission would build on it to recommend transforming mental health care. A psychologist named Tim Kelly helped pave the way.

Kelly had been Virginia's mental health commissioner between 1994 and 1997, and he was appalled by Virginia's "inadequate and ineffective mental health services" in state hospitals, which, he said, "doomed" patients.[9] He campaigned for SAMHSA to evaluate services, and he followed public service with a stint as a scholar-in-residence at George Mason University. From there he pitched ideas to the Heritage Foundation for "sweeping and comprehensive reforms."

Kelly's ideas were eclectic. He wanted accountability and better access, promoted innovative pilot programs, and endorsed consumer choice. His reformer's zeal caught the attention of Stuart Butler, head of the Heritage Foundation's health policy program, who encouraged him to contact the Bush campaign.

Candidate Bush was receptive. A college friend had struggled with depression; others had benefited from the Alcoholics Anonymous twelve-step program. Bush had resolved his own drinking problems ten years prior. Kelly convinced the campaign staff that mental health reform aligned with Bush's disability reforms. In June 2000, Bush announced a New Freedom Initiative to "ensure that Americans with disabilities, whether young or old, have every chance to pursue the American dream. Disabilities should not be a barrier to the pursuit of happiness," he said.[10] He portrayed himself the candidate for "real reform" and cast his opponent, Al Gore, as a representative of the status quo.

On behalf of the transition team, Kelly developed a platform for mental health reform.[11] He met with Laurie Flynn, who, following a bruising *Mother Jones* exposé about pharma's outsized influence polluting NAMI, would soon announce her plans to depart. Ron Manderscheid joined them occasionally and unofficially for breakfast at the Cosmos Club with catch-up conversations about reform and how to achieve it. Wanting Bush to form a national commission for this purpose, they enlisted heavyweight Republicans in their cause. As had Jimmy Carter, President Bush wasted no time in the dawn of his administration. The month after taking office, he announced a President's New Freedom Commission to study mental health.

The project awaited SAMHSA's new chief, Charles "Charlie" Curie. Trained as a social worker in Ohio, he never forgot how clients of an aftercare program answered when he asked them what they wanted. Most said "someone special in my life" or "a date." Many wanted a job to be able to answer the common question, "What do you do?"[12] As Pennsylvania's mental health commissioner for a decade, Curie's disdain for the way hospitals practiced deepened.

As SAMHSA's chief, Curie selected the director of the President's New Freedom Commission from five candidates. Four of them had been state mental health directors. The other was Flynn, then heading Columbia University's teen screening program for suicide prevention. With bipartisan support from Ohio's lawmakers, Mike Hogan got the nod.

The *Report of the Surgeon General* was Hogan's intellectual backstop for the President's New Freedom Commission. Howard Goldman came to the launch meeting in June 2002 and furnished background material from the report. Mental health, he said, was fundamental to whole health and should command the same urgency as physical health.[13] The idea aligned with Hogan's team and became the organizing principle for recommendations about transforming the mental health system.

Hogan also reached out to Rosalynn Carter. It had been twenty-five years since she had chaired a presidential commission, and he asked her to talk about nuts-and-bolts issues. Was there something important to keep in mind? Yes, she said: we now know that recovery is possible.

The President's New Freedom Commission held eleven public hearings, and at each Hogan repeated their driving premise: "A life in the community for everyone" required a delivery system to enable adults with serious mental illnesses and children "to live, work, learn, and participate fully in their communities." The final report, *Achieving the Promise: Transforming Mental Health Care in America*, championed a system-wide transformation making recovery the "common, recognized outcome of mental health services." Science supported it, and the need was urgent. Obtaining services had become so onerous that parents of 12,700 children had been forced to relinquish custody in order to get their kids Medicaid help. Transformation would be essential to fulfill Bush's executive order about implementing the Supreme Court's 1999 *Olmstead* decision. Transformation had to take place if the New Freedom Commission were to truly "envision a future when everyone with a mental illness will recover."

Curie understood the difficulties of culture change. As Pennsylvania's deputy secretary of mental health, he had tried to end seclusion and restraint. It was more than staff and patient injuries, although broken ribs, jaws, and teeth mattered. The iniquity of trauma was its own misdeed. In addition to evidence showing that eliminating seclusion and restraints dramatically cut down on injuries, they were simply not therapeutic.[14] Recovery shouldn't include force.

Attention was drawn to seclusion and restrains in 1998 when the *Hartford Courant* ran a five-day series, "Deadly Restraint." When the Senate subcommittee on appropriations opened hearings the next year, Joseph Rogers testified and brought props—straitjackets and chains.[15]

"Show us how these work," coaxed Pennsylvania senator Arlen Specter.

Rogers complied and held a straitjacket by the straps. "You pull them down and they strap to a chair or to a bench or whatever," he said. If a person "gets violent, throws themselves around, a gurney can flip over," he explained. "If they are not being observed, the gurney lands on top of them, they can literally break their neck."

Iowa senator Tom Harkin was horrified and transfixed. "You have got to be kidding me," he said. There were more questions, more disbelief, and a horror chilled the room. Harkin called them "macabre devices . . . enough to instill fright and apprehension." He compared them to "movies you see in wartime when they torture people."

Curie was hopeful that political pressure could curtail seclusion and restraints. The Judge David L. Bazelon Center for Mental Health Law had led a campaign to tighten restrictions for the euphemism "behavior management." Connecticut's senators and representatives attempted writing laws following the *Hartford Courant's* exposé, but hearings were all they could achieve. From President Clinton to local officials, even in places such as Curie's Pennsylvania, at best changes were piecemeal. Senator Joseph Lieberman called them a "dark corner of institutional life."[16] But fundamentally, they exemplified force and violated dignity and choice, and Curie would write, "Seclusion and restraint cannot co-exist with a recovery-oriented system."[17]

Even without ending seclusion and restraints, the President's New Freedom Commission called for a transformation of a system that had failed on multiple levels. It started with the fact that "the mental health delivery system is not oriented to the single most important goal of the people it serves—the goal of recovery." Partly, this was because "mental illness is the only category of illness for which state and local governments operate distinct treatment systems, making comprehensive care unavailable in the larger health care system. Ultimately the system must change."[18]

With limited authority to repair the fragmented layering of disconnected services, the commission could only make recommendations such as ending unnecessary institutionalization or better coordination of state and local services. It could recommend protecting civil rights, and it could recommend integrated services, as it did by featuring the Village in Long Beach. But it couldn't legislate, appropriate, or implement changes, leaving unrealized the expectation that "recovery will be the common recognized outcome of mental health services."[19]

Knowing that "reform is not enough," Hogan insisted that "transformation" guide next steps. They had the knowledge and now they needed the will to move the process. Curie convened advisors to create an action agenda with objectives to arrive at the day when people with mental illness will "live, work, learn and participate in their communities."

Not since the early 1980s, when Courtenay Harding and Bob Spitzer argued about prognosis while the *DSM-III* was remaking psychiatry, had recovery received more considered attention. But of what did recovery consist? The synergy flowing from the federal government's two meaty reports, and *Mental Health: A Report of the Surgeon General* (1999) and *Achieving the Promise: Transforming Mental Health Care in America* (2003) would thrum journals and conferences for the next two decades. Consumers with firsthand knowledge could point to their own experiences. Most psychiatrists and psychologists didn't have that knowledge, and many remained suspicious. For them, for everybody, it became important to answer, what exactly was recovery?

People knew what it wasn't. There were no quick fixes, and recovery wasn't synonymous with a hospital discharge. Nobody claimed recovery was cure. But did it amount to more than ameliorating symptoms? Did it require returning to a precrisis level of functioning? Was it a synonym for wellness, or the same as healthy? Articles in *Psychiatric Services* outlined the poles separating professional opinions starting in 2001. Authors Nora Jacobson and Dianne Greenley asked "What Is Recovery?" when, in the April issue, they posited a framework of "outcomes research, personal narrative, services design and provision, and system reform." Jacobson, a medical sociologist, and Greenley, a social worker before attending law school, were identified as being on the front lines of promoting a "recovery-oriented" mental health system for Wisconsin. Like others attempting to engage a new audience about recovery, they cast a wide net about a culture of healing, a process of consumer engagement, and a future propelled by hope. These elements promoted personal empowerment commensurate with swapping a social role with one defined by a disease. The new role elevated consumer agency, where people "assume more and more responsibility for themselves . . . [in] a profoundly social process" filled with collaboration, and connection with service providers to develop goals. They conclude with models of medical rehabilitation.[20]

Not everybody agreed, and *Psychiatric Services* printed a response from a New York City psychiatrist, Herbert Peyser, who challenged their premise. In his words, the patient was "taken over by the disease," leaving no room for agency in decision-making. His years of practice led him to question the core of their conceptual model and its therapeutic usefulness. Where he operated from assumptions about the downfall brought by persistent symptoms, they asked about managing symptoms in the service of a larger ambition. Peyser dismissed this. He characterized their work as "hopeful exposition and a forceful advocacy," and he worried that their beliefs could "even interfere with treatment."[21]

The new construct of recovery required reimagining time-honored verities. A generation's research had led to rethinking strategies for responding to children with worrisome behavior, averting a crisis, or establishing appropriate services. It had also made clear what training was needed to provide treatments beyond conventional medications. A new construct would accompany the demolition of obstacles, including stigma about people with a mental illness.

Recovery challenged the standard measurement tools experts used to chart symptoms while assigning a diagnosis. "Can We Measure Recovery?" asked Ruth Ralph and Kathryn Kidder, at the University of Southern Maine.[22] They had set out to publish a compilation of research tools in 2000, and they found only about twelve compared to the dozens assessing moods, depression, anxiety, self-harm, and schizophrenia. In 2002, NASMHPD published a report about the nuts and bolts of recovery programs, conceding that recovery was more than symptom relief. Two years later, SAMHSA sponsored a conference about incorporating recovery in service systems.[23]

Seasoned researchers at universities such as Dartmouth, Rutgers, the University of Illinois, and UCLA, people who had routinely studied services, continued unraveling recovery's threads. Two psychologists, Larry Davidson at Yale University's Program on Recovery and Community Health, and Arthur Evans, the head of Connecticut's Department of Mental Health and Addiction Services, bridged the town-gown divide in the service of a transformation in Connecticut. They wrote about "the recent proliferation of the concept" but said its focus had generated "confusion and debate among various constituencies within the mental health community."[24] That was primarily because recovery from serious mental illnesses was new, despite parallels to ideas in adjacent fields such as addiction services. Although heterogeneous outcomes had been documented for decades, mental illnesses had not been organized under a single umbrella with principles about reclaiming a life in which an illness was an element but not the sole driver of that person. That people had managed obstacles and tackled symptoms to achieve their goals often meant a continuous journey, a process that was life-affirming.

However exciting it seemed to have fresh ideas and new ways of thinking, more than rhetoric would be needed to effect recovery. Systems of care with dynamic programs would be essential,[25] and Davidson's team designed the Recovery Knowledge Inventory to guide staff development while navigating "a multi-dimensional concept that holds different meanings for different parties."[26] It was tantamount to a culture change, said Thomas Kirk, Connecticut's new mental health commissioner.

Parallel to emerging efforts to define recovery, in 2003 six psychiatrists tackled questions about remission in schizophrenia. They had roots in NIMH laboratories, *DSM-III* advisory committees, the FDA's clozapine hearings, and, for one of them, a drug company. The working group explored a number of medical and psychiatric conditions. They could enumerate the important social, psychosocial, pharmacological, vocational, and clinical factors relevant to treating schizophrenia. But, they wrote, "the availability of such key supports varies substantially between localities, and social and vocational interventions are seldom applied in a manner consistent with optimal clinical outcome."[27]

Reviewing the scientific and consumer models of recovery for schizophrenia, Alan Bellak noted that earlier generations would have considered recovery an oxymoron. Why no more? He thought the answer was apparent: "New data and consumer voices," he said.[28]

The century closed differently than it had begun. Kraepelin's prognostic dictum about an unrelenting decline for people with schizophrenia had been shown to be inaccurate, damaging, and obsolete. A new construct, aligned with a process including a plethora of complex interactions promoting recovery, had been carved, but incorporating it would be no small matter.

CHAPTER 18

RECOVERY
AND WELLNESS

T HE FIRST GENERATION OF EX-PATIENT ACTIVISTS shared a similar impression that their hospital experiences were oppressive. Reform was in the air, and they were part of their generation's hopefulness that protest could reveal and then improve on a flawed reality. For feminists, it was sexism; for people of color, it was institutional discrimination; for pacifists, it was war in foreign lands. For former patients, it was psychiatry's unimpeded authority and its unaccountable power. Standing on the shoulders of pioneers such as Judi Chamberlin, Howie the Harp, Su and Dennis Budd, and Sally Zinman, the next wave of activists inherited their mission and used it while building tools for a recovery-driven self-determined life.

But tools for recovery disturbed the medical establishment who expected to maintain control of a care system. The subtitle of Judi Chamberlin's now iconic book, *On Our Own*, "Patient-Controlled Alternatives to the Mental Health System," presaged the struggles that would ensue. None has spoken more eloquently about this process than Patricia "Pat" Deegan, whose pensive narratives have inspired a generation in a hard-to-budge system.

Deegan is a psychologist who rebelled against the hope-crushing diagnosis of schizophrenia she received as a Massachusetts teenager in the 1970s. While she watched her high school classmates move ahead, she chain-smoked day after day at home, and her dream, that of a gifted athlete wanting to become a gym teacher, slipped away. The side effects of medication colluded with a self-imposed stigma. Slowly, eventually, she regained a sense of purpose, building it back with small achievements.

Deegan's psychiatrist presumed that her future would be defined by a disease and told her so. His assumption was pivotal to her decision to become a psychologist, imagining that a *doctor* Deegan could rescue others from a damaging system. "It was my anger that announced the resurrection of my dignity after it had been so battered down during hospitalizations," she said.[1] Institutionalization created obstacles, and she believed they "thwart us in our efforts to regain control over our lives and the resources that affect our lives."[2]

Activists with intellectual and physical disabilities inspired her. She had met many who summoned anger to improve on the sordid residential institutions preparing them to do nothing but lead meager lives and then die. A short time at L'Arche, in nearby Ipswich, Massachusetts, and a job later at the Northeast Center for Independent Living in Lawrence impressed her. There she met founder Charlie Carr, whose diving accident at the age of sixteen left him requiring a wheelchair. But it didn't leave him without hope, goals, or abilities. And he wouldn't let authorities squash his ambition to attend college by telling him it was more than he could handle. He became a builder of programs in the disability rights movement.

Deegan was later impressed by Boston University's assignment for students studying psych rehab. They had to negotiate campus without using sight to cross busy streets. They couldn't find faculty in offices with painted numbers only, or grab lunch in a cafeteria's buffet line. They surmised it was the obstacles, not the condition of not having sight, that prevented full participation.

Deegan asked herself about the obstacles for people who, like her, heard voices. Clinicians often skirted talking about voices, audible hallucinations, to redirect patients and focus them on external factors, as if the voices weren't real. But to people who heard voices, they were real. She decided to build a tool for the field's first responders and treatment professionals.

Deegan was on the cusp of a movement, the Hearing Voices Network. NBC News reported that by 2018 there were more than one hundred such support groups in the United States. But that wasn't the case in 1994, when she constructed a device simulating four overlapping voices. How difficult this was to live with, and how real the voices were, was apparent in a 2014

CNN segment featuring Anderson Cooper. He wore earbuds with piped-in voices in a clip that was subsequently posted to YouTube.[3] Shouts, whispers, instructions, imperatives, and criticisms distracted him, making work difficult. He sat for a mock interview to answer questions that would be asked of someone admitted to a hospital. At one point, overcome by frustration, he blurted, "It's hard to concentrate." Walking around New York City became distressing. He said he had to remove the buds because he wanted to respond to the voices. "It makes you feel incredibly isolated from everyone else around you," he said.

Deegan developed a workbook, a hundred-page manual titled *Personal Medicine for Distressing Voices*. It is a step-by-step plan to manage intrusive voices with exercises establishing authority and personal agency. Each begins with the declaration, *I will*. I will practice relaxing; I will do something physical; I will shrink my voices. These and other personalized instructions accompany a list of choices for how to accomplish that goal, and then note whether that was a successful strategy.

Deegan knows that recovery requires personal drive of the sort institutions subdued or buried or crushed. Her work addresses this with an elegant fury, weaving metaphors about nature's struggles—seascapes, dunes, trees seeking light—with existential meditations from Martin Buber about a shared humanity. As she told NAMI parents at a meeting in Massachusetts in 1995, the right environment can excite internal qualities of self-worth and purpose. It embeds hope, perhaps even a "conspiracy of hope," a phrase that has become her trademark.

Deegan's recovery narratives have touched the current generation of activists. Long before hope became one of recovery's metrics, she understood it was a matter of life and death. To live without hope is to stagnate, to surrender, to give up. As a messenger, she clarifies how the journey includes an internal process that is "within and beyond the limits of a disability."[4] The recovery journey doesn't only control a symptom; it revises an identity by sculpting a vision for regaining personhood. "The goal is to embrace our human vocation of becoming more deeply, more fully human . . . to become the unique, awesome, never to be repeated human being that we are called to be." For that, "hope filled, humanized environments and relationships" must replace systems that "tried to break our spirit."

Recovery and wellness principles were jarring for clinicians who found it difficult to modify the time-honored expectation of compliance with shared decision-making. Psychiatrists turned out to be slower than other doctors to adopt this practice. It is, as Deegan notes, based "on the premise that two experts are in the consultation room: the practitioner and the client."[5] Her own doctors had said she was "non-compliant" because she refused medication. She saw it differently, as an act of self-assertion and independence, a rejection of a discouraging prognosis. When SAMHSA endorsed shared decision-making, it tactfully acknowledged that it was "a potentially radical change in current mental health practice."[6]

In 1997, Deegan cofounded the National Empowerment Center in Boston, one of SAMHSA's technical advisory centers. She worked with fellow activist Dan Fisher, a psychiatrist who had also been hospitalized and diagnosed with schizophrenia. They designed a project, funded for a year by the Center for Mental Health Services, which brought together those challenging the idea that people with mental illness didn't recover.

Following that, Deegan met with Larry Fricks and the Georgia Consumer Council, which had just discovered a pile of discarded markers from patients' graves. Thirty thousand people had been buried in Milledgeville, identified only by numbered metal sticks that had been tossed aside to mow the fields. State officials had claimed that the nameless markers respected patient confidentiality, but activists were horrified, both by the self-serving explanation and by history having robbed patients of identity and dignity in death. Georgia's activist consumers vowed to restore the cemetery.

This was not an isolated occurrence. At the Oregon State Hospital in Salem, five thousand unmarked funeral urns would be discovered in the cremains room, adjacent to the hospital's incinerator.[7] Unmarked urns and abandoned graves were found in Minnesota's state hospitals for thirteen thousand people, and in New York for fifty-five thousand people. In Massachusetts, at the Danvers State Hospital, Deegan tripped over similarly numbered metal markers. These were the individuals institutions had ignored and hidden under the category of "the mentally ill," making them equally anonymous in life and in death.

"That could have been me buried there," Deegan said in a documentary posted on YouTube. On September 25, 2002, activists read the names of 768 people Danvers had buried anonymously.[8] That day, their names were recorded, their personhood declared, and they were remembered. Deegan called it a moment for justice.

Her odyssey was slow. It required dismantling the stigma she had initially internalized while discovering her value. Deegan's pioneering narrative, her recounting of her painstaking journey, meeting one storm after another, and slowly shedding the detritus of her diagnosis,[9] has inspired audiences as far as Australia and New Zealand, and throughout Western Europe.

———————

At the same time, Peggy Swarbrick was at work at Rutgers University, where her research appointments have led to deeper understandings of the importance of integration of peer-delivered services with wellness priorities. Like Deegan, she understood the importance of hope and motivation for managing stress and symptoms. Swarbrick, who holds a doctorate in rehabilitation therapy, conceptualized a framework with eight interrelated dimensions of health and wellness that has become iconic in the field: social, spiritual, intellectual, physical, environmental, financial, occupational, and emotional. Modern medicine had overlooked some of these factors and hadn't given purchase to the synergistic relationship of others.[10] SAMHSA adopted Swarbrick's wellness model in 2007 and has produced many posters with a color wheel, intersecting circles, petals of a flower joined at the center, yoga poses—just about anything that drove home the point that these were not isolated qualities but connected to a core, making them parts of a whole.

Swarbrick was among the early researchers publishing proactive steps that lead to wellness and developing self-management and resiliency tools to manage crises. Her work would become elemental to writing curriculum training for peers whose certification was needed for Medicaid reimbursement. It turned out that incorporating peers on treatment teams, integrating professionals with streetwise people, and establishing a few peer-driven respite centers was creating a demand. In 2004, a member association, the National Association of Peer Supporters (NAPS), was formed to develop professional guidelines.[11] It took Larry Fricks and Ike Powell's Appalachian Consulting Group only a decade to train more than three thousand people with lived experience. In another decade, they would count twenty-nine states where they had trained certified peer specialists.[12] In New York City, the Howie the Harp Peer Training Program operated full throttle with classroom work amplified with on-site internships in hospitals, prisons, housing programs, crisis mobilization teams, and freestanding peer-run programs. By September 2021, RI International, headquartered in Arizona, had trained more than fifteen thousand peers from twenty-one states and five countries, plus a certified training program for veterans.[13]

Of the consumer-designed initiatives, none has been more attuned to promoting wellness or managing symptoms than Mary Ellen Copeland's Wellness Recovery Action Plan (WRAP). It was the epitome of person-centered choice, designed to meet someone's unique and specific situation.

Copeland, a psychologist living in Vermont, had herself been diagnosed with bipolar disorder in her thirties. Until toxic side effects forced her to stop, she took lithium. When she asked her psychiatrist for other strategies for regaining wellness, it turned out he had none for community-based or nonmedication options. Believing she could recover and engage, as had her mother, whose career as a dietician was begun after a hospitalization, she reached out to her local community. Copeland called it "networking recovery information," and in 1997, she published a structured system called WRAP to organize wellness in daily life.

Each of the acronym's letters matters. Wellness, not a disease or its limitations, organizes the work. Recovery is aspirational, more than the blunting of symptoms. Action requires engagement, autonomy, collaboration, and sometimes risk. Planning is purposeful and future oriented; it restores agency and enlists hope. Notably, a wellness recovery action plan—WRAP—might anticipate a crisis—who to call, what works, and what doesn't—information that gets lost when families, doctors, or emergency responders take over.

There are no imperatives, only tools for sustaining wellness and a desired life. They include medication, diet, exercise, hobbies, faith-based meetings, caring for a pet, or knowing who can go to the grocery store or the post office in an emergency. A wellness recovery action plan can also be cautionary, identifying activities that undermine the self-directed wellness its author seeks. In this way, WRAP becomes an action plan with the support of a trained peer counselor and an inventory of tools promoting recovery.

Copeland's self-directed program galloped across the United States and reached Japan, China, and six English-speaking countries in less than a decade. In 2005, she opened offices, the Copeland Center for Wellness and Recovery, in Vermont. Soon the research community was engaged. In 2006, Judith Cook, a sociologist at the University of Illinois in Chicago, studied eighty people who had enrolled in a WRAP training program; her resulting data affirmed WRAP's benefits.[14] A subsequent project of 519 people in Ohio compared those using WRAP to others in outpatient treatment programs. The authors concluded "that peer-delivered mental illness self-management training reduces psychiatric symptoms, enhances participants' hopefulness, and improved the quality of life as measured by a World Health scale."[15]

New Hampshire activist Sherry Mead organized a respite in 1997, using the model of intentional peer support that is conversation based, not focused on the solution. The power of peers was key to Alcoholics Anonymous and 12-step fellowship programs dating from the 1940s. Since then, peer support groups have helped new mothers, cancer patients, and people grieving the loss of a loved one. Peers as agents for recovery in mental health has introduced a new element, and peers have become a mainstay in the fast-growing respite movement.

Respites provide a short-term haven, a sanctuary for anywhere from twenty-four hours to three months. Studies have indicated that peers sharing a similar journey can nurture hope and confidence and inspire people in specific ways that psychiatrists or other clinicians haven't.[16]

They have been steadily growing. In New York's Hudson River Valley, People USA opened the Rose House Hospital Diversion Program in 2001; fifteen years later, it was operating four of the six regional centers. The Georgia Mental Health Consumer Network opened its first center for respite and wellness in 2008, and a decade later it was operating five.[17] Massachusetts opened a respite center in 2009.[18] Pennsylvania, Ohio, and Iowa each have a single peer-driven center. RI International, with respite centers in six states, runs the Retreat, a respite in Phoenix. Peers make up two-thirds of the paid staff and hold positions at all levels of leadership and responsibility. They greet each person on arrival and are available to them throughout their stay. As a hybrid model, RI International's Arizona license requires that a medically trained person provide clearance. Of the 13,195 people coming through this peer-support program between 2014 and 2018, not a single one ended up in the emergency room.[19] Peers are central to the respite services of RI International's Retreat, and they are essential for anybody who chooses a longer stay in the Living Room, a model of service more homelike than medical, effectively diverting people from emergency rooms as well as framing a wellness journey for clients called guests.

RI International operates one of the country's largest respite programs. David Covington, president and CEO, was aligned with RI's empowerment model when he arrived in 2016. He came from Magellan Health Services, where he had been instrumental in supporting peer-driven services.[20]

That respite programs divert admissions to hospitals or jails has not been lost on insurance companies, especially in states where a psychiatric emergency room visit leads to inpatient admission. Of the people RI International has seen in crisis, about 80 percent are brought by local law enforcement, a figure that remained steady between 2018 and 2021.[21]

Not all peer respites are the same. Some serve as alternatives to an emergency room, while others have restrictions based on suicide risk or on substances and detox needs. Every RI International respite admission is a diversion from an unneeded hospitalization or an incarceration with subsequent court proceedings. That is an opportunity to minimize additional trauma and leave behind the gratuitous baggage of a diagnosis, medication, HIPAA, waivers, and discharge planning. It becomes a way station permitting careful consideration of needs and paying equally careful attention to how to meet them, making it the first door to a recovery journey.

Mental health reform cannot be detached from politics, or politics from lobbies, or lobbies from self-interest, making grassroots reform initiatives potentially contentious. The peer-driven recovery movement elicits strong reactions when it challenges vested authorities, and at no time has this been more apparent than when politicians pin mental health reform on a mass shooting. This was apparent in March 2013, three months after twenty children and six adults died at Sandy Hook Elementary School in New-town, Connecticut, at the hands of Adam Lanza. Rep. Tim Murphy introduced the Helping Families in Mental Health Crisis Act. Murphy was a six-term Republican from Pennsylvania, the only child psychologist then sitting in Congress, and he intended to repair the system through which gunman Adam Lanza had slipped. Lanza had used a semi-automatic AR-15, a military-grade weapon on which the federal ban had expired in 2004.

As chair of the oversight subcommittee of the House Energy and Commerce Committee, Murphy had clout. Along with E. Fuller Torrey and D. J. Jaffe, he was disappointed with the direction of federal policies and programs, and he worried about violence committed by people with an untreated mental illness.

On the afternoon of March 5, 2013, Murphy planned a forum, "Mental Illness and Violence," so that members of the subcommittee could hear from parents. Earlier that day, he appeared on *Washington Journal*, a cable show with audience call-ins for politicians. During an interview with the host he described how America's mental health system bordered on dysfunctional: HIPAA's confidentiality laws had become a tangle of excuses barring families from helping a relative; poor access to services threw people into crisis before they could get an appointment. SAMHSA had estimated that about 4.3 million people, roughly 40 percent of those with a serious mental illness, reported having not received treatment.[22] Those who were in treatment were often overmedicated, or wrongly so. Others crowded jails and prisons.

Accusing the federal government of shunning its responsibilities, he blamed the health institutes, especially NIMH. Cancer's research budget was five times greater than that for mental illnesses. NIMH hadn't focused on people with the most serious mental illnesses. Now the nation was in a crisis after a mentally disturbed gunman attacked an elementary school.[23]

When the phone lines opened, the first caller, a DC resident, introduced herself by saying she had a psychiatric history. She had also finished law school and had an established career. She expressed her concern, however, that none of the panelists he had invited to appear later could speak about having a mental illness. Murphy nodded his understanding.

Why, she asked him, had his bill emphasized inpatient hospitalization and not community-based care or peer services? At the mention of peers, Murphy straightened. He threw his shoulders back, tightened his lips, and sat up. He was tall and slim, with a military haircut befitting an active member of the naval reserves who treated people at Walter Reed Hospital for PTSD. "Okay," he said irritably, telling the host that the caller was describing peer services, which, he said, "work very well with alcohol and drug abuse." But this panel, he continued, had been convened to discuss families and mental illness and violence. "When we're talking about severe mental illness and violence, there is high risk," Murphy said. Then, astonishingly, he equated people needing treatment for mental illness with felons. "I'm not going to bring a convicted felon out of prison to talk about why they kill people," he said.

An hour later, at 10:00 a.m., Murphy arrived at the Rayburn House Office Building for subcommittee meetings. Present were a couple of psychiatrists, including NIMH director Thomas Insel and E. Fuller Torrey. They joined elected representatives and three parents who had been invited to discuss their frustrations helping adult children. Their conversation was all too familiar. The system was deficient. How should it be fixed? And who should chart the course? They talked about a crisis and predicted more were likely to happen. The specter of the mad gunman hovered until Torrey put violence on the table. Assisted outpatient treatment is a remedy for violence, he emphasized, as he often did, for people who are untreated.

While Torrey repeated his ideas that mentally ill people are violent and need to be restrained, Insel disagreed. Soon he would talk about social inequities, disparities, and the need for "accurate and evidence-based information."[24] With a different framework, he turned to Torrey. "What do we have in place to make sure that people finish their education, get jobs, have families, contribute in some important way[?] . . . The package of interventions exist," he said, "but they have not been integrated in a package of care."

Murphy's critics and supporters disagreed over fundamentals, such as who should have access to HIPAA records. What parts of the federal protection and advocacy law (PAIMI) should remain for institutionalized people? What was the federal government's position on involuntary treatments?

Murphy proposed bigger hospitals, longer stays, and medication management—the antithesis of recovery priorities. His bill incentivized states to pass laws for forced treatment. As consumers had done in 1995, when Senator Nancy Kassebaum held hearings, they mounted a vigorous opposition. Leah Harris, an emerging consumer leader, lambasted court orders for involuntary treatments, "the same service approaches that have already failed to help them."[25] Writing in the *Pittsburgh Post-Gazette*, Murphy's hometown paper, she reminded readers that person-centered approaches are common elsewhere in medicine. "Why not focus instead on providing an upfront investment in voluntary housing and support services that are proven to work?" she asked.

Their differing viewpoints about established psychiatric practice focused attention on SAMHSA. Torrey's misunderstandings amplified his grave doubts about its policies supporting state programs. If six people in ten weren't getting timely services, what was the agency doing with its billion-dollar budget? Who was in charge? On what evidence were decisions made? And why, pointedly, had SAMHSA not endorsed involuntary outpatient treatments?

Another SAMHSA critic, psychiatrist Sally Satel, testified at the House oversight subcommittee's meeting in May 2013.[26] Her résumé included serving on the faculty of Yale Medical School between 1988 and 1993, and after moving to Washington, she worked in drug treatment and served on the advisory board of the Center for Mental Health Services (CMHS) under SAMHSA's authority. She considered recovery a dubious treatment model and objected to the CMHS's formal adoption of it in 2004. It was, in her estimation, "an idiosyncratic interpretation" of its mission and a policy that failed to consider "the most severely disabled." An even greater problem at SAMHSA, Satel said, was the "dearth of psychiatrists in leadership position."

SAMHSA was then helmed by a lawyer, Pam Hyde, and a self-disclosed consumer, Paolo del Vecchio, headed the CMHS. And they were at odds with those wanting greater psychiatric authority. Peer supports broadened the focus of treatment, allowing for the permutations of a recovery journey that included activities not strictly medical and hence not guided by psychiatry. The APA's immediate past president, Jeffrey Lieberman, who was then chair of Columbia University's Department of Psychiatry, described SAMHSA as "a proxy agency for the anti-psychiatry movement." At a June 2016 committee hearing, he called SAMHSA a backwater. It "has resisted the scientifically driven evidence-based approach to mental health care that psychiatric medicine has embraced since its scientific revolution began in the 1970s."[27]

Lieberman exemplified why consumer leaders worried about psychiatry's priorities.[28] He had simplified the movement's fifty-year-old complaints, grievances that were born of psychiatry's domination of a failed service. He complained that hospital beds had dwindled to forty thousand, 95 percent less than the half million in 1976—as though that were the issue. He dusted off the standard explanations about stigma and poor funding—both of which were true—as causal factors. His solution focused primarily on the workforce and recruiting more medical professionals. And it could have applied to any day or era. In 2016, it seemed out of time.

Measuring psychiatric treatment in the twenty-first century by the existence of long-term inpatient beds was like building the interstate highway system to incorporate specs for the Ford Model T. Author Anne Harrington writes in *Mind Fixers* how "in the course of narrowing its focus," psychiatry had outsourced care "to therapists, counselors, social workers, social service providers, and patient-run organizations." Still, "the fiction persists," she writes, "that all this work, regardless of the kind of patient, is carried out in the service of the same medical mission. Psychiatrists create all the diagnoses and jealously guard their prescribing rights. A general consensus remains, implicitly, that the knowledge and practice of all the nonmedically trained workers are by definition subordinate to those of the medically trained ones."[29]

While the Murphy bill focused the political conversation, venture capitalists were consolidating psychiatric services. Through the 1990s, Wall Street expanded its vision to include psychiatric services, which it described as a "fragmented industry," making it a ripe takeover target. The model for consolidation had been refined since 1968, when Tennessee mogul Jack Massey cofounded the Hospital Corporation of America (HCA). His work subsequently influenced the privatization of correctional facilities, waste facilities, immigrant detention centers, and charter schools. The disruptor in behavioral health, Psychiatric Solutions, Inc. (PSI), was founded by HCA veterans and led by Joey Jacobs.[30] Around 1996, Jacobs started buying psychiatric management services as part of the benefit programs for employees. He then acquired hospitals in North Carolina and Texas. A decade later, PSI owned fifty facilities, including the behavioral health division of Ardent Health Services. Jacobs was elated and confirmed his belief by saying, "There's a tremendous market opportunity to meet the demand for inpatient psychiatric service." By 2007, according to an ED-GAR filing with the Securities and Exchange Commission, PSI owned or operated seventy-four inpatient behavioral health facilities in twenty-nine states for a total of 8,400 beds; it managed another fifteen inpatient facilities for Horizon Health, with fifteen hundred beds in eleven states. Failed youth facilities were added next.

Service in all areas—acute, outpatient, children, adults, urban, rural— were grouped into a category called the Behavioral Rehabilitation Sector. The model presumed Medicaid would absorb the costs, the same way Medicare had for the nursing home industry. The common denominator was tapping into government funding through entitlements or grants, or writing favorable contracts, something common for correctional facilities guaranteeing bed capacity exceeding 90 percent. Freestanding psychiatric hospitals stood to benefit from the campaigns families and consumers had waged to get treatment. The 2008 Mental Health Parity and Addiction Act expanded both commercial health insurance and the customer base. The Affordable Care Act of 2010 (ACA) also brought new customers. Facilities needed only beds and staff, not expensive equipment or technology; cutting staff while increasing beds and length of stay, chain companies pitched a 25 to 30 percent growth in revenue.

PSI's profits soared, but legal woes challenged its corporate image along with its earnings. Lawsuits in California, Illinois, Virginia, Florida, and Texas charged sex abuse, poor training, understaffing, negligence, restraints causing brain damage, schemes to cover up suicide attempts, and grossly inadequate clinical records. And people died. The Department of Justice investigated complaints about PSI's substandard care of children; the Center for Medicare and Medicaid Services terminated contracts for reimbursements. A former employee noted, "It's not a client-centered approach. It's a money-centered approach."[31]

Business Week described PSI as a "pure play, public company" in 2007: "In a pattern similar to the consolidation of fast foods, breakfast cereals, or women's apparel, big business has its eye on mental health services and an estimated $20 billion market." PSI had a contract with Utah's Bureau of Indian Education to provide therapy in a Salt Lake City suburb for nearly half a million dollars.[32] Becoming philosophical, the magazine mused, "who will shape treatment and care for people needing mental health services? And who, in the long run, will benefit?"[33]

Universal Health Services (UHS) bought PSI in 2010 and thus merged two hundred facilities. In 2016, a *BuzzFeed* investigation reported dubious practices of misrepresented symptoms, exaggerated risks of self-harm, or delayed discharge.[34] In 2020, UHS, with annual revenue at $11.4 billion, including hospitals in England, ranked 168 on the list of Fortune 500 companies.[35]

Aiming to lift a federal cap on the number of patient beds qualifying for Medicaid reimbursement, Murphy's bill could boost hospital profits. Lobbyists understood this, and in 2014, the healthcare industry, including the National Association for Behavioral Healthcare, contributed more than $14 million to sitting members of the House Energy and Commerce Committee. Activists thought an injection of federal money ought to promote community integration, consistent with the Supreme Court's *Olmstead* decision affirming the ADA, not hospitals minimizing or delaying recovery.

The harshness of institutional confinement seemed less concerning to medical ethicists from the University of Pennsylvania when they proposed expanding asylums.[36] They spoke glibly about how asylums were originally "a protected place where safety, sanctuary, and long-term care for the mentally ill would be provided." But the showstopper was this: "It is time to build them—again." They continued: "For persons with severe and treatment-resistant psychotic disorders, who are too unstable or unsafe for community-based treatment, the choice is between the prison–homelessness–acute hospitalization–prison cycle or long-term psychiatric institutionalization."

The president of the APA, Renée Binder, responded to the fatuous claim about asylums being "safe, modern and humane." Return? "NEVER!" headlined her editorial in *Psychiatric News*. Her preference was "a coordinated, well-funded system of care" with "discharge planning after an acute hospitalization." What was needed was treatment, funding, diversion programs, and collaborative courts.[37]

Describing choices as limited between hospitals and prisons seemed as much an assault on recovery ideals as the romanticization of psychiatric facilities. If information about new service models or evidence about community engagement as a foundation for recovery had not been accessible in professional journals or the lay press, they might not have seemed as much of a gadfly in their ivory tower.[38] Health reporter Benedict Carey implied the divide when he noted how "lawmakers in Washington are debating large-scale reforms to the mental health care system, [while] analysists are carefully watching a handful of new first-break programs."[39]

———————

When a near-unanimous Congress passed the 21st Century Cures Act in 2016, it contained many items from Murphy's Helping Families with Mental Illness Act. Among them was the creation of an assistant secretary for mental health and substance abuse services to oversee SAMHSA. A psychiatrist named Elinore McCance-Katz, then the chief medical officer in Rhode Island, got the nod. Her rich résumé included appointments at Yale University and Brown University, and a two-year stint as SAMHSA's chief medical officer between 2013 and 2015. But she hated what she saw and accused SAMHSA of working "to the detriment of clinical care." She called for renewing conventional treatments, and in an article appearing in *Psychiatric Times*, she criticized SAMHSA's definition of recovery. She accused the Center for Mental Health Services of ignoring the treatment of mental disorders and having its own definition of recovery.[40]

Politico's Brianna Ehley predicted that McCance-Katz would "shake things up" with "a dramatic overhaul."[41] She said she wanted "a collaborative care model," but collaboration was intended for other doctors, not with peers.[42] Research about consumer-run programs of people with lived experience didn't qualify for inclusion as psychiatric treatment. Although she sugarcoated her message with science, it was overtly political, and consumers saw it as a threat.

David Oaks took seriously her intention to transform SAMHSA. He announced her appointment with the all-cap headline "TRUMP'S NEW FORCED PSYCHIATRIC DRUGGING CZAR ELLIE McCANCE-KATZ DOESN'T BELIEVE YOU SHOULD HAVE THE RIGHT TO YOUR OWN BODY."[43]

Advocates building recovery-oriented programs didn't see their work as detrimental. Nor did they think they were neglecting the most vulnerable, or lacking in evidence, or ignorant of collaboration, or overlooking treatments of mental disorders. They saw their accomplishments as engaging people whom psychiatry hadn't reached, had neglected, or had sent to social workers or psychologists for nonmedical therapies while they focused almost exclusively on tweaking medication—or those who had not even been on the radar, such as people being discharged from hospitals who needed help from peer bridging services while they resettled in the community. That credit goes to Harvey Rosenthal, a national consumer leader and executive director of the New York Association for Psychiatric Rehabilitation Services (NYAPRS).

With collaboration and conciliation in mind, Rosenthal invited McCance-Katz to keynote the 2018 annual executive seminar NYAPRS hosts in Albany.[44] But she fell flat, filling most of her hour with bland slides thick with data. She noted shortcomings: of the people receiving services, one-third only received medication; opioids accounted for two-thirds of drug overdose fatalities. Of note was the law requiring the dissemination of research findings and evidence-based practices to improve prevention and treatment services. She also endorsed involuntary outpatient treatment (assisted outpatient treatment, or AOT), the equivalent of waving a red flag, and a redesign of SAMHSA's website. True to her word, during her appointment the website changed, and most of the consumer-friendly "Recovery to Practice" pages with resources authored by Swarbrick, Deegan, Copeland, Cook, and others who were building a knowledge base about peer-operated wellness programs came down. In the fall of 2018, SAMHSA would announce that Paolo del Vecchio would no longer head the Center for Mental Health Services. *Politico* called it a "shuffle" while crediting del Vecchio with "steering the surgeon general's mental health report and multiple HHS initiatives on mental health."[45]

———————————

Psychiatry has been slow to adopt recovery programs. In 2005, five years after the surgeon general enthused that "recovery is real," *Psychiatric News* observed that the recovery model "seeks more than symptomatic relief." Five years after that, staff writer Aaron Levin noted that recovery remained "in the early stages of incorporation."[46] A research scientist, Wayne Katon, thought the snail's pace might be because ideas about recovery or wellness create "tension with a system created to treat people's illness."[47]

While some psychiatrists were talking about options for recovery in the 1980s, they remained on the fringes of a field increasingly reliant on biological dicta and the *DSM*. Activists couldn't wait, didn't wait, for the field to unwrap itself from models that threatened to entrap them in perpetual patienthood. The need was becoming urgent. It was time for action beyond protests and rhetoric about what wasn't working. The legacy of Howie the Harp, Sally Zinman, and Judi Chamberlin, who died in 2010, was action and self-help, building blocks to recovery. From California to Vermont, drop-in centers opened with welcome mats and activities. Ex-patients/survivors/consumers used their organizational skills, their internal combustion notwithstanding, to shape a movement. They borrowed where they could from psychologists, nurses, social workers, police officials, judges, bureaucrats, administrators, politicians, and psychiatrists. But they dug internally, using their skills, lives, and experiences.

When Art Bolton told Assemblyman Jesse Unruh to tear down California's hospitals, he couldn't have imagined that a broad coalition of former patients and innovators would birth a movement for recovery. It didn't take long to redirect anger or tap into networks quickly coalescing. A generation later, they had developed a multiplicity of tools for achieving wellness and social integration using community-based, person-centered, multilayered, choice-driven programs. They had created a sector of the workforce carrying hope and showing aspects of recovery previously undreamt. All this had taken place since I was told there was no hope for BJ, that my brother would be forever lost based on what was considered a wastebasket diagnosis for a condition his doctors said was immutable.

It's hard to imagine what NIMH visionary Robert Felix would think of these conversations. He had wanted a seamless "framework of service which admits of no separation of prevention, treatment, and rehabilitation."[48] He would be disappointed, alas, to see fragmentation still a challenge, and perplexed to see the contradictions in a vision he considered self-evident when he wrote a bill to revolutionize mental health care, starting with the creation of the National Institute of Mental Health. The debate about returning to asylums and the rebuilding of hospitals would surely disappoint. How would that bring the benefit of community support he knew was essential to wellness? After all, he imagined obsolete and empty hospitals would become museums, a testimony to the failures of a bygone era, and fixed in time like the pyramids. I'm guessing he would have been troubled knowing that a mental health crisis still affects one family in four, and millions still struggle with addiction, trauma, and biological and social toxins in their neighborhoods.

He would be disappointed to see that despite all we have learned, and what we now know, politics had left us with a legacy of missed opportunities.

A revolution still in the wings challenges us to act on behalf of the forty-three million citizens needing help for a mental health incident in any given year. It beckons to the nearly eight and a half million adults who care for someone with a mental illness, and to the seven and a half million people receiving government support in the public disability system. We hear the challenge for the more than three million adolescents with major depression, 60 percent of whom received no treatment in 2016.[49] And we hear it for the two million people with mental illness languishing in prison.

Reports indicate that it can take close to two decades for clinicians working with patients to incorporate research findings.[50] Twenty years ago, the surgeon general hailed recovery. Time's up. We should wait no longer.

EPILOGUE

W HAT DID TWENTY YEARS MEAN FOR MY FAMILY? For BJ? For anybody's relative? And where does recovery fit into expectations for
a loved one now?

I can't imagine how I would face a crisis today. Should I call the local
public health office to ask about resources in my community, or a psychiatrist? My family doctor, a neighbor, or the police? We call it a broken
system, but it seems there's no system at all.

Despite evidence about how to promote recovery, the moral imperatives, and the legal mandates, including the Supreme Court's 1999 *Olmstead* decision affirming the Americans with Disability Act, too many
barriers remain for someone fighting for recovery. The facts seem to conflict with today's profoundly unequal, often inaccessible, usually underfunded, and inconsistently managed patchwork system of services with
public and private entities operating in fifty different states.

Barriers must be overcome. Through the lenses of art, design, and
engineering, Sara Hendren, author of *What Can a Body Do?*, describes
how curb cuts, ramps, elevators, and the globally recognized International
Symbol of Access enable "entryways to public life, schools and transportation and workplace." These modifications to existing structures promote
"access [to] a meaningful future."[1] But the barriers to equity in behavioral
health reside not only in wood, plastic, or cardboard, but in the residue of
norms, myths, and politics.

A report jointly issued by the Group for the Advancement of Psychiatry and the National Council for Behavioral Health in March 2021 describes the "roadmap to the ideal crisis system."[2] The place to start has
been with changes in first responders whose management of a crisis can

have lasting consequences for the trajectory of a recovery. An early effort to improve opportunities for crisis intervention came in the late 1980s in Memphis, Tennessee, after a bungled police response led to the death of a mentally ill Black man. Local NAMI families collaborated with local law enforcement to develop alternatives to uniformed police with handcuffs, guns, and stun guns, the very image of force, attempting to calm someone on the emotional or behavioral edge or engaged in self-harm. Crisis intervention training (CIT), also called the Memphis Plan, developed techniques to de-escalate rather than escalate, and then help that person receive appropriate attention other than in jail or a hospital. Timing and location matter, as does the choice of a destination.

Physical ailments like stroke, heart failure, or asthma all benefit from early interventions. In each case, a delay in treatment or the wrong choice can lead to impairment or death. The same is true for people experiencing a behavioral health crisis. Careful intervention can lead to recovery. Police departments learning CIT techniques interrupted pipelines to jail, saved lives, and also saved taxpayer money. According to Alisa Roth, author of *Insane: America's Criminal Treatment of Mental Illness*, CIT in San Antonio, Texas, saved $50 million between 2008 and 2018, diverting more than sixty thousand people from the criminal justice system. Based on the work of a county mental health commissioner, Leon Evans, and with the support of a psychiatrist, Dr. Roberto Jimenez, a comprehensive service center, Restoration Center, built a program with access to multiple services under one roof. It's become both a success and a model.[3]

Yet even with lives saved, and money well spent, in 2021 fewer than 20 percent of the nation's eighteen thousand police forces were partially or fully trained in CIT. The *Washington Post*'s tracking of the deaths of people in custody show that since 2015, one-quarter of those who died in police custody had a mental illness.[4]

Knowing the chances for recruiting appropriate help for BJ were no better than one in five, I would be loath to call 911. This concern would not be mine only. The executive director of CIT International, Ron Bruno, points to the "underfunded mental health care system and a common misperception of the danger presented by people with mental illness." He adds that this has led law enforcement to "become the de facto behavioral health crisis response service."[5] Writing for *Police1*, the crisis intervention trainer Ellis Amdur recognizes the need for responses to a range of situations. "What's needed (and exists in too few places) are short-term crisis respite centers (CRC), where people are discharged as soon as they are emotionally stable. Individuals who are prone to short-term crises have a place to stay with trained staff so they can get through their immediate mental health crisis and go back to their home or a temporary shelter, rather than being hospitalized."[6]

If I had access to the FCC's new 988 emergency number for mental health crises, the replacement for 911, my concerns might be less. The 988 number came about after years of collaboration between suicide prevention activists, the Veterans Administration, and SAMHSA. Even before the alarming rise in suicides among teenage girls and transgendered youth,[7] a plan to replace the ten-digit Suicide Prevention Lifeline with people trained to understand mental health conditions was under way. The rub is that each state is responsible for financing and accountability for adequate paid staff to coordinate local needs with call centers, crisis teams, and chat lines.[8] If that can be resolved, 988 can become one of the levers easing a crisis, beginning a recovery on the streets.

The 988 line, which is set to go live in July 2022 at the time of this writing, makes me guardedly hopeful. But it is still too early to tell whether it can fulfill the promise. To roll out 988, SAMHSA worked mightily under the leadership of Assistant Secretary of Health Miriam Delphin-Rittmon to assist public and private entities and facilitate an easy transition and implementation. Opening a Center for Recovery in September 2021 signalled SAMHSA's reversal of the previous administration's approach.

Of course, in the best-case scenario, mental health care doesn't start with an acute situation. Ideally, people with behavioral health needs would not use different doors from those visiting their internist or family doctor. Robert Felix, steeped in principles of public health, intended his institute to address the segregation of mental health services from mainstream medicine while local officials addressed prevention. Today schools are also the place where children are most likely to show signs of the adverse childhood experiences (ACE) known to lead to problems needing services. This makes it imperative that skills nurturing wellness are integrated into classroom environments, while information about local patterns of substance use or attempted or completed suicides are identified for assessing a community's need for services.[9] This information can benefit planning for local health systems that have historically depended on states to arrange for services.

Recovery ideals include person-centered voluntary services, shared decision-making, community integration, intentional peer support, and peer employment. These principles have appeared in bills now moving through Congress. None of them influenced JFK's Community Mental Health Act of 1963, which intended to bypass state hospitals. They weren't mounted to challenge the Reagan-era rollbacks to the 1980 Mental Health Systems Act. But they are in evidence in the Promoting Effective and Empowering Recovery Services (PEERS) in Medicare Act of 2021 calling on Medicare to pay a living wage to peers working on coordinated teams. Meeting peers had influenced Congressman Adrian Smith (R-NE) and his co-author, Representative Judy Chu (D-CA). In the Senate, the bill's bipartisan sponsors were Bill Cassidy (R-LA) and Catherine Cortez Masto (D-NV). Their collaborations garnered endorsements from advocacy associations including the National Association of Peer Supporters (NAPS).[10]

To replicate and fund mobile crisis teams, Senator Ron Wyden (D-OR), chair of the Senate Appropriations Committee, looked to his home state of Oregon to insert CAHOOTS in President Joe Biden's 2021 American Rescue Plan (ARP). (It was similar to a bill he and Senator Masto had introduced in 2020 that was never acted upon.) CAHOOTS, which stands for Crisis Assistance Helping Out On The Streets, dates from 1989 when the White Bird Clinic in Eugene designed a mobile service to relieve the police and fire departments from health emergencies. The clinic already had been working with teens who had had bad drug trips, others living on the streets, and still others who had run out of medicine and needed immediate help. The mobile crisis teams consist of mental health counselors, medics, and peers with a lived experience. CAHOOTS is considered a prehospital program as well as a jail diversion program, and of the 24,000 calls to which CAHOOTS responded in 2019, only 150 required police assistance.[11] These numbers bolster claims that most emergencies do not need police action.

Crisis response teams, many of which credit the influence of CAHOOTS, have been spreading. Some are modest, such as Atlanta's Police Alternatives and Diversion (PAD) Initiative, which began in 2017.[12] In Colorado,

Denver's program, called STAR, began in 2020 as a pilot program, but its success diverting people from jail led the city council to fund its continuation.[13] After ARP distributed money to localities, Los Angeles announced it would use $18.5 million of its share to jump-start a diversion program it was calling Alternative Crisis Response.

Wyden wanted "to change the way this country helps those in crisis on the streets." He said these grants "are a critical first step to helping communities across America re-imagine public safety by decriminalizing mental illness, connecting people with services they need."[14]

The need to divert people with mental health problems from jails has never been greater. "Along with race and poverty, mental illness has become a salient feature of mass incarceration," writes Alisa Roth. In her book about imprisoned mentally ill men and women, she reports that perhaps as many as 30 percent of the nine thousand inmates in Chicago's Cook County jail have a mental illness. In New York City, of the seventy thousand people passing through Rikers Island in 2016, 40 percent had a mental illness. In some places, the numbers of incarcerated mentally ill people have led to the construction of specifically designed inmate hospitals. California spent $900 million building near Stockton what is with 1,700 beds the nation's largest prison hospital. In 2011, more than half the beds of Texas's public system were reserved for forensic patients, and in Virginia it was more than one-third of the beds.[15]

"The way we spend money now is ludicrous," says Steven Leifman,[16] associate administrative judge of Miami-Dade County's Eleventh Judicial Court. In Miami, one person in eleven has a diagnosable mental illness. By his own account, in 2000 he became gatekeeper to the county jail, Florida's largest psychiatric facility. When he was unable to get treatment for someone in his courtroom with marked delusions and paranoia, he set out to learn why. He discovered that Florida spent one-quarter of its $144 million mental health budget to restore the competency of 2,500 people so their cases could be tried or dismissed. "Restoring competency" was not connected to more effective treatment. Most of the cases were dismissed for time already served, and people left with no treatment.

Angry, frustrated, and impelled to end the de facto use of the jails as mental health facilities, he built a diversion program with treatment opportunities for people who would otherwise cycle through the courts.[17] With Jackson Memorial Hospital training local law enforcement to employ the Memphis CIT model, and with the blessings of local politicians, Leifman secured an interagency task force of providers. He hired a social worker steeped in rehabilitation principles, Cindy Schwartz, a veteran of Miami's oldest clubhouse, Fellowship House. Gradually and purposefully, since 2000 they have developed a comprehensive care program staffed with social workers and eight peers, four of whom had come from this same court's diversion program.[18]

Leifman has expanded the model of a jail diversion. His most recent focus has been on creating a service that includes crisis respite, housing, support services for employment and job training, and culinary training.[19] For this he acquired a seven-story onetime forensic facility and has been transforming it, making it a warm and welcoming place in which formerly incarcerated people with a mental illness can rehabilitate and recover.[20]

Work with individuals who were convicted of felonies has earned the acronym FACT: F for forensic and ACT for assertive community services. As with all mental health services, it is locally designed.[21] Unlike the original ACT, which was a voluntary program helping people move from hospital to community, FACT helps people move from incarceration to community, and it mandates medication compliance, something that's not been lost on activists. With Belgium, Canada, the Netherlands, and New Zealand leading the way, FACT is gaining attention in the United States. It's another example of how recovery aims for new frontiers.

———————————

Recovery's reach and influence could not have been imagined when Judi Chamberlin and Howie the Harp spawned a liberation movement. Their disruptions sought to bypass the institutional and professional barriers holding them back. Instead, they wanted to build self-help and drop-in centers, provide peers with paid employment, and ensure that parity and social justice were embedded in choice and hope. Over time, these would become the bricks and mortar of recovery.

Most of the field was still grappling with stretching its resources to meet service obligations when Bill Anthony said the 1990s should be the Decade of Recovery. Anthony was the epitome of a disruptor, and even Mark Ragins at the Village in Long Beach was stunned to hear Anthony say recovery would become the next frontier. Most everybody else was engrossed with biology's pursuits and the NIH's embrace of the Decade of the Brain. Anthony, trained as a psychologist, was confident that rehabilitation could offer people skills and techniques to learn self-management strategies for a more promising future. His accomplishments already included founding the *Psychiatric Rehabilitation Journal*. He had floated recovery education more formally within the halls of Boston University, where classes incorporated building life skills based on need and interests, similar to other adult education. Still, saying that recovery was possible, even for people like Ragins whose work foreshadowed a transformative model, seemed eye-opening.

Today, thinking about BJ, and how he didn't have access to resources for a recovery-oriented journey, makes me sad. I would love to say that now that we know more, we actually do a better job. And for many lucky individuals, that is true. But as a nation, until we close the gap between knowing what works and implementing the programs to effect the transformation we know can occur, the narrative is still being written. But the imperative remains, as Tipper Gore said when Surgeon General David Satcher handed her the first *Surgeon General's Report on Mental Health*: "It's time for America to act." That is still the case, and what we do will be not just our test but our legacy.

ACKNOWLEDGMENTS

I AM DEEPLY APPRECIATIVE of the many people who helped me patch this story together with interviews, follow-up conversations and correspondence, and personal records—all vital to my understanding. I am particularly saddened by the deaths of those identified with an asterisk, whose lifelong contributions to mental health reform included fighting for recovery.

In alphabetical order, I thank Bill Anthony*, Dr. Bernard Arons, Jules Asher, Dr. Jack Barchas, Eugene Bardach, Dr. Chris Beels, Paul Berry, Art Bolton, Thom Borneman, Dr. Peter Bourne, Dr. Bertram Brown*, Lynnae Brown, Neal Brown, Dr. Tom Bryant*, Dennis Budd, Su Budd, Katie Cadigan, Gina Calhoun, Sylvia Caras*, Dr. Will Carpenter, Rosalynn Carter, Lee Carty*, Steve Coe, David Covington, Charlie Curie, Pat Deegan, Paolo del Vecchio, Dr. Ron Diamond, Kathy Dobbins, Nancy Domenici, Ann Drissler, Bill Emmett, Joan Erney, David Ferleger, Mike Finkle, Dr. Becca Finn, Dr. Dan Fisher, Laurie Flynn, Larry Fricks, Dr. Louis Gerbino, Dr. Fred Goodwin*, Charles Halpern, Courtenay Harding, Fran Hoffman*, Julie Hoffman, Tony Hoffman*, Mike Hogan, Ron Honburg, Gil Honigfeld, Carole Howe*, Jim Howe*, Gail Hutchins, Sherry Tucker Jenkins, Dr. Lewis Judd*, Dr. Sam Keith, Tim Kelly, Rose King*, Marti Knisley, Dr. Richard Lamb, Judge Steven Leifman, Judge Ginger Lerner-Wren, Alan Leshner, Stephen Lieber, Jay Mahler*, Ron Manderscheid, Goldie Marx, Dr. Herbert Meltzer*, Gwill Newman*, Vi Orr, Dr. Herbert Pardes, Darby Penney*, Dave Pilon, Judge John Racanelli*, Dr. Mark Ragins, Dr. William Reid, Estelle Richman, Harvey Rosenthal, Karen Rosenthal, Leslie Scallet, Nina Schooler, Rusty Selix*, Dr. Steven Sharfstein, Dr. Louis Sokoloff*, Darrell Steinberg, Tanya Temkin, Bill TenHoor, Mary Ann Test,

Bos Todd, Dr. E. Fuller Torrey, Judy Turner-Crowson, Richard Van Horn*, Judge Patricia Wald*, Dr. Daniel Weinberg, Dan Weisburd*, Bev Young, and Sally Zinman.

A fellowship from the Logan Nonfiction Program enabled five glorious weeks at the Carey Institute for Global Good in Rensselaerville, New York. I am grateful to Carol Ash and Josh Friedman for their vision with the right mixture of solitude and community, and to Chantal Flores, Matthew Galizia, Jane Gerster, Sara Hendren, Adam Perez, and Hazel Thompson for balancing critical thinking with levity.

I owe an enormous debt to friends and colleagues who pointed me in directions I wouldn't have gone otherwise. For sharing their knowledge and insights, and for their fact-checking, I am grateful to Chris Beels, Steve Coe, Courtenay Harding, Sam Keith, Ron Manderscheid, and Harvey Rosenthal. On more than one occasion, they saved me from errors. Mistakes remain mine alone.

Friends have shown patience and wisdom beyond reasonable expectation, and I thank Jean Arnold, Carole Artigiani, Margaret Newmark Beels, Basia Kinglake, David Lerner, Andrew Levin, Betty Medsger, Linda Moot, Arlene Notoro Morgan, Denise Rosenberg, Joan Rubinstein, and Bob Scott.

I have heartfelt appreciation for Katie Cadigan and Laura Murray who planted a seed many years ago when they were working on *When Medicine Got It Wrong*; Lisanne Finston, executive director of Gould Farm, where I have been privileged to serve on the board of directors, for modeling how unparalleled leadership promotes recovery; and for thoughtful conversations with Penny Wolfson, whose demand for clarity moved me forward.

Archivists and librarians, guardians of a past undiscovered, took me under their wings to give me access to material even before it was archived. I am grateful to and salute the late Lee Carty at the Judge David L. Bazelon Center for Mental Health Law, to Jules Asher at the National Institute of Mental Health, to Marcia Meldrum at UCLA's Collection of Material on Mental Health Advocacy in California at the Louise M. Darling Biomedical Library History and Special Collections for the Sciences, and to the late Rob Cox at the Special Collections Archives of the W. E. B. Du Bois Library at UMass Amherst. Research assistants in Georgia and Washington have cut through bureaucracies to my benefit, and I thank

Tracey Waldeck at NIMH and Lynn Watson Powers at the Jimmy Carter Presidential Library and Museum.

Friends and family turned research trips into culinary adventures with late-night meditations or early-morning walks, and I appreciate the gracious hospitality of Susan Jaffe, and Marlee and Kenton Clymer in Washington, DC; Megan and Scott Haddock in Rockville, Maryland; Sandi and Shel Rosenblum and Jennifer, Paul, and Elizabeth Nock in Northern California; Sid and Marilyn Pink in Southern California; Chuck and Lorraine Rabideaux in Madison, Wisconsin; and Sam and Susan Keith in Albuquerque, New Mexico, and San Diego, California.

My agent, Anne Edelstein, has provided unstinting encouragement and support to make sure this story is told. At Beacon Press, Amy Caldwell posed just the right question to guide me through more than one impasse, and I am grateful to the entire team for their careful contributions: Marcy Barnes, Perpetua Charles, Nicole-Anne Keyton, Susan Lumenello, Pam MacColl, and Catherine Tung.

My biggest and most profound debt is to my family for giving me the love and the space to make this journey. They know that I know I couldn't have done it without them, starting with my husband Gary who cleared the way, as did our children, Matthew, with Anisha, and Molly, with Kevin, and Teagan. And of course, to BJ, my brother Brian Joel Vine.

A NOTE ON SOURCES

R ESEARCH AND INTERVIEWS for my book *Families in Pain* (1982) generated a trove of records in my personal possession: news clips, white
papers, meeting agendas and handouts, and official and unofficial reports
from numerous organizations. The collection of material grew during the
years I published the site MentalIllnessWatch.org, and it deepened while
researching this book. I am citing these as "courtesy of" the person who
provided them. Some of the official documents are probably in state archives or libraries. For example, Arthur Bolton forwarded material in his
personal files that are surely somewhere in California's vast historical records. In those instances, I provide the document title, date, and all other
material for the treasure hunt. The following people generously provided
these personal records, whether or not they might also be found elsewhere:

Jean Arnold

Arthur Bolton

Neal Brown

Katie Cadigan

Steve Coe

Mike Finkle

Fran Hoffman

Ron Honberg

Laura Murray

Gwill Newman

Eve Oliphant

Vi Orr

Darby Penney

Joseph Rogers

Dan Weisburd

ORGANIZATIONS

Family and former patient groups formed, merged, and changed names.
To simplify, there are places where I have swapped in the generic phrase
"activists" rather than clog the narrative with explanations each time an

organization's name changed. Where the purpose of the organization changed, or a different leadership or constituency evolved, the new name is used.

PEOPLE

Some people changed their name because of divorce, the discovery of birth parents, or a change in personal identity. In those instances, I have included the names by which someone might have been known in parentheses the first time that person appears.

JOURNALS

Throughout I have cited the journal *Psychiatric Services*. When the American Psychiatric Association started publishing this journal in the 1950s, it was called *Mental Hospitals*. Later the name was changed to *Hospital and Community Psychiatry*. In 1995, it became *Psychiatric Services*.

Archives of General Psychiatry was folded into the Journal of the American Medical Association—Psychiatry.

ARCHIVAL RESOURCES AND LIBRARIES

Collection of Material on Mental Health Advocacy in California (Collection 510), Louise M. Darling Biomedical Library History and Special Collections for the Sciences, University of California, Los Angeles: Julie Hoffman Papers

California State Archives, Sacramento, California: Lanterman Papers; Petris Papers; State Government Oral History Program

Special Collections of University Archives, Du Bois Library, University of Massachusetts at Amherst: Behrendt Papers; Chamberlin Papers; Cynthia Miller Papers

National Library of Medicine, Bethesda, Maryland: Bertram S. Brown, MD; Robert Felix, MD

National Institutes of Health and Stetten Museum, Bethesda, Maryland: Minutes of the National Advisory Mental Health Council, 1948–2005; The NIH Record

Jimmy Carter Presidential Library and Museum, Atlanta, Georgia: President's Commission on Mental Health; First Lady's Office; Peter Bourne Papers

Community Access, New York, New York: Howie the Harp Papers
(references to the Harp Papers are courtesy of Community Access
and its former executive director, Steve Coe)
New York Public Library: *Madness Network News* (In 2003, activist
David Gonzalez reprinted the eight volumes that had been published
between 1972 and 1986 to make them available broadly.)

INTERVIEWS

Information attributed to the following people comes from interviews and
conversations that took place over several years for different projects, from
2007 to 2020. Once I focused on a book-length project, interviews took
place over the phone, by way of Skype or Zoom, or in person, often in
restaurants, an office, or a private home. All were recorded with the permission of the informant. Once I started researching this book, initial interviews were commonly followed up with more than one conversation. I
also relied on material drawn from interviewees' personal files and records.

Bill Anthony: August 2009, August 2010 (Boston, MA)
Bernard "Bernie" Arons, MD: March 2010 (Washington, DC), May
2011 (phone)
Jules Asher: June 2009, July 2011 (Rockville, MD)
Eugene Bardach, PhD: March 2020 (phone)
C. Christian Beels, MD: January 2018 (New York City)
Arthur Bolton: August 2008 (phone)
Thom Bornemann: April 2010 (Atlanta, GA)
Peter Bourne, MD: October 2010 (phone)
Bertram Brown, MD: January 2016 (Philadelphia, PA), September 2015,
March 2016, November 2016 (phone)
Lynnae Brown: May 2019 (New York City)
Neal Brown: December 2014 (Rockville, MD), June 2017, October 2019
(phone)
Tom Bryant, MD: January 2010 (Washington, DC)
Dennis Budd and Su Budd: August and September 2014 (phone)
Sylvia Caras: January 2007 (Berkeley, CA)
Gaye Carlson, MD: July 2018 (phone)

William C. Carpenter, MD: November 2009 (phone)
Rosalynn Carter: February 2011 (Atlanta, GA)
Steve Coe: May 2016, April 2019 (New York City)
David Covington: June 2019 (Washington, DC)
Charlie Curie: June 2009 (Washington, DC)
Pat Deegan, PhD: July 2021 (phone)
Ron Diamond, MD: April 2010 (Madison, WI)
Anne Drissel: July 2010 (Washington, DC), December 2016 (phone)
David Ferleger: September and October 2017 (phone)
Mike Finkle: May 2014 (phone), July 2019 (Washington, DC)
Dan Fisher, MD: May 2013, and March and October 2018 (phone)
Laurie Flynn: January 2012 (New York City), October 2012, June
    2015 (phone)
Larry Fricks: August 2011 (Milledgeville, GA)
Lou Gerbino, MD: September 2009 (New York City)
Liz Glass: June 2019 (phone)
Fred Goodwin, MD: January 2009 (Chevy Chase, MD); December 2009,
    July 2011 (phone)
Courtenay Harding, PhD: October 2017 (New York City)
Julie Hoffman: August 2009 (phone)
Mike Hogan, PhD, May 2009 (New York City), January 2011 (phone)
Ron Honberg: March 2010 (Arlington, VA), November 2011 (phone)
Gil Honigfeld, PhD: June 2009, May 2017 (New Jersey)
Lewis Judd, MD: May 2013 (San Diego, CA)
Sam Keith, MD: October 2008, May 2009, June 2009, June 2015 (phone),
    November 2013 (Albuquerque, NM)
Rose King: February 2007, May 2009 (Sacramento, CA)
Martha "Marti" Knisley: November 2019 (phone)
Richard Lamb, MD: September 2013 (Pasadena, CA)
Alan Leshner, PhD: August 2012 (Washington, DC), September 2015 (phone)
Jay Mahler: January 2017 (phone)
Ron Manderscheid, PhD: August and December 2012, November 2014,
    October 2016 (Washington, DC), August 2012 (phone)

Goldie Marx: August 2011 (St. Simons Island, GA)

Gwill Newman: August 2008 (Albuquerque, NM)

Lucy Ozarin, MD: December 2014, (Rockville, MD)

Herbert Pardes, MD: April 2008 (New York City)

Jackie Parrish: December 2010 (phone)

Delores Parron-Ragland, PhD: September 2011 (Rockville, MD)

Darby Penney: July and August 2019 (phone)

Ike Powell: July 2019 (phone)

Judge John Racanelli: July 2017 (New York City)

Mark Ragins, MD: March 2011 (Long Beach, CA)

William Reid, MD: May 2017 (phone)

Estelle Richman, PhD: June 2012 (Washington, DC)

Joseph Rogers: May 2013 (phone)

Harvey Rosenthal: March 2010, June 2018 (phone)

DeWitt Sage: February 2011 (Greenwich, CT)

Leslie Scallet: July 2010 (Washington, DC)

Louis Sokoloff, MD: January 2014 (Rockville, MD)

Lisa St. George: September 2000 (phone)

Steven Sharfstein, MD: May 2009 (Baltimore, MD)

Leonard Stein, MD: April 2010 (phone)

Tanya Temkin: August 2011 (phone)

William TenHoor: August 2010 (phone)

Mary Ann Test, PhD: June 2010 (Madison, WI)

Boswell "Bos" Todd: October 2008 (phone)

E. Fuller Torrey, MD: March 2020 (phone)

Judith Turner-Crowson: July 2013 (Skype)

Richard Van Horn: April 2009, December 2008, December 2010 (phone)

Dan Weisburd: January 2010 (Toluca Lake, CA), December 2010 (phone)

Roger Williams: April 2010 (Madison, WI)

Bev Young: April 2010 (Verona, WI)

Sally Zinman: April 2011, June 2017 (phone)

NOTES

INTRODUCTION
1. *Diagnostic and Statistical Manual of Mental Disorders*, 2nd ed. (Washington, DC: APA Press, 1967), 33.
2. Robert H. Hanna interview by Eli Rubinstein, May 27, 1975, National Institute of Mental Health Oral History Collection, National Library of Medicine, Bethesda, Maryland.
3. John F. Kennedy, "Special Message to Congress on Mental Illness and Mental Retardation," Feb. 5, 1963, President's Office Files, Presidential Papers, John F. Kennedy Library, Boston, Massachusetts.
4. Quoted in Gerald N. Grob and Howard H. Goldman, *The Dilemma of Federal Mental Health Policy: Radical Reform or Incremental Change?* (New Brunswick, NJ: Rutgers University Press, 2006), 36.
5. Robert H. Felix, "Community Mental Health—1963," *American Journal of Orthopsychiatry* 33, no. 5 (1963): 789–95.
6. John Talbott, *The Death of the Asylum* (New York: Grune & Stratton, 1978), 163.
7. Talbott, *Death of the Asylum*, 125, 126, 160.
8. *Psychiatric News* 10, no. 16 (Aug. 20, 1975): 15, 16.
9. Siddhartha Mukherjee, *The Emperor of All Maladies* (New York: Scribner, 2010), 400.
10. Felix, "Community Mental Health—1963."
11. Substance Abuse and Mental Health Services Administration, National Survey on Drug Use and Health Data Review, "Receipt of Services for Substance Use and Mental Health Issues among Adults: Results from the 2016 National Survey on Drug Use and Health," Sept. 2017, https://www.samhsa.gov/data/sites/default/files/NSDUH-DR-FFR2-2016/NSDUH-DR-FFR2-2016.pdf.
12. Jean Addington et al., "Duration of Untreated Psychosis in Community Treatment Settings in the United States," *Psychiatric Services* 66 (July 2015): 753–56; Healthcare Cost and Utilization Project (HCUP), 2014, Agency for Healthcare Research and Quality, www.hcupnet.ahrq.gov.
13. Fred Osher, testimony before the US Senate Committee on the Judiciary, "Breaking the Cycle: Mental Health and the Criminal Justice System," 114th Congress, 2nd session, Feb. 10, 2016, https://www.judiciary.senate.gov/imo/media/doc/02-10-16%20Osher%20Testimony.pdf.
14. Warren Susman, "History and the American Intellectual: Uses of a Usable Past," *American Quarterly* 16, no. 2, part 2 Supplement (Summer 1964): 243–63.
15. Howard Zinn, *A People's History: 1492 to the Present* (New York: HarperPerennial, 1995), 11.
16. Jill Lepore, *These Truths: A History of the United States* (New York: W. W. Norton, 2018), xvi.
17. "Release of the Surgeon General's Report," C-SPAN, Dec. 13, 1999, https://www.c-span.org/video/?154147-1/surgeon-general-report-mental-health.

CHAPTER 1: TEAR 'EM DOWN
1. Earl Warren, *The Memoirs of Chief Justice Earl Warren* (New York: Doubleday, 1977), 175–82; Biennial Report for 1950–1952 State of California Department of Mental Hygiene, California State Library, Sacramento.

2. Special Message on mental illness and mental retardation, Feb. 5, 1963, Papers of John F. Kennedy, Presidential Papers, President's Office Files, Legislative Files, JFK Library, Boston.

3. For a discussion of the association of hospital administrators' meeting in Dallas in 1964, see Albert J. Glass, "The Future of Large Public Mental Hospitals," *Mental Hospitals* (now *Psychiatric Services*) (Jan. 1965): 9–19.

4. Bill Boyarsky, *Big Daddy: Jesse Unruh and the Art of Power Politics* (Berkeley: Regents of the University of California, 2008), 152–62.

5. This and all other unattributed remarks from Arthur Bolton come from conversations and my recorded interview with Arthur Bolton.

6. Hospital conditions are described in Biennial Report for 1950–1952.

7. Disability Rights California, "California Memorial Project, Press Release," Sept. 20, 2010.

8. Author interview with Bolton.

9. This account comes from Arthur Bolton, "Confidential Staff Report Visit to Dewitt State Hospital, July 23, 1964, prepared for Assembly Ways and Means Committee," DeWitt State Hospital, Mental Health Files, Frank D. Lanterman Papers, California State Archives.

10. These descriptions were expanded by author interview with Bolton, and those by Katie Cadigan and Laura Murray, producers of *When Medicine Got It Wrong* (2010), https://itvs.org/films/when-medicine-got-it-wrong.

11. Author interview with Bolton.

12. Cadigan and Murray interview with Bolton.

13. Cadigan and Murray interview with Bolton.

14. California Legislature. Assembly Interim Committee on Ways and Means, Subcommittee on Mental Health Services, Arthur Bolton, et al., *The Dilemma of Mental Health Commitments in California, a Background Document, November 1966*, in author's possession, 3, 5.

15. Bolton, *The Dilemma of Mental Health Commitments in California*, 19.

16. Karl W. Kreplin, "Mental Illness Commitment: A Study of the Decision-Making Process" (PhD diss., University of California at Berkeley, Jan. 1966), 50–51, quoted in Bolton, *The Dilemma*, 35–37.

17. Bolton, *The Dilemma of Mental Health Commitments in California*, 19, 28, 30–31, 40, 105, 126.

18. Author interview with Bolton; Cadigan and Murray interview with Bolton.

19. Author interview with Judge John Racanelli (ret.).

20. Bolton, *The Dilemma of Mental Health Commitments in California*, 43.

21. "Illinois, New York Build Courtrooms in Hospitals," *Psychiatric News* 2, no. 8 (Aug. 1967): 8.

22. Bolton, *The Dilemma of Mental Health Commitments in California*, 11.

23. Dorothy Miller and Michael Schwartz, "County Lunacy Commission Hearings: Some Observations of Commitments to a State Mental Hospital," *Social Problems* 14, no. 1 (Summer 1966): 26–35.

24. Author interview with Bolton.

25. F. Theodore Reid Jr., MD, and Leon Kuhs, MD, "Training a Ward Team in a Therapeutic Community," *Psychiatric Services* 17, no. 12 (Dec. 1966): 349–54.

26. Bolton, *The Dilemma of Mental Health Commitments in California*, 84–85.

27. "New California Commitment Law," *Psychiatric News* (Oct. 14, 1967).

28. Bardach, *Skill Factor*, 101.

29. *Rouse v. Cameron*, 373 F2d 451, US Court of Appeals District of Columbia Circuit, Apr. 4, 1967.

30. Charles Halpern, *Making Waves and Riding the Currents: Activism and the Practice of Wisdom I* (San Francisco: Berrett-Koehler, 2008), 10–24.

31. Patricia M. Wald, "Warehousing vs. Dumping—an Absurd Debate," *Mental Health Law Project Newsletter*, June 1975, in author's possession.

32. *Rouse v. Cameron*.

33. Bardach, *The Skill Factor*, 203.

34. Richard Schmuck, PhD, and Mark Chesler, MA, "Superpatriot Opposition to Community Mental Health Programs," *Community Mental Health Journal* 3, no. 4 (Winter 1967): 382–88.

35. Eugene Bardach, *The Implementation Game: What Happens After a Bill Becomes Law* (Cambridge, MA: MIT Press, 1977), 13.

36. Harry Nelson, "Civil Rights Bill on Mental Health Sets High Goals," *Los Angeles Times*, June 11, 1967.

37. NIMH Director Stanley Yolles to Arthur Bolton, Mar. 13, 1969, Mental Health Files, Lanterman Papers.

38. Jerry Gillam, "Reagan Disputed on Mental Health Care," *New York Times*, Apr. 16, 1967; "Reagan Backs Local Mental Health Plans," *Los Angeles Times*, May 10, 1967; *San Francisco Chronicle*, June 1, 1966, quoted in Bardach, *The Skill Factor*, 31, 143.

39. "We're Here to Speak for Justice: Founding California's Regional Centers," Golden Gate Regional Center, 1999, in author's possession.

40. Quoted in Bardach, *The Skill Factor*, 144.

41. Press release, "Citizen Committee for Improved Treatment in Our State Hospitals," June 13, 1967, Mental Health Files, Psychiatrists, 1967–68, Lanterman Papers. The psychiatry faculty at Stanford University School of Medicine outlined the untoward effects of cutbacks in the first year of Reagan's tenure. A plea for a review and correction was signed by eighteen faculty members on Feb. 1, 1968. Mental Health Files, Psychiatrists, 1967–68, Lanterman Papers.

42. See, for example, *Modesto Bee and News-Herald*, Nov. 19, 1967.

43. Bardach, *The Implementation Game*, 288.

CHAPTER 2: "NOTHING ABOUT US WITHOUT US"

1. Judi Chamberlin, *On Our Own: Patient-Controlled Alternatives to the Mental Health System* (New York: Hawthorne Books, 1978); Shukao Tomao, "The Politics of Psychiatric Experience," master's thesis, University of Massachusetts Amherst, 2014.

2. Chamberlin, *On Our Own*, 22–62.

3. Chamberlin, *On Our Own*, 41.

4. Judi Chamberlin, "Confessions of a Non-Compliant Patient," Chamberlin Papers, Special Collections of University Archives, University of Massachusetts Amherst (SCUA).

5. Chamberlin describes her inpatient experiences in *On Our Own*.

6. Judi Chamberlin "Client Run Alternative Care Models: A Special Workshop with Patients," American Psychiatric Association Conference, May 13, 1986, typescript, Harp Papers, CA.

7. Steve Coe, slide presentation, Utrecht 2013, Harp Papers.

8. Howard Smith, "Scenes," *Village Voice*, June 3, 1971.

9. The discussion of Frank's hospitalization comes from the records he published in *Madness Network News* 2, no. 5 (Dec. 1974): 109–14. In 2003, David Gonzalez issued the eight volumes that were originally published between 1972 and 1986, available at Madnessnetworknews.com. Leonard Roy Frank, "The Crime of Forced 'Treatment,'" presented at the Conference on Refusing Mental Health Treatment: Values in Conflict, Sept. 11, 1981, San Francisco, in Chamberlin Papers.

10. Carl Taub, "Distribution of Psychiatric Beds by Geographic Division, 1970," *Statistical Notes* 45, Department Health, Education, Welfare (DHEW), Apr. 1971; Richard W. Redick, "Changes in the Age, Sex, and Diagnostic Composition of Additions to State and County Mental Hospitals," *Statistical Notes* 117, DHEW, June 1975.

11. "How Madness Network News Came to Be," *Madness Network News* 1 (1974): 2.

12. Sherry Hirsh et al., eds., *Madness Network News Reader* (San Francisco: Glide Publications, 1974), 11.

13. Frank organized the American Association for the Abolition of Involuntary Mental Hospitalization in 1969, which sponsored lawyers, jurists, and Szasz for a panel in San Francisco attended by three hundred people on Oct. 21, 1972. See Leonard Roy Frank, "Thomas Szasz: Freedom Fighter," *Madness Network News* 1, no. 2 (Nov. 1972): 12–13.

14. Leonard R. Frank, "Peter Breggin Visits the Bay Area, " *Madness Network News* 2, no. 1 (1973): 12.

15. Leonard Roy Frank, "The Frank Papers," *Madness Network News* 2, no. 5 (Dec. 1974): 13–17.

16. "Shock Doctor Roster," *Madness Network News* 2, no. 4 (Sept. 1974): 19; "Shock Doctor Roster," *Madness Network News* 5, no. 4 (Spring 1979): 18–19.

17. Edward Shorter and David Healey, *Shock Therapy: A History of Electroconvulsive Treatment in Mental Illness* (New Brunswick, NJ: Rutgers University Press, 2007), 223.

18. Kitty Dukakis and Larry Tye, *Shock: The Healing Power of Electroconvulsive Therapy* (New York: Avery, 2006), 195–210.

19. Subsequently, this technology acquired greater credibility when it was applied to a nonresponsive heart to bring patients back to life (cardiac defibrillation). For a review of ECT, see Laura Hirshbein and Sharmalie Sarvananda, "History, Power, and Electricity: American Popular Magazine Accounts of Electroconvulsive Therapy, 1940–2005," *Journal of the History of the Behavioral Sciences* 44, no. 1 (Winter 2008): 1–18, http://deepblue.lib.umich.edu/bitstream/handle/2027.42/57903/20283_ftp.pdf?sequence=1.

20. Arthur Bolton et al., *The Dilemma of Mental Health Commitments in California, a Background Document*, Nov. 1966, in author's possession, 67–68.

21. This was reported by the American Psychiatric Association. See Jean Dietz, "ECT Study Reveals Disparity Between Public, Private Units," *Psychiatric News* 10, no. 15 (Aug. 6, 1975): 1.

22. "NAPA Notes," *Madness Network News* 3, no. 1 (Apr. 1975): 18–19.

23. See Frank's interview with Bruce Ennis in *Madness Network News* 2, no. 2 (Feb. 1974): 10–15.

24. Harry Nelson, "Psychiatrists to Fight Shock Therapy Law," *Los Angeles Times*, Dec. 19, 1974; "California Enacts Rigid Shock Therapy Controls," *Psychiatric News* 10, no. 3 (Feb. 5, 1975): 1.

25. Vasconcellos's bill required full disclosure of risks, informed consent, exclusion of involuntary patients, and prior approval of a committee of three physicians. Similar criteria applied to medication. It was far more extensive than any reform to date.

26. Paul Fredric Slawson, MD, "Psychiatric Malpractice: The California Experience," *American Journal of Psychiatry* 136, no. 5 (May 1979): 650–54.

27. Nearly three thousand people responded. See APA Task Force 14, *ECT, Electroconvulsive Therapy* (1978), http://www.ectresources.org/ECTscience/APA_ECT_Task_Force_1978_3_-4.pdf.

28. APA Task Force, *ECT*, 3.

29. See Robert Whitaker, *Anatomy of an Epidemic: Magic Bullets, Psychiatric Drugs, and the Astonishing Rise of Mental Illness in America* (New York: Broadway Paperbacks, 2010).

30. Frank D. Allman to Editors, *Madness Network News* 2, no. 3 (June 1974): 20.

31. Judi Chamberlin, Janet Gotkin, Anthony Brandt, and Wade Hudson testimony, Senate Subcommittee of the Committee of the Judiciary, "Abuse and Misuse of Controlled Drugs in Juvenile Institutions," 94th Congress, 1st session, Aug. 18, 1975, 166–84.

32. Department of Health, Education, and Welfare, National Commission for the Protection of Human Subjects of Biomedical and Behavioral Research, *Report and Recommendations Psychosurgery* (Washington, DC: Government Printing Office, 1977).

33. V. H. Mark, MD, W. H. Sweet, MD, and F. R. Ervin, MD, "Role of Brain Disease in Riots and Urban Violence," *Journal of the American Medical Association* 201, no. 11 (Sept. 11, 1967): 895.

34. The stories appeared in local as well as national media: David Holmstron, "Psychosurgery: New Doubts," *Christian Science Monitor*, May 4, 1972; in the *Los Angeles Times*: "Proposals for Surgery on Convicts Rejected," Dec. 26, 1971; "Brain Surgery for Criminals," Dec. 28, 1971; Harry Nelson, "Psychosurgery Controversy Triggers Protest," Apr. 16, 1973; Stuart Auerbach, "VA Surgery to Alter Behavior Done 16 Times, Despite Warning," June 12, 1973; Jane Brody, "Psychosurgery Myriad Tough Questions," *New York Times*, Mar. 18, 1973; "Is a Convict's Brain Really His Own?," Apr. 2, 1972, *Washington Post*.

35. "Dangers of Violence Center," *Madness Network News* 1, no. 6 (n.d.): 1, 3.

36. Williford Stanley, "Blacks Figure in Struggle over UCLA Center," *Los Angeles Times*, Aug. 2, 1973.

37. The APA weighed in early. See Jeffrey Gillenkirk, "Lehmann Defends Psychosurgery, Blasts Critics," *Psychiatric News* 7, no. 16 (Aug. 16, 1972): 1; Senate Subcommittee on Health, Committee on Labor and Public Welfare, Quality of Health Care, Human Experimentation, 1972, 93_91 (Feb. 23 and Mar. 6, 1973).

38. Harry Nelson, "Psychosurgery Controversy Triggers Protest," *Los Angeles Times*, Aug. 16, 1973.

39. Walter Freeman claimed personal responsibility for 3,500 of the 50,000 lobotomies in the years after World War II. By the 1970s, he had become a source of embarrassment, not pride. For a panel discussion about Freeman, see PBS transcripts at http://www.pbs.org/wgbh/american experience/features/transcript/lobotomist-transcript.

40. On the results of the procedure, see the review article by Edward Hitchcock and Varier Cairns, "Amygdalotomy," *Postgraduate Medical Journal* (Dec. 1973): 49, 894–904. More extensive discussion justifying the procedure can be found in M. Hunter Brown, "Brain Surgery Can Help Rehabilitate Criminals," *Los Angeles Times*, Jan. 22, 1972; Lothar B. Kalinowsky, MD, "Psychosurgery Said to Help in Certain Neuroses," *Psychiatric News* 6, no. 7 (Apr. 7, 1971): 3; "Psychosurgery Hailed in Experimental Texas Study," *Psychiatric News* 5, no. 18 (Dec. 16, 1970): 1; Tanya Temkin, "Psychosurgery Approved," *Madness Network News* 5, no. 3 (Winter 1979): 6.

41. Constance Holden, "Psychosurgery: Legitimate Therapy or Laundered Lobotomy?" *Science* 179, no. 4078 (Mar. 16, 1973): 1109–12. By the 1970s, phenothiazines, heavy tranquilizers, had replaced lobotomies to manage out-of-control emotions of ward patients.

42. HEW, Protection of Human Subjects, *Federal Register* 42, no. 99 (May 23, 1977): 26321.

43. Senate Subcommittee on Health and Scientific Research of the Committee on Human Resources, "Project MKULTRA, the CIA's Program of Research in Behavioral Modification," 95th Congress, 1st session, Aug. 3, 1977.

44. Temkin, "Psychosurgery Approved," 6, 10, 22.

45. Author interviews with Su Budd and Dennis Budd.

46. Flyer, typescript, Chamberlin Papers.

47. Author interviews with Su Budd and Dennis Budd.

48. Don Weitz, "I Will Be Me," *Madness Network News* 2, no. 5 (Dec. 1974): 125–27.

49. David Ferleger, "Loosing the Chains: In-Hospital Civil Liberties of Mental Patients," 13 *Santa Clara Lawyer* 447 (1973), http://digitalcommons.law.scu.edu/lawreview/vol13/iss3/5.

50. Author interviews with David Ferleger.

51. Author interviews with David Ferleger. The local Philadelphia press covered this extensively.

52. *Downs v. Department of Public Welfare*, trial transcript, quoted in David A. Ferleger and Patrice M. Scott, "Rights and Dignity: Congress, the Supreme Court, and People with Disabilities after Pennhurst," *Western New England Law Review* 55, no. 3 (1982–83): 327–61. Also see interview by Lisa Sonneborn, Temple University Institute on Disabilities, "Visionary Voices: David Ferleger," Jan. 13, 2013, https://disabilities.temple.edu/voices/interviews/ferleger.

53. *Rogers v. Okin*, 478 F. Supp. 1342 (1979).

54. "The Boston Conference," *Madness Network News* 4, no. 1 (Oct. 1976): 1–7; Neil Miller, "Marchers Seek Mental Patients' Rights," *Gay Community News*, n.d., Chamberlin Papers; Janet Gotkin, "Fourth Nat'l Conference on Human Rights & Psychiatric Oppression," *Radical Therapist* (Sept. 1976).

55. [Griffith Park] Conference on Human Rights and Psychiatric Oppression, 1977, series 2, box 6, Chamberlin Papers.

56. "The L.A. Conference . . . Su Budd," *Madness Network News* 4, no. 5 (Winter 1978): 10.

57. Judi Chamberlin testimony, Senate Judiciary Subcommittee to Investigate Juvenile Delinquency, 93rd Congress, 2nd session, Aug. 18, 1975, 166–84.

58. Typescript MPLF, "Statement from the Mental Patients' Liberation Front Regarding the Department of Mental Health Regulation 7.03, 'confidentially of records'—Public Hearings—January 28, 1976," box 34, Chamberlin Papers.

59. "Ex-Mental Patient Denied Records by Brooklyn Judge," *New York Times*, July 25, 1974.

60. "DMH Hearing—June 10, 1977," box 34, Chamberlin Papers.

61. The 1978 correspondence between Chamberlin and Roy Menninger and Karl Menninger is in Chamberlin Papers.

62. Author telephone interview with Sally Zinman.

63. "The L.A. Conference . . . Sally Zinman," *Madness Network News* 4, no. 5 (Winter 1978): 11.

64. Chamberlin to Temkin, Apr. 17, 1978, box 4, Chamberlin Papers.

65. Chamberlin to Temkin, Apr. 19, 1978, and "APA Annual Meeting," Chamberlin Papers.

66. "Reports from APA: Psychiatrists Listen to Mental Health Consumers," *ADAMHA News*, June 15, 1978.

67. Author interview with Tanya Temkin.

68. "Reports from APA."

CHAPTER 3: BUILDING OPPORTUNITIES FOR COMMUNITY CARE

1. Author interview with Mary Ann Test.

2. Paul Polak, "The Irrelevance of Hospital Treatment to the Patient's Social System," *Psychiatric Services* (Aug. 1971): 255-56; Richard M. Eisler and Paul Polak, "Social Stress and Psychiatric Disorder," *Journal of Nervous and Mental Disease* 153, no. 4 (Oct. 1971): 227-33. Fort Logan received considerable attention between 1961 and 1974 when politics redirected money to other programs in Colorado. This description comes from Frederick A. Lewis and Alan M. Kraft, "Fort Logan: A Community-Oriented Program," *Psychiatric Services* 13, no. 3 (Mar. 1962): 154-57; "The Versatile Program at Fort Logan Mental Health Clinic," *Psychiatric Services* 15, no. 10 (Oct. 1964): 552-54; Alan M. Kraft et al., "The Community Mental Health Program and the Longer-Stay Patient," *Archives of General Psychiatry* 16, no. 1 (Jan. 1967): 64-70.

3. Jack Zusman, "Some Explanations of the Changing Appearance of Psychotic Patients: Antecedents of the Social Breakdown Syndrome," *Milbank Memorial Fund Quarterly* 44, no. 1, part 2 (Jan. 1966): 363-94; George R. Metcalf, "The English Open Mental Hospital: Implications for American Psychiatric Services," *Milbank Memorial Fund Quarterly* 39, no. 4 (Oct. 1961): 579-93.

4. Felix's thinking is apparent in his many articles and conference presentations. See "Mental Disorders as a Public Health Problem," *American Journal of Psychiatry* 106, no. 6 (Dec. 1949): 401-6. Felix's 1956 address to the American Psychiatric Association meetings discussed NIMH's responsibility to assist the states. See "Evolution of Community Mental Health Concepts," *American Journal of Psychiatry* 113, no. 8 (Feb. 1957): 673-79.

5. Leo Srole et al., *Midtown Manhattan Study* (New York: McGraw Hill, 1962). This study became a landmark for its methodology of surveying families at home, as well as for its findings about the prevalence of psychiatric disturbance based on social class. The study's originator, a psychiatrist named Thomas C. Rennie, had been mentored by Adolph Meyer at Johns Hopkins, as had Robert Felix. At the time of his death, at the age of fifty-two, Rennie was becoming the foremost proponent of community psychiatry at New York's Cornell Hospital.

6. Daniel M. Fox, "The Significance of the Milbank Memorial Fund for Policy: An Assessment at Its Centennial," *Milbank Quarterly* 84, no. 1 (2006): 5-36; Melly Simon, Dorothy G. Wiehl, Katharine Berry, and Ernest M. Gruenberg, "Inquiries to a Mental Health Association Concerning Treatment Facilities," *Milbank Memorial Fund Quarterly* 38, no. 4 (Oct. 1960): 301-61.

7. Public Health Service [NIMH] National Advisory Mental Health Council, Minutes of the Thirty-Sixth Meeting, Nov. 1958, Office of NIH History and Stetten Museum, Bethesda, Maryland.

8. J. F. Wilder, G. Levin, and I. Zwerling, "A Two-Year Follow-up Evaluation of Acute Psychotic Patients Treated in a Day Hospital," *American Journal of Psychiatry* 122Sc (1966): 1095-1101; C. Christian Beels, "Family and Social Management of Schizophrenia," *Schizophrenia Bulletin* 1, no. 13 (Summer 1975): 97-118. Also see Frank R. Scarpitti et al., "Home versus Hospital Care," *Archives of General Psychiatry* 187, no. 3 (Feb. 1964): 143-54.

9. National Advisory Mental Health Council, Minutes of the 42nd Meeting, Nov. 28-30, 1960.

10. See National Advisory Mental Health Council, Minutes of the 39th Meeting, Nov. 16-18, 1959; Forty-Second Meeting, Mar. 7-8, 1960; Forty-First Meeting, June 20-22, 1960.

11. Robert H. Felix interview by Eli Rubinstein, May 27, 1975, National Institute of Mental Health Oral History Collection, National Library of Medicine, Bethesda, Maryland.

12. Paul R. Binner, "Evaluating the Effectiveness of Mental Health Services," and Paul Polak, "Unclean Research and Clinical Change," in Ernest Greunberg, ed., "Evaluation of the Dutchess County Services," *Milbank Memorial Fund Quarterly* 44, no. 1 (1966): 1-193, http://www.jstor.org /stable/3349068.

13. Author interview with Mary Ann Test.

14. Arnold M. Ludwig and Frank Farrelly, "The Code of Chronicity," *Archives of General Psychiatry* 15, no. 6 (Dec. 1966): 562–68. For background to chronicity, see Zusman's discussion in "Some Explanations." The most prominent of these studies is by Erving Goffman, who wrote about the mechanisms producing this adaptability, based on research conducted at St. Elizabeths Hospital. See Goffman, *Asylums: Essays on the Social Situation of Mental Patients and Other Inmates* (New York: Anchor, 1961).

15. Ludwig and Farrelly, "The Code of Chronicity." Also see Zusman, "Some Explanations of the Changing Appearance of Psychotic Patients."

16. Ludwig and Farrelly, "The Code of Chronicity"; Sue Estroff, *Making It Crazy: An Ethnography of Psychiatric Clients in an American Community* (Berkeley: University of California Press, 1981), discusses the social learning of patients.

17. "Prevention of Chronicity Through 'Community Treatment,'" typescript, State Division of Mental Health Research Grant, Fall 1970, courtesy of Mary Ann Test.

18. Arnold M. Ludwig, MD, and Arnold J. Marx, MD, "Influencing Techniques of Chronic Schizophrenics," *Archives of General Psychiatry* 18, no. 6 (June 1968): 681–88.

19. Author interview with Mary Ann Test. Also see "Reflections on 'PACT' and Intensive Community-Based Care," *Journal of the California Alliance for the Mentally Ill* 9, no. 1 (1998): 31–33.

20. Test, "Reflections on 'PACT.'"

21. For a good summary of the literature, see Mary Ann Test and Leonard Stein, "Community Treatment of the Chronic Patient: Research Overview," *Schizophrenia Bulletin* 4, no. 3 (1978): 350–64.

22. William A. Anthony, Mikal R. Cohen, and Ray Vitalo, "The Measurement of Rehabilitation Outcome," *Schizophrenia Bulletin* 4, no. 3 (1978): 365–83.

23. Polak, "The Irrelevance of Hospital Treatment," 554.

24. See George Fairweather, ed., Social Psychology in Treating Mental Illness: An Experimental Approach (New York: John Wiley & Sons, 1964).

25. Mary Ann Stein and Leonard Test pointed to some of the thinking that influenced their work in 1976. B. Weinman, R. Sanders, R. Kleiner, and S. Wilson, "Community-Based Treatment of the Chronic Psychotic," *Community Mental Health Journal* 6 (1970): 13–21.

26. Arnold J. Marx, Mary Ann Test, and Leonard I. Stein, "Extrahospital Management of Severe Mental Illness," *Archives of General Psychiatry* 29 (Oct. 1973): 505–11. Stein describes this growing awareness and change in perceptions in Leonard I. Stein and Alberto B. Santos, *Assertive Community Treatment of Persons with Severe Mental Illness* (New York: Norton, 1998). See also Geraldine M. Koonce, "Social Work with Mental Patients in the Community," *Social Work* 18, no. 3 (May 1973): 30–34.

27. Marx et al., "Extrahospital Management."

28. Leonard I. Stein and Mary Ann Test, "Retraining Hospital Staff for Work in a Community Program in Wisconsin," *Psychiatric Services* 27, no. 4 (1976): 266–68: Stein and Santos, *Assertive Community Treatment of Persons with Severe Mental Illness.*

29. Stein and Santos, *Assertive Community Treatment of Persons with Severe Mental Illness*, 24.

30. Comptroller General's Report to Congress, *Returning the Mentally Disabled to the Community: Government Needs to Do More* (Washington, DC: Government Printing Office, 1977), 22.

31. Author interview with Bev Young.

32. *Making It Crazy* was based on Estroff's doctoral dissertation.

33. Estroff, *Making It Crazy*, chap. 4, 48.

34. "APA Gold Award," *Psychiatric Services* 25, no. 10 (1974): 660.

35. "The Impact of Redeployment of Funds on a Model State Hospital," *Psychiatric Services* 26, no. 9 (Sept. 1975): 554–56.

36. Ford used his veto power so frequently and aggressively that majority leader Thomas P O'Neill Jr. (D-MA) quipped that he was proud of them. See Richard D. Lyons, "Congress Overrides Ford's Veto of Bill on Social Services," *New York Times*, Oct. 1, 1976.

37. For example, see the National Advisory Mental Health Council, Minutes of the Ninety-Sixth meeting, Dec. 2–3, 1974, and the Ninety-Seventh Meeting, Mar. 17–18, 1975.

38. Lucy C. Ozarin, "Community Mental Health Center Activity in Rehabilitation," *International Journal of Mental Health* 3, nos. 2–3 (Summer–Fall 1974): 147–52.

39. Committee on Interstate and Foreign Commerce Subcommittee on Health and the Environment, "Community Support for Mental Patients," 96th Congress, 1st session, Oct. 11, 1979, 77–115.

40. Saul Feldman, "Community Mental Health Centers: A Decade Later," in "Community Mental Health: Problems and Prospects," ed. Phillip E. Jacobs and Saul Feldman, special issue, *International Journal of Mental Health* 3, nos. 2–3 (Summer–Fall 1974): 19–34, http://www.jstor.org /stable/41343995.

41. The conference informed the articles appearing in John Talbott, ed., *The Chronic Mental Patient: Problems, Solutions, and Recommendations for a Public Policy* (Washington, DC: American Psychiatric Association, 1978).

42. Judith Clark Turner and William J. TenHoor, "The NIMH Community Support Program: Pilot Approach to a Needed Social Reform," *Schizophrenia Bulletin* 4, no. 3 (Jan. 1978): 328.

43. Author interview with Anne Drissel (known at the time as Anne McCuan), 2016.

44. Author interview with Judy Turner-Crowson.

45. Draft report of NIMH working conference on "Community Support for the Mentally Disabled," Arlington, Virginia, typescript, Jan. 13–15, 1976, 12, courtesy of Bill TenHoor.

46. Author interview with Mary Ann Test.

47. Jeffrey L. Geller, "The Last Half-Century of Psychiatric Services as Reflected in Psychiatric Services," *Psychiatric Services* 51, no. 1 (Jan. 2000): 41–67.

48. Draft report, "Community Support for the Mentally Disabled."

49. *Government Needs to Do More*, 26, i.

50. *Government Needs to Do More*, i.

51. *Government Needs to Do More*, 22–23.

52. Dixon v. Weinberger, 405 F Supp. 974 (D.D.C. 1975).

53. Department of Health and Human Services, "Alternatives to Hospitalization," in *A Network for Caring: Summary Proceedings of Four National Conferences, 1978–79* (Washington, DC: Government Printing Office, 1982), 83–84.

54. Bryce MacLennan, "A Week's Worth," *GAO Review* (Fall 1980): 55–57.

55. B. Stone, B. TenHoor, and J. Turner, Draft: Report of the HIP/HSD Task Force to DMHSP (NIMH), Dec. 12, 1976, courtesy of Bill TenHoor.

56. Author interview with Anne Drissel, 2016.

57. See *A Network for Caring*, 2–3.

58. Joseph P. Morrissey and Howard H. Goldman, "Cycles of Reform in the Care of the Chronically Mentally Ill," *Psychiatric Services* 35, no. 8 (Aug. 1984): 785–93.

59. Paul Polak, Michael Kirby, and Walter Deitchman, "Treating Acutely Psychotic Patients in Private Homes," *New Directions for Mental Health Care* 1 (1979): 62.

60. Turner and TenHoor, "The NIMH Community Support Program."

61. Department of Health and Human Services, ADAMHA, National Advisory Mental Health Council, Mar. 2–3, 1981, National Institutes of Health and Stetten Museum, Bethesda, Maryland.

62. Mary Ann Test and Leonard Stein, "Use of Special Living Arrangements—A Model for Decision Making," typescript, NIMH Conference, Sept. 22–24, 1976, box 20, PCMH, Carter Library.

63. Quoted in Turner and TenHoor, "The NIMH Community Support Program."

64. Leonard Stein and Mary Ann Test, "The Evolution of the Training in Community Living Model," *New Directions* 26 (1985): 7–16.

65. Gary Bond et al., "Assertive Community Treatment: Correcting Some Misconceptions," *American Journal of Community Psychology* 19, no. 1 (1991): 41–51.

66. Health and Human Services, "Alternatives to Hospitalization," 83.

67. Morrissey and Goldman, "Cycles of Reform in the Care of the Chronically Mentally Ill"; William A. Anthony and Andrea Blanch, "Research on Community Support Services: What Have We Learned," *Psychosocial Rehabilitation Journal* 12, no. 2 (Jan. 1989): 55–81.

CHAPTER 4: BECAUSE OF OUR SONS

1. *When Medicine Got It Wrong* (2010), https://itvs.org/films/when-medicine-got-it-wrong. The chronology of Brett Oliphant's treatment throughout this chapter comes from his mother's interview with Katie Cadigan and Laura Murray, and from Eve Oliphant's typescript chronology, [1973], in the Collection of Material on Mental Health Advocacy in California (Collection 510), Louise M. Darling Biomedical Library History and Special Collections for the Sciences, University of California, Los Angeles. I had also interviewed PAS leaders, including Eve Oliphant and Fran and Tony Hoffman, for my book *Families in Pain: Children, Siblings, Spouses, and Parents of the Mentally Ill Speak Out* (New York: Pantheon, 1982). The Hoffmans subsequently sent me material from which this is also drawn, identified as "author's private collection."

2. "San Mateo AMI," typescript, History of Mental Health, UCLA Archives.

3. Author phone interview with Julie Hoffman.

4. Vine, *Families in Pain*, 222.

5. Katie Cadigan and Laura Murray interview with Marian Russell in *When Medicine Got It Wrong*.

6. Fran Hoffman, PAS Newsletter, History of Mental Health, UCLA Archives.

7. "San Mateo AMI."

8. Tony Hoffman interview Mar. 1975 with author for *Families in Pain*.

9. Tony Hoffman interview.

10. PAS position paper, Feb. 19, 1975, History of Mental Health, UCLA Archives.

11. Richard Lamb, "The APA Conference on the Chronic Mental Patient: A Defining Moment," *Psychiatric Services* 51, no. 7 (2000): 874–78.

12. Tony Hoffman, application for Ad-Hoc Faculty for Madison Conference, Hoffman Papers, UCLA Archives.

13. PAS to George Pickett, MD, Director of Public Health and Welfare (San Mateo), Nov. 20, 1974, in author's possession.

14. PAS Newsletter, Dec. 1975, History of Mental Health, UCLA Archives.

15. Advertisement for Mateo Lodge, n.d., History of Mental Health, UCLA Archives.

16. PAS Newsletter, Nov. 1975, History of Mental Health, UCLA Archives.

17. Mrs. Frances Hoffman, Mar. 6, 1974, in "Case Histories," History of Mental Health, UCLA Archives.

18. H. R. Lamb, "The New Asylums in the Community," *Archives of General Psychiatry* 36, no. 2 (1979): 129–34.

19. H. Richard Lamb, "Alternatives to Hospitals," in John A. Talbott, MD., ed., *The Chronic Mental Patient Five Years Later* (New York: Grune & Stratton, 1984), 215–33.

20. Richard Lamb, Tony Hoffman, Fran Hoffman, and Eve Oliphant, "No Place for Schizophrenics—The Unwelcome Consumer Speaks Out," *Psychiatric Annals* 6 (Dec. 1976): 39–47; *When Medicine Got It Wrong*. See also Hoffman Papers, UCLA Archives.

21. Vera Graham, "Peninsula's 'Little Lady,'" *San Mateo Times*, Aug. 25, 1977. Oliphant and PAS owed these opportunities to Lamb who was steadfast in his support for families throughout his career.

22. Author interview with Bev Young.

23. Author interview with Young.

24. Author interview with Ron Diamond, MD.

25. Author interview with Diamond.

26. Young to Oliphant, Aug. [22], 1978, History of Mental Health, UCLA Archives.

27. Lamb to Menninger, n.d., History of Mental Health, UCLA Archives.

28. Author interview with Young.

29. Harriet Shetler, ed., "A History of the National Alliance for the Mentally Ill" (NAMI, 1986), in author's possession.

30. Agnes Hatfield, "Keynote: The Family and the Chronically Mentally Ill," Madison, Wisconsin, Sept. 1979, in author's possession.

31. C. Christian Beels, "Social Networks, the Family, and the Schizophrenic Patient," *Schizophrenia Bulletin* 4, no. 4 (1978): 512–21.

32. Hatfield, interview in *When Medicine Got It Wrong.*
33. Hatfield, interview in *When Medicine Got It Wrong.*
34. Author interview with Young.
35. Judi Chamberlin, "The National Alliance for the 'Mentally Ill': Parents' Groups as Advocates," *Madness Network News* 5, no. 6 (Winter 1980): 5–6.
36. Author interview with Vi Orr, Nov. 2008; email communication from Vi Orr, Mar. 4, 2010; interview with Young.
37. Chamberlin, "The National Alliance for the 'Mentally Ill': Parents' Groups as Advocates."
38. Harriet Shetler to Judi Chamberlin, n.d., Chamberlin Papers.
39. Herbert Pardes, "NIMH Initiatives for the Chronically Mentally Ill," in *Proceedings of a National Conference: Advocacy for Persons with Chronic Mental Illness: Building a Nationwide Network,* ed. Roger T. Williams and Harriet M. Shetler, typescript, Sept. 7–9, 1979, 51–57, in author's possession.
40. Author interview with Young.
41. From Missouri came George Hecker, NAMI's newly chosen board president; and from New York, Irving Blumberg, an activist parent, rounded out the threesome.
42. Starr describes the visit in Shetler, "A History of the National Alliance for the Mentally Ill," 11.
43. Shetler, "A History of the National Alliance for the Mentally Ill," 9.
44. Pardes, "Looking for New Initiatives," in Department of Health and Human Services, *A Network for Caring,* 25–26.

CHAPTER 5: A FIRST LADY'S LAW
1. Rosalynn Carter, *First Lady from Plains* (Boston: Houghton Mifflin, 1984). Also see her later book, with Susan K. Golant, *Helping Someone with Mental Illness: A Compassionate Guide for Family, Friends, and Caregivers* (New York: Times Books, 1999), chap. 1.
2. Descriptions of Georgia Central State come from Peter Cranford, *But for the Grace of God: Milledgeville! The Inside Story of the World's Largest Insane Asylum,* repr. (Atlanta: Georgia Consumer Council, 2005).
3. Author interview with Goldie Marx.
4. Carter, *First Lady from Plains,* 95–97; Rosalynn Carter's Special Projects and Events Files, box 131, memo, Office of the Governor, Weds., Sept. 8, 1971, Georgia Department of Public Health, box 134 (July 26, 1971), Jimmy Carter Presidential Library (hereafter Carter Library).
5. Rosalynn Carter to Mrs. Eugene Adams, Feb. 16, 1971; Mrs. Amelia Barn memo, May 20, 1971, box 131, First Lady's Office (FLO), Central State Hospital, Carter Library.
6. "Rosalynn Carter's Statement on Mental Health" (draft), Oct. 15, 1976, Bakersfield, California, Peter Bourne Papers, Carter Library.
7. "Wife Says Carter Will Set Up Mental Health Panel," *New York Times,* Nov. 20, 1976.
8. Thomas E. Bryant, MD, to Dr. Peter G. Bourne, Feb. 9, 1977, box 28, Bourne Papers, Carter Library.
9. See Peter Bourne, *Jimmy Carter: A Comprehensive Biography from Plains to Post-Presidency* (New York: Scribner, 1997), 241–42, 412–35.
10. Author interview with Peter Bourne.
11. Tom Bryant to Peter Bourne, "Organizing the President's Commission on Mental Health," Feb. 21, 1977, box 28, Bourne Papers, Carter Library.
12. Bryant to Bourne, "Organizing the President's Commission."
13. There are several nominating letters Dr. Bert Brown received in February 1977 while he was director of NIMH. See box 139, Bertram Brown Papers, History of Medicine Division, NLM.
14. "Firing of NIMH Director Bert Brown Reflects Califano Policy and Style," *Science* 199, no. 4326 (Jan. 20, 1978): 218–80.
15. Coates Redmond to Mary Hoyt, Apr. 1, 1977, box 8, FLO-Cade, Carter Library; "Meeting of the President's Commission on Mental Health," Apr. 19, 1977, box 1, PCMH files, Carter Library. Also see Gerald Grob, "Public Policy and Mental Illness: Jimmy Carter's Presidential Commission," *Milbank Memorial Quarterly* 83, no. 3 (Sept. 2005): 425–56.

16. [Beatrix "Betty" Hamburg, MD], "Mental Health in America: Scope and Limits of the Challenge," typescript, n.d., box 1, PCMH files, Carter Library.

17. Priscilla Allen, "Meeting of the President's Commission on Mental Health," Mar. 29, 1977, box 8, FLO-Cade, PCMH, Carter Library.

18. Chamberlin, "President's Commission on Mental Health," *Madness Network News* 4, no. 3 (Summer 1977): [n.p.].

19. Robert Mackay, "Mental Hospital Is One Without Bars," *Journal and Guide* (Norfolk, VA), May 14, 1977.

20. Priscilla Allen to Tom Bryant, Apr. 26, 1977, box 20, FLO-Cade, PCMH, Carter Library.

21. President's Commission on Mental Health, Tucson, Arizona, transcripts, June 20, 1977, Ricardo A. Samaniego, 139–48, box 11, FLO-Cade, PCMH Hearings, Carter Library.

22. President's Commission on Mental Health, Tucson, Arizona, transcripts, June 20, 1977, Joy Tuxford, 157–64.

23. President's Commission on Mental Health, Philadelphia, transcripts, May 24, 1977, Bob Harris, 41–49, box 10, FLO-Cade, PCMH Hearings, Carter Library.

24. President's Commission on Mental Health, Nashville, transcripts, May 25, 1977, Judi Chamberlin, transcripts, box 12, PCMH, 275–89, Carter Library.

25. Judi Chamberlin, "Resolution to President Carter," *Madness Network News* 4, no. 5 (Winter 1978): 21.

26. The President's Commission heard from George Moscone, Tanya Temkin, Ted Chabasinski, Frank Morain, and Frank Lanterman. All references to the San Francisco hearings come from June 21–22 transcripts in box 17, PCMH Hearings, Carter Library.

27. "Organization of Interim Report, September 1, 1977," box 8, FLO-Cade, PCMH, Carter Library.

28. John M. was the first person the commission discussed when it met January 18–20, 1978, at the Wingspread Conference in Wisconsin to iron out the health service issues before delivering the report to President Carter. See "Outline Long Term/Short Term," box 16, PCMH, Carter Library; *Report to the President from the President's Commission on Mental Health*, vol. 1 (Washington, DC: Government Printing Office, 1978), 12.

29. For detailed analysis of the President's Commission on Mental Health and the work of the task panels, see Henry A. Foley and Steven S. Sharfstein, *Madness and Government: Who Cares for the Mentally Ill* (Washington, DC: American Psychiatric Press, 1983); Gerald N. Grob and Howard H. Goldman, *The Dilemma of Federal Mental Health Policy: Radical Reform or Incremental Change?* (New Brunswick, NJ: Rutgers University Press, 2007); Richard G. Frank and Sherry A. Glied, *Better but Not Well: Mental Health Policy in the United States Since 1950* (Baltimore: Johns Hopkins University Press, 2006).

30. All the networks carried this story—Bill Lynch on NBC, Peter Jennings on ABC, and Robert MacNeil and Jim Lehrer on PBS, Apr. 27, 1978.

31. [1] Marjorie Hunter, "Carter Backs a $500 Million Plan to Improve Mental Health Care," *New York Times*, Apr. 27, 1978.

32. National Advisory Mental Health Council, Minutes of the 107th Meeting, Jan. 24–25, 1977. A study of foreign-born psychiatrists in January 1975 showed the greatest number had come from the Philippines, followed by India, Cuba, and South Korea. See Joan Jenkins, PhD, and Michael Witkin, "Foreign Medical Graduates Employed in State and County Mental Hospitals," Division of Biometry and Epidemiology, *Mental Health Statistical Note* 13 (July 1976); Herbert Pardes, Address to the Psychiatric Research Society, Sept. 27, 1980, box 2, FLO-Cade, Carter Library.

33. President's Commission on Mental Health, *Report to the President from the President's Commission on Mental Health*, vol. 1 (Washington, DC: Government Printing Office, 1978), 26, 22.

34. Tom Bryant to Stuart Eizenstat, Oct. 9, 1978, box 2, PCMH, Carter Library.

35. Matt Clark, Mary Hager, Elsie B. Washington, Michael Reese, and Pamela Ellis Simons, "The New Snake Pits," *Newsweek*, May 15, 1978, 93–94; Rosalynn Carter, "Mental-Illness Myths," Letters, *Newsweek*, date unknown, both clips in box 2, FLO-Cade, Carter Library.

36. For Kennedy's perception of the tensions with the Carter administration, including differences about national health insurance, see Edward M. Kennedy, *True Compass: A Memoir*

(New York: Twelve, 2009), chap. 18. For Carter's, see Jimmy Carter, *White House Diary* (New York: Farrar, Straus & Giroux, 2010), 325.

37. Memo, Kathy [Cade] to RSC, Nov. 14, 1978; Tom Bryant, memorandum for Mrs. Rosalynn Carter, Oct. 31, 1978, box 41, Domestic Policy Staff: Eizenstat; Kathy [Cade] to RSC, "Call to Secretary Califano," Oct. 9, 1978, all in box 2, FLO-Cade, Carter Library.

38. Tom Bryant to Stuart Eizenstat, Dec. 13, 1978, box 1, FLO-Cade; Tom Bryant to Stuart Eizenstat, Oct. 9, 1978, and Kathy [Cade] to RSC, "Meeting with Secretary Califano," Oct. 26, 1978, box 2, FLO-Cade; Tom Bryant, memorandum for Mrs. Rosalynn Carter, Oct. 31, 1978, box 41, Domestic Policy Staff: Eizenstat, all Carter Library.

39. Tom Bryant to Stuart Eizenstat, Mental Health Budget for FY 1980, box 1, FLO-Cade, Carter Library.

40. Bourne, memorandum for the president, National Health Insurance, Dec. 12, 1977, Peter Bourne Papers, Carter Library.

41. David S. Broder, "Kennedy Exposed Gaping Weakness," *Washington Post*, Dec. 13, 1978; Edward Walsh, "Lackluster," *Washington Post*, Dec. 10, 1978.

42. "John Herling's Labor Letter," vol. 28, no. 51, box 13 (Kennedy), Staff Office-speechwriters, Carter Library; Adam Clymer, "Carter's Clash with Kennedy," *New York Times*, Dec. 13, 1978.

43. Peter Bourne to Hamilton Jordan, Jan. 28, 1979, Peter Bourne Papers, Carter Library. In *White House Diary* Carter described wanting Califano to block Kennedy in Congress because "Kennedy's proposals would be excessively expensive and impossible to pass" (Feb. 23, 1979, 295).

44. Senate Subcommittee on Health and Human Services of the Committee on Labor and Human Resources, "Examination of the Recommendations of the President's Commission on Mental Health: Reappraisal of Mental Health Policy, 1979," 96th Congress, 1st session, Feb. 7, 1979.

45. Marjorie Hunter, "Mrs. Carter, in Capitol Debut, Praised by Kennedy," *New York Times*, Feb. 8, 1979.

46. For a discussion of Rosemary Kennedy's lobotomy, see E. Fuller Torrey, *American Psychosis: How the Federal Government Destroyed the Mental Illness Treatment System* (Oxford: Oxford University Press, 2014), 10–14.

47. House Sub-Committee on Health and the Environment to consider H.R. 4156, "The Mental Health Systems Act," 96th Congress, 1st session, June 14, 1979.

48. Kathy Cade memorandum, "Discussion of the 3/30/79 Draft of the Mental Health Systems Act," box 2, FLO-Cade, Carter Library; Tom Bryant to All Concerned, "New Mental Health Legislation," Apr. 6, 1979, box 18, FLO-Cade, Carter Library.

49. Author interview with Anne Drissel (2016). Also see Foley and Sharfstein, *Madness and Government*.

50. Rosalynn Carter discusses the encounter with a reporter in a C-SPAN interview. See http://firstladies.c-span.org/FirstLady/41/Rosalynn-Carter.aspx. Three drafts of the first lady's speech contain her marginal corrections plus Tom Bryant's comments. This comment comes from the draft titled "APA, May 16, 1979," box 18, FLO-Cade, Carter Library.

51. Sharfstein announced having named Anne McCuan Drissel for this post at the 118th meeting of the National Advisory Mental Health Council, Sept. 18–19, 1979.

52. Mrs. Carter's Scheduling Office, Fact Sheet, Briefing/Reception, Apr. 4, 1979, Cade–Mental Health, box 2, Carter Library.

53. Kathy [Cade] to RSC, "Briefing for the President's Commission . . . ," June 6, 1979; Tom Bryant to RSC, Feb. 23, 1979; Kathy Cade to Mrs. Carter, "Call to Mr. Waxman," June 12, 1979; Kathy [Cade] to RSC, "Status of the Mental Health Systems Act," Aug. 31, 1979, all in box 4, FLO-Cade, Carter Library.

54. Rick Hertzberg, Memorandum for the President, Oct. 7, 1979, box 57, Speechwriters Chronological Files, Carter Library.

55. Kathy [Cade] to RSC, "Mental Health Systems Act," Sept. 28, 1979, box 4, FLO-Cade, Carter Library.

56. Beverly S. Long to Rosalynn [Carter], Oct. 26, 1979; Beverly Long to Kathy [Cade], Oct. 29, 1979; Allan Moltzen to Sen. Kennedy, Nov. 1, 1979, all in box 3, FLO-Cade, Carter Library.

57. Harry Schnibbe to Tom Bryant, Cathy [sic] Cade, Gerry Conner, Oct. 30, 1979, box 3, FLO-Cade, Carter Library.

58. Al McDonald, "Legislative Priorities," Jan. 17, 1980, box 2, FLO-Cade, Carter Library.

59. Kathy [Cade] to RSC, Feb. 22, 1980, box 4, FLO-Cade, Carter Library.

60. Director [Steven Sharfstein], Division of Mental Health Service Programs to Gerry Connor, Special Assistant Office of Health Legislation, Aug. 6, 1980, box 4, FLO-Cade, Carter Library.

61. US Congress, *Congressional Record*, 96th Congress, July 22, 1980, 18952–18957; see also *Congressional Quarterly*, July 1980. A side-by-side comparison of the bills was completed by Steven S. Sharfstein, MD, Director, Division of Mental Health Service Programs, NIMH, "Comparison . . . ," June 12, 1980, 56–60, box 3, FLO-Cade, Carter Library. Many of the fifteen items enumerated in the draft of S. 1177, the Senate's bill, have still not been adopted. For a discussion of the background legal issues as well as the redrafting by the Senate subcommittee, see Leslie Scallet, "Mental Health Law and Public Policy," *Psychiatric Services* 31, no. 9 (Sept. 1980): 614–17; Harrison Donnelly, "Senate Fight Expected over 'Bill of Rights' for Mental Patients," *Congressional Quarterly*, July 12, 1980, 1949. Also see Foley and Sharfstein, *Madness and Government*.

62. White House Schedule for Signing of the Mental Health Bill, box 4, Staff Office, Carter Library.

63. Peter [Bourne] to Rosalynn [Carter], Oct. 3, 1980, Bourne Collection, Carter Library.

CHAPTER 6: WITH BLINDERS ON

1. Rosalynn Carter, *First Lady from Plains* (Boston: Houghton Mifflin, 1984), 340–52.

2. Author interview with Steven Sharfstein, MD.

3. Details about this process involving Drissel, Jacqueline Rosenberg, and Antoinette "Dolly" Gattozzi come from conversations, interviews, and follow-up email with Anne Drissel.

4. The examples and statistical information in this section come from US Department of Health and Human Services, *Toward a National Plan for the Chronically Mentally Ill* (Washington, DC: Government Printing Office, 1980), A95, A9–A11, A74–A79.

5. Garry Wills, *Reagan's America: Innocents at Home* (Garden City, NY: Doubleday, 1987), 366–67; William Grieder, "The Education of David Stockman," *Atlantic*, Dec. 1981.

6. Walter Shapiro, "The Stockman Express," *Washington Post*, Feb. 8, 1981.

7. Shapiro, "Stockman Express"; author interview with Herbert Pardes, MD.

8. Author interview with Pardes.

9. Senate Subcommittee on Labor, Health and Human Services, and Education, "Departments of Labor, Health and Human Services, Education, and Related Agencies Appropriations, FY82, Part 2," 97th Congress, 1st session, Feb. 19, 1981, 1083–1120.

10. "Departments of Labor . . . Appropriations," Feb. 19, 1981, 919–27.

11. "Departments of Labor . . . Appropriations," Feb. 19, 1981, 816.

12. Author interview with Pardes.

13. Katie Cadigan and Laura Murray interview with Dr. Herbert Pardes, New York City, n.d., courtesy of Cadigan and Murray.

14. John Gunther statement on behalf of United States Conference of Mayors, Hearing before the Senate Subcommittee on Labor and Human Resources, "Health Services and Preventive Health Block Grants, 1981," 97th Congress, 1st session, Apr. 2, 10, 1981, 413.

15. Ron Dellums testimony at Hearings before the Subcommittee on Fiscal Affairs and Health of the Committee on the District of Columbia, "Deinstitutionalization of the Mentally Ill," 97th Congress, 1st session, Nov. 2, 17, 18, 1981, iv–vii.

16. Sen. Orrin Hatch, opening statement before the hearing of the Senate Committee on Labor and Human Resources, "Health Services and Preventive Health Block Grants, 1981," 97th Congress, 1st session, Apr. 2, 1981, 1–5.

17. James Reston, "How Byrd Sees the Future," *New York Times*, Feb. 18, 1981.

18. Mary E. Hombs testimony, Hearing before House Subcommittee on Housing and Community Development, "Homelessness in America," 97th Congress, 2nd session, Dec. 15, 1982, 12–22.

19. Steven Rose testimony at Hearings, US House Committee on District of Columbia, "Deinstitutionalization of the Mentally Ill," 97th Congress, 1st session, Nov. 2, 1981, 86–117.

20. John Talbott testimony, Day 2, "Deinstitutionalization of the Mentally Ill," Nov. 18, 1981, 115–87.

21. Martin Tolchin, "Senate Rejects Bid to Restore Welfare Funds," *New York Times*, Apr. 1, 1981.

22. Robert Pear, "Fairness of Reagan's Cutoffs of Disability Aid Questioned," *New York Times*, May 9, 1982.

23. Howard Goldman and Antoinette Gattozzi, "Murder in the Cathedral Revisited: President Reagan and the Mentally Disabled," *Psychiatric Services* 39, no. 3 (May 1988): 505–9.

24. US Senate Committee on Finance, "Social Security Disability Insurance Program," 97th Congress, 2nd session, Aug. 18, 1982, 13–15.

25. Quoted in *PAIA*, National Mental Health Association's newsletter, n.d..

26. Quoted in Pear, "Fairness of Reagan's Cutoffs."

27. Pear, "Fairness of Reagan's Cutoffs."

28. Mental Health Association of Minn. v. Schweiker, US District Court, District of Minnesota, Fourth Division (case No. 4–82-Civ. 83), http://law.justia.com/cases/federal/district-courts/FSupp/554/157/1629069.

29. Select Committee on Aging, 98th Congress, June 20, 1983.

30. US Senate Finance Committee, "Impact of the Omnibus Reconciliation Act," 97th Congress, 2nd session, Aug. 1982.

31. Martin Tolchin, "Conferees Decide on $37 Billion Tax Cut in Federal Budget," *New York Times*, July 29, 1981.

32. National Advisory Mental Health Council, Minutes of 125th Meeting, May 18, 19, 20, 1981.

33. Email communication, Drissel to author, July 30, 2016.

34. Robert Cohen, "Annual Report of the Division of Clinical and Behavioral Research," *Mental Health Intramural Research Program of NIMH*, Oct. 1, 1980–Sept. 30, 1981, 7.

35. Marilyn Sargent, "Pardes Discusses NIMH Changes, Directions, Priorities," *ADAMHA News* 8, no. 19 (Oct. 15, 1982).

36. Paul Freddolino and Paul Applebaum, "Rights Protection and Advocacy: The Need to Do More with Less," *Psychiatric Services* 35, no. 4 (Apr. 1984): 319–20.

37. "Mentally Ill Bearing Brunt of SSA Cuts, APA Tells Senate," *Psychiatric News* 18, no. 9 (May 6, 1983): 1.

38. "Government May Suspend Disability Benefit Reviews," Associated Press, Mar. 23, 1984, https://advance-lexis-com.ezproxy.cul.columbia.edu/api/document?collection=news&id=urn:contentItem:3SJ4-JGN0-0011-64B2-00000-00&context=1516831.

39. Author interview with Anne Drissel (2016).

CHAPTER 7: FINDING A STRATEGIC VISION

1. David Obey, "Address to the Third Annual NAMI Conference," *NAMI News* (Arlington, VA, 1981), 47.

2. National Advisory Mental Health Council, Minutes of the 134th Meeting, Sept. 19–21, 1983.

3. Report on CSP Project Directors, Jan. 25–27, 1982, courtesy of Neal Brown.

4. US Department of Health and Human Services, *A Network for Caring: Proceedings of the Sixth National Conference 1983* (Boston: Center for Rehabilitation Research and Training in Mental Health, Boston University, 1984), 49, 54.

5. Author interview with Joseph Rogers.

6. Joseph A. Rogers, "'The Self-Help Alternative," typescript, [1985], courtesy of Joseph Rogers.

7. Joseph Rogers testimony, Hearings of the Senate Committee on Labor and Human Resources, "Barriers to Health Care for the Mentally Ill," 99th Congress, 1st session, Oct. 9, 1985, 137.

8. US Congress, Senate Subcommittee of the Committee on Appropriations, "Schizophrenia: The Plight and the Promise . . . Special Hearing," 99th Congress, 2nd session, Nov. 20, 1986, 67–72.

9. A Network for Caring, Sixth Annual Conference, 52–63.

10. Judi Chamberlin, "The Ex-Patients' Movement: Where We've Been and Where We're Going," *Journal of Mind and Behavior* 11, nos. 3–4 (Summer/Autumn 1990): 323–36.

11. Project Release v. Prevost, 551 F. Supp. 1298 (E.D.N.Y. 1982) District Court, E.D. New York, filed Nov. 24, 1982, https://law.justia.com/cases/federal/appellate-courts/F2/722/960/51279.

12. Marcia Lovejoy, "Recovery from Schizophrenia: A Personal Odyssey," *Psychiatric Services* 35, no. 8 (Apr. 1984): 809–12.

13. Chamberlin, "The Ex-Patients' Movement."

14. Judi Chamberlin, "Fifth Learning Community Conference," typescript, n.d., Chamberlin Papers, Special Collections and University Archives, University of Massachusetts Amherst.

15. Chamberlin, "The Ex-Patients' Movement."

16. Howie the Harp, "A Crazy Folks Guide to Reasonable Accommodation," [1990], Harp Papers, Community Access; Richard Severo, "Mental Patients Seeking a Voice in Determining Their Therapies," *New York Times*, Dec. 11, 1978.

17. Leonard Roy Frank, "Peter Breggin," *Madness Network News* 1, no. 4 (Mar. 1973): 10.

18. Chamberlin, "Fifth Learning Community Conference."

19. Vermont Department of Mental Health, "Community Support Program Accomplishment Summary, Marcy 15, 1983," NIMH Summaries, courtesy of Neal Brown.

20. Dorfner describes this in Sally Zinman, Howie the Harp, and Su Budd, eds., *Reaching Across: Mental Health Clients Helping Each Other* (Riverside: California Network of Mental Health Clients, 1987), 173–76.

21. Zinman, Howie the Harp, and Budd, *Reaching Across*.

22. "Client-Run Alternative Care Models," APA Workshop with Su Budd, Judi Chamberlin, Mike Finkle, Howie the Harp, and Wendy Kapp, May 13, 1986, typescript, Harp Papers, CA.

23. Paul J. Carling, "The NIMH Community Support Program: Emerging Issues, a Report of the NIMH/CSP Program Review," prepared under purchase order #84MO52538901D, typescript, Jan. 1984, courtesy of Neal Brown.

24. A Network for Caring: Sixth National Conference, 1983, 52–53.

25. Teleconference minutes, Jan. 22 and Feb. 14, 1985, courtesy of Joseph Rogers.

26. Teleconference minutes, Mar. 14, 1985, courtesy of Joseph Rogers.

27. "Conference Report: First National Consumer Conference," On Our Own Center of Baltimore, typescript, Mar. 1987, courtesy of Mike Finkle, On Our Own.

28. Summary of Alternatives '85, courtesy of Mike Finkle.

29. "Conference Report: First National Consumer Conference," *Madness Network News* 8, no. 1 (Fall 1985): 4–12.

30. Petitions to the Conference, signed by 21 [anonymous] people, "13th Annual International Conference for Human Rights and Against Psychiatric Oppression," *Madness Network News* 8, no. 1 (Fall 1985): 10.

31. Kate Millett, *The Loony-Bin Trip* (New York: Simon & Schuster, 1990), 312.

32. See articles by John C. Allen, Sue Doell, Morgan Firestar, John Judge, and Lenny Lapon in *Madness Network News* 8, no. 1 (Fall 1985). Two groups sponsored Pottstown: Boston University's Center for Rehabilitation and Training in Mental Health, where Chamberlin was affiliated, and a new group under the name Project SHARE, a clearinghouse for self-help groups, in Philadelphia, which Rogers had just founded.

33. Nancy C. Carter to Joe Rogers, Nov. 13, 1984, courtesy of Joseph Rogers.

34. Joe Bevilacqua to Joe Rogers, June 27, 1985, courtesy of Joseph Rogers.

35. Patrick Irick, "Constructive Criticism [1986]," courtesy of Joseph Rogers.

36. [Rae Unzicker], "NAMP in the Media," [1986], Chamberlin Papers.

37. Howie the Harp, "Dear Sisters and Brothers," [1986], Chamberlin papers.

38. Chamberlin to Sally [Zinman], Su [Budd], George, Wendy, and Rae [Unzicker], Jan. 26, 1986, Chamberlin Papers.

39. Howie the Harp, "On Forced Treatment and the National Organizations: An Open Letter to the NAMP Membership," Chamberlin Papers.

40. Su Budd to Richard Stanley, June 3, 1986, Chamberlin Papers.

41. Harriet P. Lefley, "The Role of Family Groups in Community Support Systems," issue paper for the Seventh NIMH-CSP Learning Community Conference, Rockville, Maryland, Apr. 28–May 1, 1985, courtesy of Neal Brown.

42. Carling, "The NIMH Community Support Program," 24–25.

43. Su Budd, "A History of the Mental Health Consumer/Survivor Movement," SAMHSA ADS Center Training Teleconference, Dec. 17, 2009, in author's possession.

44. Chamberlin, "The Ex-Patients' Movement."

45. Sally Zinman, "History of the Consumer Focus on the Beginnings," unpublished presentation, courtesy of Sally Zinman.

46. Author interview with Sally Zinman.

47. Joseph Rogers, "Milestones of the Consumer/Survivor/Ex-patient (C/S/X) Movement for Social Justice," typescript, n.d., courtesy of Joseph Rogers.

48. Author interview with Jacqueline Parrish.

49. Author interview with Neal Brown.

50. *Community Support Network News* 4, no. 2 (Oct. 1987), courtesy of Neal Brown.

CHAPTER 8: THIS IS AMERICA'S SHAME

1. US Senate Subcommittee on the Handicapped, Committee on Labor and Human Rights, Hearings, "Enforcement of Section 504 of the Rehabilitation Act; Institutional Care and Services for Retarded Citizens," 98th Congress, 1st session, Nov. 17, 1983, 111–43.

2. [Jan] Heininger interview with Lowell Weicker, Presidential Oral Histories, Miller Center, University of Virginia, June 19, 2009, https://millercenter.org/the-presidency/presidential-oral -histories/lowell-p-weicker-jr-oral-history-senator-connecticut.

3. Heininger interview with Weicker.

4. US House Committee on the Judiciary, "Civil Rights of Institutionalized Persons Act," 98th Congress, 1st session, Dec. 7, 1983, 98th Congress, 2nd session, Feb. 8, 1984, 170–74.

5. "Civil Rights of Institutionalized Persons Act," 43.

6. "Civil Rights of Institutionalized Persons Act," 52.

7. "Civil Rights of Institutionalized Persons Act," 89.

8. Juan Williams, "In His Heart but Not in His Mind," *Washington Post*, Jan. 10, 1986.

9. "Civil Rights of Institutionalized Persons Act," 231.

10. Teleconference minutes, Mar. [1985], courtesy of Joseph Rogers.

11. US Senate Subcommittee on the Handicapped, Committee on Labor and Human Resources, "Care of Institutionalized Mentally Disabled Persons," 99th Congress, 2nd session, Apr. 1 and 2, 1985, part 2.

12. Sandra Boodman, "The Mystery of Chestnut Lodge," *Washington Post*, Oct. 8, 1989.

13. "Care of Institutionalized Mentally Disabled Persons," 12, 214, 222–23.

14. Ravenel to Henry McMaster, Mar. 30, 1983, reprinted in "Care of Institutionalized Mentally Disabled Persons," 221–23.

15. Lowell Weicker, "Care of Institutionalized Mentally Disabled Persons," US Senate Subcommittee on the Handicapped, Committee on Labor and Human Resources, 99th Congress, 2nd session, Apr. 1, 1985, 1.

16. "[Notice of senate committee report]," *Madness Network News* 8, no. 1 (Fall 1985): 8.

17. Trial transcript, quoted in David A. Ferleger and Patrice M. Scott, "Rights and Dignity: Congress, the Supreme Court, and People with Disabilities After Pennhurst," *Western New England Law Review* 55, no. 3 (1982–83): 327–61. Also see Ferleger's account in his interview with Lisa Sonneborn, Temple University Institute on Disabilities, "Visionary Voices: David Ferleger," Jan. 13, 2013, https://disabilities.temple.edu/voices/interviews/ferleger.

18. Trial transcript.

19. *The Drummer*, Apr. 26–May 3, 1977, in author's possession.

20. David Ferleger, "Care of Institutionalized Mentally Disabled Persons," 27.

21. "Care of Institutionalized Mentally Disabled Persons," 28–29.

22. Paul Applebaum, "The Rising Tide of Patients' Rights Advocacy," *Psychiatric Services* 37, no. 1 (Jan. 1986): 9–10.

23. Judi Chamberlin and Joseph Rogers, "Planning a Community-Based Mental Health System: Perspective of Service Recipients," *American Psychologist* 45, no. 11 (Nov. 1990): 1241–44.

24. Laura Van Tosh, Joseph Rogers, and William Snavely, testimony at hearings of Senate Subcommittee on the Handicapped, Committee on Labor and Human Resources, "Protection and Advocacy for Mentally Ill Individuals Act (PL 99–319)," 100th Congress, 2nd session, May 10, 1988, 10–42.

25. "Protection and Advocacy for Mentally Ill Individuals Act," 8.

26. Williams, "In His Mind but Not His Heart."

CHAPTER 9: THE GENTLEMEN FROM KENTUCKY

1. All the descriptions, anecdotes, and direct quotes come from conversations or memos, notes, and memorabilia in Bos Todd's personal collection.

2. US House Committee on Appropriations, "Departments of Labor, Health, Education, and Welfare, and Related Agencies Appropriations for 1981, Part 11," 96th Congress, 2nd session, Apr. 15–16, 1980, 458–75.

3. In 1963, Jonathan Bingham was electrocuted while working at home on his family's estate. In 1966, another of Barry Bingham Sr.'s sons died in a freak automobile accident involving a surfboard. See "Barry Bingham, Jr., Publisher Is Dead at 72," *New York Times*, Apr. 4, 2006, http://www.nytimes.com/2006/04/04/business/media/barry-bingham-jr-louisville-publisher-is-dead-at-72.html.

4. Bosworth Todd Jr., "Bingham and Schizophrenia," (Louisville, KY) *Courier-Journal*, June 3, 1988.

5. Department of Health and Human Services, National Institute of Mental Health, National Advisory Mental Health Council, Minutes of the 126th Meeting, Sept. 1981.

6. Lasker Foundation "[14C] Deoxyglucose Method for Measuring Brain Function," 1981 Albert Lasker Clinical Medical Research Award, http://www.laskerfoundation.org/awards/show/14cdeoxyglucose-method-for-measuring-brain-function.

7. Author interview with Dr. Louis Sokoloff.

8. Claudia Wasserman interview with Dr. Louis Sokoloff, Mar. 3, 2005, Oral History Program, Office of NIH History and Stetten Museum, National Library of Medicine; interview with Louis Sokoloff, Society for Neuroscience, filmed May 26, 1996, deposited with YouTube, July 5, 2012, https://www.youtube.com/watch?v=LzOOzfOC2j4.

9. US Department of Health and Human Services, *ADAMHA News on Alcohol, Drug Abuse and Mental Health* 9, [no. 14] (Aug. 1983), describes the hopes scientists carried.

10. Department of Health and Human Services, Public Health Service, National Institutes of Health, "Annual Report of Program Activities of NIMH Research, 1982," part 2, pp. 18, 179, 359, 443, 446, Office of NIH History and Stetten Museum. The unpublished annual in-house reports, with rich details about activities under way at each of the NIMH labs, are digitally accessible at the Internet Archives: https://archive.org/search.php?query=creator%3A%22National+Institute+of+Mental+Health+%28U.S.%29.+Division+of+Intramural+Research+Programs%22.

11. Author phone interview with Robert Trachtenberg.

12. Author interview with Dr. Louis Sokoloff.

13. Wasserman interview with Sokoloff.

14. Sharon Begley, John Carey, and Ray Sawhill, "The Human Computer: How the Brain Works," *Newsweek*, Feb. 7, 1983, 40–47.

15. *Annual Report of the Mental Health Intramural Research Program Activities of the NIMH, 1980*, Office of NIH History and Stetten Museum, National Library of Medicine, Bethesda, Maryland.

16. National Advisory Mental Health Council, Minutes of the 123rd Meeting, Dec. 1–2, 1980, 22; 125th Meeting, May 2–3, 1981, 30; 128th Meeting, Mar. 1–2, 1982, 20, Office of NIH History and Stetten Museum, Bethesda, Maryland.

17. Robert Cohen, director, Division of Behavioral Research, *Annual Report, 1980*, vol. 1, p. 7.

18. "Needed: A 'Critical Mass' of Clinical Researchers," *ADAMHA News*, Sept. 5, 1980.

19. See Katharine Graham, *Personal History* (New York: Vintage, 1998), 243–44.

20. Graham invitation, courtesy of Gwill Newman.

21. Donald Graham, personal communication with author, Feb. 9 and 10, 2017. Katharine Graham's son wrote that the wooden wringer was purchased "at an antique shop and presented to her, signed, by Bob Woodward and Carl Bernstein." When Attorney General John Mitchell heard that the *Washington Post* intended to publish a story exposing his connections to the criminal break-in, he warned Bernstein that "Katie Graham's gonna' get her tit caught in a big fat wringer if that's published." She describes this in *Personal History*, 465.

22. Gwill Linderme York Newman, *My Son's Name Was Fred* (Santa Fe, NM: Artwork International, 2006).

23. Notes, Boswell Todd Jr. to Gwill Newman, July 10, 1984, courtesy of Boswell Todd.

24. Notes, Boswell Todd Jr. to Gwill Newman, July 10, 1984.

25. Notes, Boswell Todd Jr. to Gwill Newman, July 10, 1984.

26. "Congress Gets Message during Mental Illness Awareness Week," *Psychiatric News* 20, no. 21 (Nov. 1, 1985): 1.

27. The organizations shared a goal to find a cure or successful treatments for mental illnesses. NAMI's leaders joined the earliest efforts to set up NARSAD. The two groups held joint meetings while NAMI continued lobbying Congress on behalf of NIMH's priorities. NAMI's family membership had actually donated more than $300,000 explicitly for NARSAD's agenda. It stopped short of relinquishing its membership list of the 739 local affiliate groups that NARSAD wanted for direct solicitation. NAMI struggled to resolve how much of its resources should go into research. For a short period, the organizations were able to transcend personalities and priorities, but neither group was willing to subordinate to the other's mission, and they abandoned earlier ambitions to merge. Some families wanted full-throttled research while others needed services simply to survive.

28. Erik Eckholm, "Schizophrenia's Victims Include Strained Families," Mar. 17, 1986; Harold M. Schmeck Jr., "Schizophrenia Focus Shifts to Dramatic Changes in Brain," Mar. 18, 1986; Phillip M. Boffey, "Schizophrenia: Insights Fail to Halt Rising Toll," Mar. 19, 1986, all in *New York Times*.

29. Herbert Pardes, MD, "The Benefits of Schizophrenia Research," *New York Times*, Apr. 8, 1986.

30. Author interview with Dr. Herbert Pardes.

31. "Administration Backing Cuts for Research at Universities," *New York Times*, Mar. 20, 1986.

32. UCLA, Case Western Reserve University, Johns Hopkins University, Washington University in St. Louis, University of Maryland, Harvard University, Columbia University (2), and Duke University.

33. Todd, "Bingham and Schizophrenia."

CHAPTER 10: DUELING DIAGNOSES

1. Courtenay Harding, "Yale Symposium: New Data and New Hopes Call for New Practices in Clinical Psychiatry," July 2015, https://www.youtube.com/watch?v=5Nww8bwp70w.

2. William E. Bunney interview by Heinz E. Lehmann, in Thomas A. Ban and Edward Shorter, eds., *An Oral History of Neuropsychopharmacology*, vol. 1: *Starting Up, Peer Interviews* (Brentwood, TN: American College of Neuropsychopharmacology, 2011), 81–91.

3. Edward Shorter, "The Q-T Interval and the Mellaril Story: A Cautionary Tale," *International Network for the History of Neuropsychopharmacology*, n.d., http://inhn.org/controversies/edward-shorter-the-q-t-interval-and-the-mellaril-story-a-cautionary-tale.html (accessed Dec. 18, 2021).

4. James Claghorn et al., "The Risks and Benefits of Clozapine versus Chlorpromazine," *Journal of Clinical Psychopharmacology* 7, no. 6 (1987): 377–84.

5. Rupert V. Chittick, George W. Brooks, Francis Irons, and William Deane, *The Vermont Story: Rehabilitation of Chronic Schizophrenic Patients* (Burlington, VT: Office of Vocational Rehabilitation, 1961), 30.

6. George W. Brooks, "Speculation on New Perspectives in Schizophrenia," *Psychiatric Journal of the University of Ottawa* 3, no. 3 (Sept. 1978): 194.

7. George Brooks and William Deane, "Rehabilitation of Severely Disabled Hospitalized Mental Patients," *Journal of Rehabilitation* 28, no. 5 (Sept. 1962): 13–14.

8. Chittick et al., *The Vermont Story*, 16–20.

9. Brooks, "Speculation on New Perspectives," 194–95.

10. Chittick et al., *The Vermont Story*, 16.

11. Chittick et al., *The Vermont Story*, 50–57.

12. Chittick et al., *The Vermont Story*, 84, 85–97.

13. "NIMH Activities: Schizophrenia-Related Research Grants—Fiscal Year 1977," *Schizophrenia Bulletin* 5, no. 1 (Jan. 1979): 138–72.

14. George Brooks, "Reflections on the Vermont Story, or Foresights, Insight, and Hindsight," *Psychiatric Journal of the University of Ottawa* 13, no. 1 (1988): 21–24.

15. Chittick et al., *The Vermont Story*, 16.

16. Courtenay M. Harding, George Brooks, and George Albee, "Twenty Year Follow-Up of 253 Schizophrenic Patients Originally Selected for Chronic Disability: Pilot Study," *Psychiatric Journal of the University of Ottawa* 2, no. 3 (Sept. 1977): 129–32.

17. Brooks, "Reflections on the Vermont Story"; author interview with Courtenay Harding.

18. Jack Drescher, "An Interview with Robert L. Spitzer, MD," *Journal of Gay and Lesbian Mental Health* 7, no. 3 (Feb. 2003): 97–111, https://www.researchgate.net/publication/244889348_An_interview_with_Robert_L_Spitzer_MD.

19. Robert L. Spitzer et al., "Mental Status Schedule: Comparing Kentucky and New York Schizophrenics," *Archives of General Psychiatry* 12, no. 5 (May 1965): 448–55.

20. Robert L. Spitzer, Joseph L. Fleiss, Jean Endicott, and Jacob Cohen, "Mental Status Schedule: Properties of Factor-Analytically Derived Scales," *Archives of General Psychiatry* 16, no. 4 (Apr. 1967): 479–93.

21. Robert L. Spitzer and Jean Endicott, "DIAGNO: A Computer Program for Psychiatric Diagnosis Utilizing the Differential Diagnostic Procedure," *Archives of General Psychiatry* 18, no. 6 (June 1968): 746–56.

22. David Rosenhan, "On Being Sane in Insane Places," *Science* 179, no. 4070 (Jan. 19, 1973): 250–58.

23. Robert L. Spitzer, "On Pseudoscience in Science, Logic in Remission, and Psychiatric Diagnosis: A Critique of Rosenhan's 'On Being Sane in Insane Places,'" *Journal of Abnormal Psychology* 84, no. 5 (1975): 442–52.

24. Spitzer, "On Pseudoscience," 447.

25. Raymond M. Glasscote, "Homosexuality and APA—The Issues Are Joined," *Psychiatric News* 8, no. 11 (June 6, 1974): 18–19; Raymond M. Glasscote, "Homosexuality and APA—The Aftermath," *Psychiatric News* 8, no. 13 (July 4, 1973): 4–5, 28; Charles Hite, "APA Rules Homosexuality Not Necessarily a Disorder," *Psychiatric News* 9, no. 1 (Jan. 2, 1974): 1, 6, 16. Also see Ronald Bayer, *Homosexuality and America Psychiatry* (New York: Basic Books, 1981).

26. Alix Spiegel, "The Dictionary of Disorder: How One Man Revolutionized Psychiatry," *New Yorker*, Jan. 3, 2005.

27. Robert L. Spitzer, "Letters to the Editor: Rosenhan (Again!)," *Psychiatric News* 10, no. 12 (June 18, 1975): 2, 18.

28. Theodore Millon, "The DSM-III," *American Psychologist* (July 1983): 804–14.

29. John P. Feighner, Eli Robins, Samuel B. Guze, Robert A. Woodruff Jr., George Winokur, and Rodrigo Muñoz, "Diagnostic Criteria for Use in Psychiatric Research," *Archives of General Psychiatry* 26, no. 1 (Jan. 1972): 57–63.

30. Kenneth S. Kendler, MD, Rodrigo A. Muñoz, MD, and George Murphy, MD, "The Development of the Feighner Criteria: A Historical Perspective," *American Journal of Psychiatry* 167, no. 2 (Feb. 2010): 134–42.

31. Robert L. Spitzer, Nancy C. Andreasen, and Jean Endicott, "Schizophrenia and Other Psychotic Disorders in DSM-III," *Schizophrenia Bulletin* 4, no. 4 (1978): 489–509; Robert L. Spitzer, Jean Endicott, and Eli Robins, "Clinical Criteria for Psychiatric Diagnosis and DSM-III," *American Journal of Psychiatry* 132, no. 11 (Nov. 1975): 1187–92.

32. Author interview with Dr. Gaye Carlson.

33. John M. Nardo, 1BoringOldMan.com.

34. Mitchell Wilson, MD, "DSM-III and the Transformation of American Psychiatry: A History," *American Journal of Psychiatry* 150, no. 3 (Mar. 1993): 399–410.

35. Allan V. Horwitz, *Creating Mental Illness* (Chicago: University of Chicago Press, 2002), 66. See also Gerald N. Grob, "Origins of DSM-I: A Study in Appearance and Reality," *American Journal of Psychiatry* 148, no. 4 (Apr. 1991): 421–31; Gary Greenberg, *The Book of Woe: The DSM and the Unmaking of Psychiatry* (New York: Blue Rider Press, 2013); Jonathan M. Metzl, *The Protest Psychosis: How Schizophrenia Became a Black Disease* (Boston: Beacon Press, 2009); Rick Mayes and Allan V. Horwitz, "DSM-III and the Revolution in the Classification of Mental Illness," *Journal of the History of the Behavioral Sciences* 41, no. 3 (Summer 2005): 249–67.

36. Ron Bayer and Robert L. Spitzer, "Neurosis, Psychodynamics and DSM-III: A History of Controversy," *Archives of General Psychiatry* 42, no. 2 (Feb. 1986): 187–96.

37. Quoted in Greenberg, *Book of Woe*, 66, 40.

38. *Diagnostic and Statistical Manual of Mental Disorders*, 3rd ed. (Washington, DC: APA Press, 1980), 186. Hereafter cited as *DSM-III*.

39. Christopher Lane, *Shyness: How Normal Behavior Became a Sickness* (New Haven, CT: Yale University Press, 2007), 80–90.

40. *DSM-III*, 310–18.

41. "Schizophrenic Disorders," *DSM-III*, 181, 186.

42. Metzl, *The Protest Psychosis*, 148–49.

43. Metzl, *The Protest Psychosis*, 185. Historian Hannah Decker's exhaustive study *Making of the DSM-III: A Diagnostic Manual's Conquest of American Psychiatry* (Cambridge: Oxford University Press, 2013) notes this ignored earlier research doubting that schizophrenia which resolves well is not a mild case of schizophrenia but something entirely different. See discussion on 135–37 and 362n27.

44. Anne Harrington, *Mind Fixers: Psychiatry's Troubled Search for the Biology of Mental Illness* (New York: W. W. Norton, 2019), 247.

45. Harrington, *Mind Fixers*, 267.

46. Fink to Lester Grinspoon, quoted in Lane, *Shyness*, 47. Also see Christopher Lane, "The Problem of Heroizing Robert Spitzer," *Psychology Today*, Jan. 22, 2016, https://www.psychologytoday.com/us/blog/side-effects/201601/the-problem-heroizing-robert-spitzer.

47. Allan V. Horwitz and Gerald N. Grob, "The Troubled History of Psychiatry's Quest for Specificity," *Journal of Health Politics, Policy and Law* 41, no. 4 (Aug. 2016): 521–39.

48. "DSM-III: The Shift," 1 Boring Old Man, May 17, 2011, https:// 1BoringOldMan.com/index.php/2011/05/17/dsm-iii-the-shift.

49. Nancy C. Andreasen, *The Broken Brain: The Biological Revolution in Psychiatry* (New York: Harper & Row, 1985), 155.

50. Nancy C. Andreasen, "The DSM and the Death of Phenomenology," *Schizophrenia Bulletin* 33, no. 1 (2007): 108–12.

51. Author interview with Courtenay Harding. Harding graciously shared a draft of her manuscript to be published by Oxford University Press.

52. Jeffrey Gillenkirk and Charles Hite, "The Concept of Schizophrenia—Still Elusive, Still Controversial," *Psychiatric News* 9, no. 1 (Jan. 2, 1974): 8–9, 12.

53. See John S. Strauss and William T. Carpenter, "The Prognosis of Schizophrenia: Rationale for a Multidimensional Concept," *Schizophrenia Bulletin* 4, no. 1 (1978): 56–67. For a summary of the findings of Carpenter and Strauss, see W. T. Carpenter Jr. and J. S. Strauss, "The Interaction of Diagnostic and Outcome Variables in Schizophrenic Patients," *Journal of Psychiatric Research* 13, no. 1 (1976): 61.

54. Strauss and Carpenter, "The Prognosis of Schizophrenia."

55. Larry Davidson, Jaak Rakfeldt, and John Strauss, *The Roots of the Recovery Movement in Psychiatry: Lessons Learned* (New York: John Wiley & Sons, 2010), 104.

56. Author interview with Courtenay Harding.

57. A discussion of methodology can be found in two pivotal articles. See Courtenay M. Harding, George W. Brooks, Takamaru Ashikaga, John Strauss, and Alan Breier, "The Vermont Longitudinal Study of Persons with Severe Mental Illness, I: Methodology, Study Sample, and Overall Status 32 Years Later," and "II: Long-Term Outcome of Subjects Who Retrospectively Met DSM-III Criteria for Schizophrenia," *American Journal of Psychiatry* 144 (June 6, 1987): 718–26, 727–35.

58. Luc Ciompi, "The Natural History of Schizophrenia in the Long Term," *British Journal of Psychiatry* 136, no. 5 (May 1980): 413–20.

59. Author interview with C. Christian Beels, MD.

60. Laurie Flynn, "John Talbott's Association with NAMI," *Psychiatric Services* 55, no. 10 (Oct. 2004): 1162–63.

61. Author interview with Courtenay Harding.

62. Flynn, "John Talbott's Association."

63. "Schizophrenics Can Lead Normal Lives, Recover, 30-Year Study Concludes," *Psychiatric News* 20, no 12 (June 21, 1985): 23.

64. Michael DeSisto, Courtenay M. Harding, Rodney V. McCornick, Takamaru Ashikaga, and George W. Brooks, "The Maine and Vermont Three-Decade Studies of Serious Mental Illness: I. Matched Comparison of Cross-Sectional Outcome," and "II: Longitudinal Course Comparisons," *British Journal of Psychiatry* 167, no. 3 (Sept. 1995): 331–38, 338–41.

65. Author interview with Harding.

66. American Psychiatric Association, *Diagnostic and Statistical Manual of Mental Disorders*, 4th ed. (Washington, DC: APA Press, 1995), 283.

67. Courtenay M. Harding and James H. Zahniser, "Empirical Correction of Seven Myths About Schizophrenia with Implications for Treatment," *ACTA Psychiatrica Scandinavia*, supplement 3849 (1994): 140–46.

CHAPTER 11: THE SOUL'S FRAIL DWELLING HOUSE

1. Richard T. Greer, Legislative Issues Report, National Alliance for the Mentally Ill, typescript, July 1984, in author's possession.

2. Constance Holden, "NIMH Emphasizes the Basics," *Science* 228, no. 4698 (Apr. 26, 1985): 474–75.

3. Author interview with Laurie Flynn.

4. Minutes of the 139th Meeting, NAMHC, Dec. 1984, NIH Library, Rockville, MD.

5. Shervert H. Frazier, "NIMH Reorganization Focuses on Specific Disorders, Basic Science, and Research Training," *Psychiatric Services* 36, no. 12 (Dec. 1985): 1265–70.

6. Samuel J. Keith and Susan M. Matthews, "A National Plan for Schizophrenia Research," *Schizophrenia Bulletin* 14, no. 3 (1988): 1.

7. Holden, "NIMH Emphasizes the Basics."

8. Daniel Weinberger, "Richard Jed Wyatt, 1939–2002," *Neuropsychopharmacology* 27, no. 4 (Oct. 2002): 687–89.

9. Constance Holden, "NIMH to Reorganize Extramural Research," *Science* 229, no. 4711 (July 26, 1985): 362.

10. Author interview with Laurie Flynn.

11. US Senate Committee on Appropriations hearings, "Departments of Labor, Health and Human Services, Education, and Related Agencies Appropriations, FY86 Part 4: Nondepartmental Witnesses," 99th Congress, 1st session, May 30, 1985, 788.

12. Valerie P. Hans and Can Slater, "John Hinckley, Jr. and the Insanity Defense: The Public's Verdict," *Public Opinion Quarterly* 47, no. 2 (Summer 1983), Cornell Law Faculty Publications paper 334, http://scholarship.law.cornell.edu/facpub/334.

13. George F. Will, "Obliterating the Idea of Responsibility," *Los Angeles Times*, June 23, 1982.

14. Patrick Young, "A Conversation with Richard Jedd Wyatt," *Psychology Today*, Aug. 1983, 30–42.

15. Philip Hilts, "The Race Is On to Develop New Drugs for Raising Intelligence," *Washington Post*, Sept. 7, 1982.

16. Richard Restak, *The Brain* (Toronto: Bantam Books, 1984), 2.

17. Related to the author by Dewitt Sage.

18. Related to the author by Dewitt Sage.

19. Memo, "Chamberlin for the Mental Patients' Liberation Front to Producer of *The Brain*," Aug. 13, 1984, Chamberlin Papers, Special Collections and University Archives, University of Massachusetts Amherst (SCUA).

20. *MacNeil-Lehrer News Hour*, July 25, 1984, transcript in author's possession.

21. US Senate Committee on Appropriations hearings, "Departments of Labor, Health and Human Services, Education, and Related Agencies Appropriations, FY86 Part 4: Nondepartmental Witnesses," 99th Congress, 1st session, May 1985, 930–37.

22. Don Richardson, "NAMI Board Urges Return of NIMH to NIH," *NAMI News* 8, no. 2 (Apr–May 1987).

23. Author interview with Fred Goodwin.

24. National Advisory Mental Health Council, Minutes of the 153rd Meeting, Feb. 1988.

25. Constance Holden, "ADAMHA Still Seeking to Consolidate Its Identity," *Science* 241, no. 4867 (Aug. 12, 1988): 782–83.

26. Author interview with Laurie Flynn.

27. Quoted in Scott LaFee, "Lewis Judd to Step Down After 36 Years as Chair of Department of Psychiatry," *This Week @UC San Diego*, June 13, 2013, https://ucsdnews.ucsd.edu/feature/lewis_judd_to_step_down_after_36_years_as_chair_of_department_of_psychiatry.

28. Author interview with Alan Leshner; National Advisory Mental Health Council, Minutes of the 160th Meeting, Nov. 1989.

29. National Advisory Mental Health Council, Minutes of the 153rd Meeting, Feb. 1988.

30. "Agenda Item: ADAMHA Administrator's Report, Transcript of Administrator's Report," Feb. 1992, in author's possession.

31. Author interview with Delores Parron-Ragland.

32. Jeffrey Mervis, "Goodwin Stumbles," *Nature* 356, no. 6 (1992): 6.

33. "Black Caucus Expresses Concern over Remarks by Health Official," *New York Times*, Feb. 27, 1992.

34. See the editorial comments in *Psychiatric News* (Apr. 3, 1992).

35. Juan Williams, "Violence, Genes, and Prejudice," *Discover*, Nov. 1, 1994.

36. Frederick K. Goodwin, MD, to the President [George H. W. Bush], Feb. 27, 1992, Resignation Files, White House Office of Personnel, George H. W. Bush Presidential Library and Museum Records.

37. *Dendron: Psychiatric Survivors and Allies Independent Media*, May 1, 1992, Judi Chamberlin Papers, MS 768, Special Collections and University Archives, University of Massachusetts Amherst.

38. "Board Considers Goodwin Flap," *Psychiatric News* (Apr. 3, 1992): 1, 24.

39. "The Speech Police," *Wall Street Journal*, Mar. 9, 1992.

40. "Psychiatrists Say No . . . ADAMHA," *Psychiatric News* (May 1, 1992): 1, 22–23.

41. Report of the Secretary's Blue Ribbon Panel on Violence Prevention, typescript, Jan. 15, 1993.

CHAPTER 12: THE CLOZAPINE STORY

1. Baron Shopsin et al., "Clozapine, Chlorpromazine, and Placebo in Newly Hospitalized, Acutely Schizophrenic Patients," *Archives of General Psychiatry* 36 (June 1979): 657–84.

2. R. W. Griffith and K. Saameli, "Clozapine and Agranulocytosis," *Lancet* (Oct. 4, 1975): 657. The authors use the reporting figure of 0.27 per 1000.

3. Melody Petersen, *Our Daily Meds* (New York: Farrar, Straus & Giroux/Sarah Crichton Books, 2008), 126–28.

4. C. Thomas Gualtieri, Robert L. Sprague, and Jonathan O. Cole, "Tardive Dyskinesia Litigation and the Dilemmas of Neuroleptic Treatment," *Journal of Psychiatry and the Law* 14, nos. 1–2 (Mar. 1, 1986): 187–216.

5. Author interview with Lou Gerbino, MD.

6. Author interview with Gerbino.

7. John Crilly, "The History of Clozapine and Its Emergence in the US Market: A Review and Analysis," *History of Psychiatry* 18, no. 1 (Mar. 2007): 39–60.

8. Department of Health and Human Services, Food and Drug Administration, "Psychopharmacologic Drugs, FDA Advisory Committee, Twenty-Sixth Meeting," vol. 1, Thursday, Feb. 23, 1984, I-16.

9. Paul Leber, "Adverse Drug Reactions," *Psychopharmacology Bulletin* 17, no. 3 (July 1981): 6–9.

10. FDA Advisory Committee, Twenty-Sixth Meeting, I-16, 25.

11. FDA Advisory Committee, Twenty-Sixth Meeting, 12.

12. FDA Advisory Committee, Twenty-Sixth Meeting, I-9–I-15.

13. Author interview with Lou Gerbino, MD.

14. FDA Advisory Committee, Twenty-Sixth Meeting, 107.

15. FDA Advisory Committee, Twenty-Sixth Meeting, 153–64.

16. FDA Advisory Committee, Twenty-Sixth Meeting, 170.

17. FDA Advisory Committee, Twenty-Sixth Meeting, 169–74.

18. FDA Advisory Committee, Twenty-Sixth Meeting, 175.

19. Thomas Ban interview of Paul Leber, December 15, 1999, in *An Oral History of Neuropsychopharmacology: The First Fifty Years, Peers Interviews*, vol. 8: *Diverse Topics*, ed. Carl Salzman (Brentwood, TN: ACNP, 2011), 219–43.

20. FDA Advisory Committee, Twenty-Sixth Meeting, 135–37.

21. The original study enrolled 319 people but with drop-outs, 268 remained. John Kane et al., "Clozapine for the Treatment-Resistant Schizophrenic," *Archives of General Psychiatry* 45 (Sept. 1988): 789–96.

22. Crilly, "History of Clozapine," 49.

23. Department of Health and Human Services, Food and Drug Administration, "Psychopharmacologic Drugs, Advisory Committee Thirtieth Meeting, Apr. 26, 1989, 13.

24. Stephen R. Marder and Theodore Van Putten, "Who Should Receive Clozapine?," *Archives of General Psychiatry* 45 (Sept. 1988): 865–67.

25. Kane et al., "Clozapine for the Treatment-Resistant Schizophrenic."

26. FDA Advisory Committee, Thirtieth Meeting (1989), 9–21.

27. Ban interview of Leber.

28. FDA Advisory Committee, Thirtieth Meeting (1989), 128–29.

29. "Advertisement: Psychiatry Today: Breakthrough," *Psychiatric News* 41, no. 1 (Jan. 5, 1990).

30. Gail Toff Berman, "Clozapine: Will States Ration Care?" *State Health Reports* 57 (May 1990), typescript.

31. Statement of Laurent S. Lehmann, MD, before Senate Judiciary Committee on Antitrust Monopolies and Business Rights, "Marketing of Clozaril," 102nd Congress, 1st session (Mar. 5, 1991), 50–58.

32. Quoted in William Reid, "Access to Care: Clozapine in the Public Sector," *Psychiatric Services* 41, no. 8 (Aug. 1990): 870–74.

33. Daniel Goleman, "Schizophrenia Drug Hailed, Except for Cost," *New York Times*, May 15, 1990.

34. Jay Centifani to Gilbert Honigfeld, Feb. 15, 1991, exhibit #3, "Marketing of Clozaril," 110–11.

35. Reid, "Access to Care."

36. Vera Hassner to Directors of Psychiatry/Administrative Directors of Out-Patient Clinics, Oct. 25, 1991, in author's possession.

37. Carl Salzman, MD, "Notes from a State Mental Health Directors' Meeting on Clozapine," *Psychiatric Services* 41, no. 8 (Aug. 1990): 838–42.

38. *NAMI Advocate*, July 1990, Sept. 1990, in author's possession.

39. Claudia Wallis and James Willwerth, "Awakening Schizophrenia," *Time*, July 6, 1992.

40. Milt Freudenheim, "Sandoz Caremark in Suit Settlement," *New York Times*, Sept. 4, 1992; Mark A. Hurwitz, "Bundling Patented Drugs and Medical Services: An Antitrust Analysis," *Columbia Law Review* 91, no. 5 (June 1991): 1188–1220.

41. Author interview with William E. Reid.

42. John S. Strauss and William T. Carpenter, "The Diagnosis and Understanding of Schizophrenia, Part III. Speculations on the Processes That Underlie Schizophrenic Symptoms and Signs," *Schizophrenia Bulletin* (Winter 1974): 61–69.

43. See for example, John Strauss's chapter, "The Everday Interpersonal Context of Recovery," in, Davidson, Rakfeldt, and Strauss, *The Roots of the Recovery Movement*, chap. 4.

44. Tribute was paid by Richard R. J. Lewin, "Negative Symptoms in Schizophrenia: Editor's Introduction," *Schizophrenia Bulletin* 11, no. 3 (1985): 361–63; Lewin credited Strauss and Carpenter's pivotal article "The Diagnosis and Understanding of Schizophrenia, Part III."

45. Douglas W. Heinrichs, "Recent Developments in the Psychosocial Treatment of Chronic Psychotic Illnesses," in John Talbott, ed., *The Chronic Mental Patient Five Years Later* (New York: Grune & Stratton, 1984), 124.

46. L. A. Opler, "Clozapine Treatment of Negative Schizophrenics Symptoms," in Vera Hassner, ed., *Clozapine Perspectives: Doctors Share Their Experience* (New York: Alliance for the Mentally Ill of New York State, 1992), 10–13.

47. FDA Advisory Committee, Thirtieth Meeting, 110.

48. Herbert Meltzer et al., "Effects of Six Months of Clozapine Treatment on the Quality of Life of Chronic Schizophrenic Patients," *Hospital and Community Psychiatry* 41, no. 8 (Aug. 1990): 892–97.

49. H. Y. Meltzer et al., "A Prospective Study of Clozapine in Treatment-Resistant Schizophrenic Patients, I: Preliminary Report," *Psychopharmacology* 99 (1989): S68–72.

50. Herbert Y. Meltzer, "Commentary: Defining Treatment Refractoriness in Schizophrenia," *Schizophrenia Bulletin* 16, no. 4 (1990): 563–656.

51. Clozapine didn't bind to two of the major receptors, D1 and D2, but it did bind to different receptors.

CHAPTER 13: BUILDING A VILLAGE

1. Howard Padwa and Kevin Miller interview with Dan Weisburd, Apr. 29 and July 8, 2010, History of Public Mental Health Archives, UCLA, https://hpmh.semel.ucla.edu/people/weisburd-dan.

2. Howard Padwa interview of Rose King, June 16, 2010, History of Mental Health Archives, UCLA, https://hpmh.semel.ucla.edu/people/king-rose.

3. Padwa interview of King, UCLA.

4. One of the subjects is available on YouTube. See "The Most Important Person: Without Saying a Word" (1972), https://www.youtube.com/watch?v=mpnNDtCRzYI.

5. *A System in Shambles*, Eldan Productions, 1986, in author's possession, courtesy of Dan Weisburd.

6. Interview with Dan Weisburd and Elaine Weisburd, "The Story of a Schizophrenic," *All Things Considered*, National Public Radio, 1986.

7. Dan E. Weisburd, "Planning a Community-Based Mental Health System: Perspective of a Family Member," *American Psychologist* 45, no. 11 (Nov. 1990): 1245–48.

8. Padwa and Miller interview with Weisburd.

9. Leo McCarthy, Speech at the California Alliance for the Mentally Ill, Apr. 3, 1987, quoted in preface to Task Force for the Seriously Mentally Ill, "An Integrated Service System for People with Serious Mental Illness: A Preliminary Proposal, June 1987," courtesy of Art Bolton.

10. Arthur Bolton, "Ambling Through the Shambles Through the Years," *The Journal* 4, no. 2 (1993): 6–9.

11. "An Integrated Service System for People with Serious Mental Illness: A Preliminary Proposal, June 1987."

12. Author interview with Richard Van Horn. Also see Marcia Meldrum and Amanda Nelligan, interview with Richard Van Horn, Mental Health Advocacy in California, Oral Histories, Louise M. Darling Biomedical Library History and Special Collections for the Sciences, University of California, Los Angeles, https://hpmh.semel.ucla.edu/people/van-horn-richard.

13. Sandra Goodwin, memo to California Conference of Local Mental Health Directors to Governor George Deukmejian, Aug. 24, 1988, California State Archives.

14. Marcia Meldrum and Howard Padwa interview of Mark Ragins, Mental Health Advocacy in California, Oral Histories, https://hpmh.semel.ucla.edu/people/ragins-mark.

15. Mark Ragins, "Transforming Staff/Client Relationships—1994," *Exploring Recovery: The Collected Village Writings of Mark Ragins*, http://static1.1.sqspcdn.com/static/f/1084149/15460835

/1323128610140/13TransformingStaffClientRelationships.pdf?token=R7EVzackLlgjC11sGaWSpKA
%2FPKM%3D.

16. The story appears in Clara Alvarez, "The Story of Libertad," in the issue "Integrated Service Agency," *The Journal* 4, no. 2 (1993): 26–27.

17. Ragins, "Transforming Staff/Client Relationships."

18. Mary Ann Test, "The Elements of Effective Community Care in Action," *The Journal* 9, no. 2 (1993): 53–56.

19. Mark Ragins, "Recovery: Changing from a Medical Model to a Psychosocial Rehabilitation Model," 1995, from *The Collected Village Writings of Mark Ragins*, http://static1.1.sqspcdn.com/static/f/1084149/15460167/1323120276660/06RecoverySevereMI.pdf?token=S9LQT2GN9QM%2FDthOSLrXQfSJ7L4%3D.

20. William A. Anthony, Mikal Cohen, and William Kennard, "Understanding the Current Facts and Principles of Mental Health Planning," *American Psychologist* 45 (Nov. 1990): 1249–52.

21. William A. Anthony, "Psychiatric Rehabilitation: Key Issues and Future Policy," *Health Affairs* (Fall 1992): 164–71.

22. William A. Anthony, "Programs That Work: Issues of Leadership," *The Journal* 9, no. 2 (1993): 51–53.

23. William A. Anthony, "Editorial: Decade of Recovery," *Psychosocial Rehabilitation Journal* 16, no. 4 (Apr. 1993): 1. Anthony was the editor of this issue, which also included his article "Recovery from Mental Illness: The Guiding Vision of the Mental Health Service System in the 1990s" (11–23).

24. Anthony, "Editorial," 1.

25. Ragins, "Recovery."

26. Mark Ragins, "Partners in Medication Collaboration," *The Journal* 4, no. 2 (1993): 19–20.

27. Mark Ragins, "Twenty Lessons from the Village in Year 1," 1991, *Village Recovery Writings*, https://drive.google.com/file/d/10QOh-FheRj1VgKNSEIHdx_sWlrugsxhX/view.

28. The third program, Ventura County, received separate consideration for their children's services.

29. Lewin-VHI, "AB 3777 System Reforms: The Integrated Service Agency Model. A Summary Report to the California Department of Mental Health, August 1995," History of Public Mental Health Archives, UCLA.

30. Senate Labor and Human Resources Committee, "Mental Health Benefits," Nov. 8, 1993, C-SPAN, https://www.c-span.org/video/?52193-1/mental-health-benefits.

31. Weisburd, "Planning a Community-Based Mental Health System."

CHAPTER 14: LEADERSHIP IN THE SERVICE OF PEERS

1. "You Are Not Alone," typescript, n.d., Harp Papers. References to the Harp Papers are courtesy of Community Access and Steve Coe.

2. "You Are Not Alone," 64.

3. Sally Zinman, Howie the Harp, and Su Budd, eds., *Reaching Across: Mental Health Clients Helping Each Other* (Riverside: California Network of Mental Health Clients, 1987).

4. Zinman et al., *Reaching Across.*

5. Howie the Harp to Steve Coe, Sept. 30, 1992, Harp Papers.

6. Harp to Stastny, Apr. 22, 1992, Harp Papers.

7. George Jurrow, "Financing Long Term Care for the Chronically Mentally Impaired in New York State: An Issue Analysis," June 4, 1979, typescript, prepared for the State Communities Aid Association Institute on Care of the Mentally Impaired in the Long Term Care System, in author's possession; John Riley, "Mentally Ill Don't Fit in Cuomo's Fiscal Plans," *Newsday*, July 2, 1993.

8. This, and all other remarks not otherwise attributed, come from my interviews with Steve Coe.

9. Vincent Canby, "Mindless Drugs: Tranquilizers for Disturbed Patients Are Scored in Documentary at Whitney," *New York Times*, May 5, 1976.

10. Celia W. Dugger, "Giuliani to Call for Curtailing Services for Some Homeless," *New York Times*, Sept. 17, 1993.

11. A discussion of the Oakland Independence Support Center (OISC) can be found in Laura Van Tosh and Paolo del Vecchio, Consumer/Survivor-Operated Self-Help Programs: A Technical Report (Rockville, MD: US Center for Mental Health Services, 2000), 23–26.12. Steve Coe, email to author, June 4, 2019.

12. Steve Coe, email to author, June 4, 2019.

13. Coe to Harp, May 7, 1992, Harp Papers.

14. "Coming Home: Ex-Patients View Housing Options and Needs," Proceedings of a National Housing Forum, Center for Psychiatric Rehabilitation, Boston, MA, Apr. 18, 1988, Chamberlin Papers, Special Collections and University Archives, University of Massachusetts Amherst (SCUA).

15. Howie the Harp to Steve Coe, Sept. 11, 1992; Steve Coe to Howie the Harp, Nov. 18, 1992, Harp Papers.

16. Harp to Coe, Mar. 1, 1993; Coe back to Harp, n.d., Harp Papers.

17. Howie the Harp, "A Crazy Folks Guide to Reasonable Accommodation," 1990, Harp Papers.

18. Author interviews with Steve Coe; author interview with Liz Glass.

19. "Testimony of Howie T. Harp, Office of Mental Health's 1994–1998 Comprehensive Plan for Mental Health Services," typescript, n.d., Harp Papers.

20. "Client Run Alternative Care Models: A Special Workshop with Patients," American Psychiatric Association Conference, May 13, 1986, typescript, Harp Papers.

21. Howie the Harp, "Taking a New Approach to Independent Living," *Psychiatric Services* 44, no. 5 (May 1993): 413.

22. Lawrence Van Gelder, "Howard Geld, 42," *New York Times*, Feb. 14, 1995.

23. Zinman et al., *Reaching Across*, 69.

24. "Testimony of Howie T. Harp on the Office of Mental Health's 1994–1998 Comprehensive Plan," Harp Papers.

25. Support Coalition International, *Dendron* 36 (Spring 1995), Cynthia Miller Papers (MS 869), SCUA.

26. Howard Geld, 1995, series 1, box 2, Judi Chamberlin Papers (MS 768), SCUA.

27. Sally Zinman, "The Legacy of Howie the Harp Lives On," *National Empowerment Center Newsletter* (Spring–Summer 1995).

28. This account is taken from Richard Cohen, *Strong in the Broken Places* (New York: Harper Collins, 2008), 247–97.

29. From *The Journal of Dual Diagnosis*, quoted in Cohen, *Strong in the Broken Places*, 277.

30. Cohen, *Strong in the Broken Places*, 288.

31. Larry Fricks, keynote address, 20th GMHCN Conference, Aug. 2016, St. Simon's Island, Georgia.

32. Fricks, keynote address.

33. [Darby Penney], "Preliminary Thoughts on Best Practices for Establishing State Offices of Consumer/Ex-Patient Affairs," typescript, Apr. 1993, Human Resources Association of the Northeast National Association of Consumer/Survivor Mental Health Administrators; Peer Specialist Job Description, Grade 9, OMH [1993], courtesy of Darby Penney.

34. Author interviews with Darby Penney.

35. Peer Specialist Job Description.

36. [Penney], "Preliminary Thoughts."

37. Laura Van Tosh, Recommendations on the Development of an Office of Consumer Affairs, submitted to Stuart B. Silver, Director of Mental Hygiene Administration, typescript, Apr. 11, 1994, Harp Papers.

38. Van Tosh, Recommendations on the Development of an Office of Consumer Affairs.

39. Marc Roberts and Nancy Kates, "Pam Hyde and Ohio Mental Health: Shifting Control of Inpatient Care," Case Program Kennedy School of Government, Jan. 1, 1987, https://case.hks.harvard.edu/pam-hyde-and-ohio-mental-health-shifting-control-of-inpatient-care/.

40. "Final Asylum: The Closing of Philadelphia State Hospital (Part 1) [a.k.a. Byberry]," YouTube, Dec. 17, 2011, https://www.youtube.com/watch?v=qJ3_hXLp4vo.

41. "Mental-Health Message for Cuomo," *Newsday*, Aug. 10, 1993.

42. "Supporters of Mental Illness Bill," *New York Voice*, Aug. 25, 1993; Jim Puzzanghera, "Mental Health Net Flawed," *Newsday*, Aug. 15, 1993.

43. Author interview with Harvey Rosenthal (June 2019).

44. Author interview with Harvey Rosenthal (June 2019).

45. Kevin Sack, "Pataki, in Switch," *New York Times*, Mar. 21, 1995.

46. Sack, "Pataki, in Switch"; Lisa Foderaro, "Health Advocates Assail Pataki," Mar. 6, 1996, *New York Times*.

CHAPTER 15: STAND ON CUE

1. Department of Health and Human Services, Office of Inspector General, *Revitalizing the Community Support Program* (June 1993), 7.

2. "Consumers/Survivors Walk Out of National CSP Meeting," *On Our Own Newsletter*, courtesy of Mike Finkle.

3. This, and all other remarks not otherwise attributed, come from my interviews with Darby Penney.

4. Max Schneier to All NAMI Board Members, Mar. 18, 1991, box 1:44, Tom Behrendt Papers (MS 870), Special Collections and University Archives, University of Massachusetts Amherst (SCUA).

5. "Consumers/Survivors Walk Out of National CSP Meeting," *On Our Own Newsletter*, courtesy of Mike Finkle.

6. US Senate Labor and Human Resources Committee, "Examining the Administration's Proposed Health Security Act, to Establish Comprehensive Health Care for Every American," part 2, Nov. 8, 1993, https://www.c-span.org/video/?52193-1/mental-health-benefits.

7. Author interviews with Laurie Flynn (January 2012).

8. H. Richard Lamb, MD, and Roderick Shaner, MD, "When There Are Almost No State Hospital Beds Left," *Psychiatric Services* 44, no. 10 (Oct. 1993): 973–76.

9. Bernard S. Arons, CMHS to Interested Parties, "Re: Electroconvulsive Therapy (ECT) Involuntary Treatment," n.d., http://www.ect.org/resources/cmhs/ect.html; Laurie Flynn to Dr. Arons, Apr. 27, 1995, http://www.ect.org/resources/cmhs/nami.html. This correspondence was obtained under the Freedom of Information Act by Support Coalition.

10. Support Coalition International, *Dendron* 36 (Spring 1995), Cynthia Miller Papers (MS 869), SCUA, http://credo.library.umass.edu/view/full/mums869-b001-f030-i001.

11. Author interview with Bernie Arons.

12. Daniel Fisher, MD, PhD, and Patricia Deegan, PhD, "Recovery Project," *Service of CMHS Ken Bulletin* 2, no. 2 (1997), [Internet Archive Wayback Machine] http://www.mentalhealth.org /publications/allpubs/CMH97-5015/recovery.htm.

13. Wayback Archives, *Ken Bulletin* 1, no. 2 (Winter 1997–1998), on Internet Archive Wayback Machine: http://www.mentalhealth.org/publications/allpubs/KEN98-0057/playrole.asp.

14. Gayle Bluebird, "Participator Dialogues: A Guide, Health and Human Services," *Ken Bulletin* 2, no. 2 (1997), https://web.archive.org/web/20000202001119/http://www.mentalhealth.org /publications/allpubs/CMH97-5015/dialogue.htm.

15. US Department of Health and Human Services, Substance Abuse and Mental Health Services, CMHS National Advisory Council meeting minutes, Apr. 11 and 12, 1996, https://web .archive.org/web/20020312020118/http://www.mentalhealth.org/cmhs/AdvisoryCouncil/minutes /MIN0496.asp.

16. Jean Campbell, "Federal Multi-Site Study Finds Consumer-Operated Service Programs Are Evidence-Based Practices," Missouri Institute of Mental Health (2009), Dec. 18, 2013, https:// www.mhselfhelp.org/clearinghouse-resources/2013/12/18/federal-multi-site-study-finds-consumer -operated-service-pro.html.

17. Gregory B. Teague et al., "MHSIP Mental Health Report Card," *Evaluation Review* 21 (June 1997): 330–41.

18. US Department of Health and Human Services, Substance Abuse and Mental Health Services, CMHS National Advisory Council Meeting Minutes, Dec. 7, 1995, https://web.archive.org /web/20020312020702/http://www.mentalhealth.org/cmhs/AdvisoryCouncil/minutes/MIN1295.asp.

19. Campbell, "Federal Multi-Site Study."

20. "SAMHSA Awards New Consumer-Focused Grants," *Consumer Affairs Bulletin* 4, no. 1 (Spring 1999), https://web.archive.org/web/20000816213338/http://www.mentalhealth.org/publications/allpubs/cmh99-5023/cabvo499.htm#Changes.

21. Campbell, "Federal Multi-Site Study."

22. Author interview with Fricks.

CHAPTER 16: THE IMPRACTICALITIES OF THE SITUATION

1. American Psychiatric Association, "Dialogue with Patients: Client-Run Alternative Care Models," May 13, 1986, Association for the Preservation of Anti-Psychiatric Artifacts Transcripts, box I:8, Tom Behrendt Papers, SCUA, UMass-Amherst.

2. "Self-Help: The Wave of the Future," *Psychiatric Services* 37, no. 3 (Mar. 1986): 213.

3. Sally Zinman, interview with Paul Engels, 1990, White Light Communications Collection, Show 55 and 56, SCUA. The list of extant organizations is included in Sally Zinman, Howie the Harp, and Su Budd, eds., *Reaching Across: Mental Health Clients Helping Each Other* (Riverside: California Network of Mental Health Clients, 1987), 206–37.

4. E. Fuller Torrey, MD, *The Death of Psychiatry* (Radnor, PA: Chilton Book Company, 1974), 75, 86, 115.

5. Torrey, *The Death of Psychiatry*, 75.

6. Michael Winerip, "Schizophrenia's Most Ardent Foe," *New York Times*, Feb. 2, 1998.

7. Jules H. Masserman, MD, *American Journal of Psychiatry* 132, no. 6 (June 1975): 672–73.

8. Bayard Webster, "Science Library," book review of *Psychiatry at the Crossroads*, ed. John Paul Brady, MD, and H. Keith H. Brodie, MD, *New York Times*, Feb. 3, 1981.

9. Kenneth Lynn, "The Roots of Treason: Ezra Pound and the Secret of St. Elizabeths, by E. Fuller Torrey," *Commentary*, Jan. 1984, https://www.commentary.org/articles/kenneth-lynn/the-roots-of-treason-ezra-pound-and-the-secret-of-st-elizabeths-by-e-fuller-torrey.

10. E. F. Torrey, *Surviving Schizophrenia: A Family Manual* (New York: Harper & Row, 1985).

11. Donald F. Klein, "Surviving Schizophrenia," *Psychiatric Services* 35, no. 5 (May 1984): 500.

12. E. Fuller Torrey, MD, Eve Bargmann, MD, and Sidney M. Wolfe, MD, "Washington's Grate Society: Schizophrenics in the Shelters and on the Street," *Public Citizen Health Research Group* 1010 (Apr. 23, 1985).

13. E. Fuller Torrey, *Nowhere to Go: The Tragic Odyssey of the Homeless Mentally Ill* (New York: Harper & Row, 1988), xiv.

14. E. F. Torrey, "Forced Medication Is Part of the Cure," *New Physician* 35 (Dec. 1986): 33–37, 44–45.

15. Susan Stefan, "The Psychiatric Cure for Homelessness: Wrong Diagnosis, Wrong Treatment," *New Physician* 35 (Dec. 1986): 44–45.

16. Torrey, "Forced Medication Is Part of the Cure."

17. Joseph P. Morrissey et al., "Local Mental Health Authorities and Service System Change: Evidence from the Robert Wood Johnson Foundation Program on Chronic Mental Illness," *Milbank Quarterly* 72, no. 1 (1994): 49–80.

18. "Involuntary Commitment and Court-Ordered Treatment, Approved by NAMI Board of Directors on October 7, 1995," NAMI press release, in author's possession.

19. "NAMI Approves New Policy on Involuntary Commitments," *Psychiatric News* 30, no. 21 (Nov. 3, 1995): 10.

20. *Dendron: Voice of Support Coalition International*, nos. 37/38 (1996), Judi Chamberlin Papers (MS 768), SCUA.

21. *Dendron: Voice of Support Coalition International* 35 (Summer 1994), Chamberlin Papers.

22. William B. Lawson, Nancy Helper, Jack Holladay, and Brian Cuffel, "Race as a Factor in Inpatient and Outpatient Admissions and Diagnosis," *Psychiatric Services* 45, no. 1 (Jan. 1994): 72–74.

23. "APA Details Drug Industry Support for Consumer Group," *Psychiatric News* (Sept. 15, 1995): 1, 12.

24. Melody Petersen, *Our Daily Meds: How the Pharmaceutical Companies Transformed Themselves into Slick Marketing Machines and Hooked the Nation on Prescription Drugs* (New York: Farrar, Straus & Giroux, 2008), 24.

25. John A. Chiles, MD, et al., "The Texas Medication Algorithm Project: Development and Implementation of the Schizophrenia Algorithm," *Psychiatric Services* 50, no. 1 (Jan. 1999): 69–74.

26. Statement of Allen Jones, downloaded from Psychrights: http://psychrights.org/Drugs /AllenJonesTMAPJanuary20.pdf#page=3.

27. [David Oaks], "National Organization Escalates a Chemical Crusade, Angering Human Rights Advocates," *Dendron* 37–38 (Summer 1996): 8.

28. D. J. Jaffe, "How to Reduce Both Violence and Stigma," *Newsletter to Staten Island AMI*, Dec. 1994, in author's possession.

29. Jaffe, "How to Reduce Both Violence and Stigma."

30. E. Fuller Torrey, "Taking Issue: Psychiatric Survivors and Nonsurvivors," *Psychiatric Services* 48, no. 2 (Feb. 1997): 143.

31. "Taking Issue with Taking Issue: Psychiatric Survivors Reconsidered," *Psychiatric Services*, 48, no. 5 (May 1997): 601–3.

32. "Taking Issue with Taking Issue."

33. E. F. Torrey to author, Mar. 27, 2020.

34. Laura Van Tosh and Paolo del Vecchio, *Consumer/Survivor-Operated Self-Help Programs: A Technical Report* (Rockville, MD: US Center for Mental Health Services, 2000).

35. Carol Mowbray and Cheribeth Tan, "Consumer-Operated Drop-in Centers: Evaluation of Operations and Impact," *Journal of Mental Health Administration* 20, no. 1 (Spring 1993): 8–19.

36. NAMI press release, "NAMI Ranked Among Top 10 Charitable Organizations Nationwide," NAMI archive, Dec. 5, 1997, https://www.nami.org/Press-Media/Press-Releases/1997/NAMI -Ranked-Among-Top-10-Charitable-Organizations.

37. Ketchum Public Relations, "Risperdal 1997 U.S. Strategic Offense Plan," in Steven Brill, "America's Most Admired Lawbreaker," *Huffington Post*, 2015, https://highline.huffingtonpost.com /miracleindustry/americas-most-admired-lawbreaker/assets/documents/2/ris-strategic-offense -1997.pdf?build=02281049.

38. The website of the Law Project for Psychiatric Rights, PsychRights, hosts the Zyprexa Papers, Allen Jones's whistleblower allegations, and the lawsuits in which he was involved with different pharmaceutical companies. See http://psychrights.org/Issues/ZPapers/ZPaperActions.pdf.

39. Ken Silverstein, "Prozac.org," *Mother Jones*, Nov./Dec. 1999, https://www.motherjones .com/politics/1999/11/prozacorg.

40. NAMI press release, "In Our Own Voice," Jan. 17, 2002, https://www.nami.org/Press -Media/Press-Releases/2002/In-Our-Own-Voice.

41. NAMI press release, "New Report Shows Costs of Medications for Severe Mental Illnesses Significantly Higher in United States, than in Europe," July 15, 1998, https://www.nami.org/Press -Media/Press-Releases/1998/New-Report-Shows-Costs-of-Medications-for-Severe-M.

42. NAMI press release, "Nation at Crossroads of Success or Failure, Declare Advocates for the Mentally Ill," July 17, 1998, https://www.nami.org/Press-Media/Press-Releases/1998/Nation -at-Crossroads-of-Success-or-Failure,-Declar.

43. Milt Freudenheim, "Psychiatric Drugs Are Now Promoted Directly to Patients," *New York Times*, Feb. 17, 1998. Also see Ralph King Jr., "Science Medical Journals Rarely Disclose Researchers' Ties," *Wall Street Journal*, Feb. 2, 1999, in which King wrote, "Although scientists are increasingly supported by for-profit companies, a new study finds that those ties are seldom revealed in published research; the finding, presented at a meeting of the American Assn. for the Advancement of Science, raises questions about the independence of researchers and the credibility of their results in an era of creeping commercialization in science."

44. NAMI press release, "New Atypical Antipsychotic Drugs Recommended as First-Line Medications for People with Serious Brain Disorders," Dec. 31, 1997, https://www.nami.org/Press -Media/Press-Releases/1997/-New-Atypical-Antipsychotic-Drugs-Recommended-As-F.

45. D. J. Jaffe, "Janssen Program May Help or Hurt Risperdal Users," www.schizophrenia.com, Apr. 1997 (no longer available online).

46. Laurie M. Flynn, "In Support of Janssen Pharmaceutical's Person-to-Person Initiative," Apr. 18, 1997, NAMI press release, https://www.nami.org/Press-Media/Press-Releases/1997/In -Support-Of-Janssen-Pharmaceutica-s-Person-To-Pe.

47. Laurie M. Flynn, "National Alliance for the Mentally Ill Assails PacifiCare for Restricting Access to Effective Medications," NAMI press release, May 22, 1977, https://www.nami.org/Press -Media/Press-Releases/1997/National-Alliance-for-the-Mentally-Ill-Assails-Pac.

48. NAMI press release, "NAMI Applauds Governor Bush and Texas Legislature for Ending Insurance Discrimination in Coverage for Severe Mental Illness," June 23, 1997, https://www.nami .org/Press-Media/Press-Releases/1997/NAMI-Applauds-Governor-Bush-and-Texas-Legislature.

49. A. F. Lehman and D. Steinwachs et al., "At Issue: Translating Research into Practice: The Schizophrenia Patient Outcomes Research Team (PORT) Treatment Recommendations," *Schizophrenia Bulletin* 24, no. 1 (Jan. 1998): 1–10.

50. Brill, "America's Most Admired Lawbreaker."

51. Susan L. Jones, "NAMI: A Convention Worth Noting," *Archives of Psychiatric Nursing* 13, no. 1 (Feb. 1999): 1–2.

52. Silverstein, "Prozac.org."

53. Ketchum Public Relations, "Risperdal 1997 US Strategic Offense Plan."

54. Everything attributed to Torrey comes from "Proposal for NAMI's Future," Mar. 2, 1996, https://web.archive.org/web/19990224011402/http://www.nami.org/about/about2.htm.

55. Torrey, "Stop the Madness," *Wall Street Journal*, July 18, 1997.

56. NAMI press release, "Legal Advocacy Project Established to End Barriers to Care for Millions," Nov. 5, 1997, https://www.nami.org/Press-Media/Press-Releases/1997/Legal-Advocacy -Project-Established-to-End-Barriers.

57. See the online Treatment Advocacy Center post for August 17, 2000, https://web.archive .org/web/20000817002747/http://www.psychlaws.org/General%20Resources/Fact4.htm.

58. *Catalyst* 1, no. 1 (Sept.–Oct. 1999). The earliest editions of *Catalyst* are not web-based, but starting with the 15th edition, they are online at https://www.treatmentadvocacycenter.org/press -room/catalyst-newsletters.

59. *Catalyst* 1, no. 1 (Sept.–Oct. 1999).

60. US Department of Justice, John M. Dawson and Patrick A. Langan, "Murder in Families," *Bureau of Justice Statistics Special Report* for (July 1994).

61. Torrey's explanation of the methodology was inconsistent. In his book *Out of the Shadows: Confronting America's Mental Illness Crisis* (New York: John Wiley & Sons, 1996), he references six local reports. He later told Dan Weisburd this was a "guestimate." See Dan E. Weisburd, "Publisher's Note: Mental Illness and the Law," *The Journal* 11, no. 3 (Sept. 28, 2001): 12.

62. Torrey quoted in "Schizophrenia and Poverty, Crime and Violence," Schizophrenia.com, http://schizophrenia.com/poverty.htm (accessed Jan. 30, 2022); Treatment Advocacy Center, *Catalyst* 2, no. 1 (Jan.–Feb. 2000), https://web.archive.org/web/20020731002923/http://treatment advocacycenter.org/JoinUs/CatalystArchive/CatalystV2N1.htm.

63. "News of the Week," Stigmanet, Nov. 28, 1999, https://stigmanet.org/NEWS%20ARCHIVE %20%281999%29.htm#28nov99.

64. "News of the Week."

65. "NIMH Corrects Inaccurate Reporting of Its Findings by TAC," *MadNation*, https://web .archive.org/web/20000620094430/http://madnation.org/citations/nimh.htm (accessed Jan 17, 2022).

66. Henry J. Steadman et al., "Response to the *National Review*," *National Review*, July 20, 1998, reprinted by *MadNation*, https://web.archive.org/web/20000305091929/http://madnation .org/citations/macarthur.htm (accessed Dec. 21, 2021).

67. D. J. Jaffe, "'Stigma' Can't Be Eliminated Without Addressing 'Violence,'" 2000, in author's possession.

68. Phyllis Vine, "Mindless and Deadly: Media Hype on Mental Illness and Violence," *FAIR* (May 2001): 28–30.

69. Dan E. Weisburd, "Publisher's Note," 1.

70. MindFreedom International, "Psychiatric Rights Censored NAMI 'Unglued,'" *Support Coalition International Hot News*, Feb. 1, 2001, no longer available online.

71. Author interview with Torrey.

72. MindFreedom International provides letters and follow-up news about the incident. *Support Coalition International Hot News*, June 17, 2001 no longer available online.

CHAPTER 17: A VINTAGE YEAR

1. "Release of the Surgeon General's Report," C-SPAN, Dec. 13, 1999, https://www.c-span.org /video/?154147-1/surgeon-general-report-mental-health.

2. "Release of the Surgeon General's Report."

3. Author interview with Mrs. Rosalynn Carter.

4. Setting the Stage for Surgeon General Report, Fifth Annual Rosalynn Carter Symposium on Mental Health Policy, Nov. 17-18, 1999, Carter Center, Atlanta, https://www.cartercenter.org /resources/pdfs/pdf-archive/settingstageforsurgeongeneralrpt-11011999.pdf (accessed Jan. 29, 2022).

5. The survey research team asked respondents to agree or disagree with the following statement: "Effective treatments exist for the majority of mental disorders and we are finding new treatments all the time." See Celinda Lake, "The Balanced Life," in *Setting the Stage for Surgeon General Report*, 17-22.

6. "Release of the Surgeon General's Report."

7. Federal News Service, National Press Club Luncheon Speaker Tipper Gore, National Press Club Ballroom, July 26, 1994, https://www.c-span.org/video/?59006-1/mental-health-care-reform.

8. All of this account comes from author interview with Larry Fricks.

9. Testimony of Timothy A. Kelly, "Dealing with Fragmentation in the Service Delivery System," Dec. 4, 2002, meeting of the President's Commission on Mental Health, courtesy of Tim Kelly.

10. Timothy A. Kelly, "Healing the Broken Mind," in *Transforming America's Failed Mental Health System* (New York: NYU Press, 2009), 47.

11. "Mental Health System Reform with the New Congress and Administration," courtesy of Tim Kelly.

12. Author interview with Charlie Curie.

13. President's New Freedom Commission on Mental Health, Meeting Minutes, "Dealing with Fragmentation in the Service Delivery System," President's New Freedom Commission, Arlington, Virginia, June 18-19, 2002, https://govinfo.library.unt.edu/mentalhealthcommission /minutes/june02.htm.

14. Charles Curie, "SAMHSA's Commitment to Eliminating the Use of Seclusion and Restraint," *Psychiatric Services* 56, no. 9 (Sept. 2005): 1139-40.

15. Joseph Rogers testimony, Hearings of the Senate Appropriations Labor, Health and Human Services, and Education Committee, "Deaths from Restraints at Psychiatric Facilities," 106th Congress, 1st session, Apr. 13, 1999, 35-38. The following account comes from this source.

16. Eric M. Weiss and Michael Remez, "Three Bills Target Restraints in Mental-Health Facilities Nationwide," *Hartford Courant*, Mar. 25, 1999.

17. Curie, "SAMHSA's Commitment."

18. Substance Abuse and Mental Health Services Administration, US Department of Health and Human Services, *Transforming Mental Health Care in America: Federal Action Agenda: First Steps*, DHHS Pub. No. SMA-05-4060 (Rockville, MD: Department of Health and Human Services, 2005), 86.

19. SAMHSA, *Transforming Mental Health Care*, 4.

20. Nora Jacobson and Dianne Greenley, "What Is Recovery: A Conceptual Model and Explication," *Psychiatric Services* 52, no. 4 (Apr. 2001): 482-85.

21. Herbert Peyser, "What Is Recovery? A Commentary," *Psychiatric Services* 52, no. 4 (Apr. 2001): 486-87.

22. Ruth O. Ralph, Kathryn Kidder, and Dawna Phillips, "Can We Measure Recovery? A Compendium of Recovery and Recovery-Related Instruments," Human Services Research

Institute, June 2000, https://www.hsri.org/publication/Can_We_Measure_Recovery_A
_Compendium_of_Recovery_and_Recovery-Related_.
23. Steven J. Onken et al., "An Analysis of the Definitions and Elements of Recovery: A Review of the Literature," *Psychiatric Rehabilitation Journal* 31, no. 1 (2007): 9–22.
24. Larry Davidson et al., "Recovery in Serious Mental Illness: A New Wine or Just a New
Bottle?," *Professional Psychology Research and Practice* 36, no. 5 (2005): 480–87.
25. Maria O'Connell et al., "From Rhetoric to Routine: Assessing Perceptions of Recovery-
Oriented Practices," *Psychiatric Rehabilitation Journal* 28, no. 4 (Spring 2005): 378–86.
26. Luis E. Bedregal, Maria O'Connell, and Larry Davidson, "The Recovery Knowledge Inventory: Assessment of Mental Health Staff Knowledge and Attitudes about Recovery," *Psychiatric
Rehabilitation Journal* 30, no. 2 (Fall 2006): 96–103.
27. Nancy C. Andreasen, MD, PhD, William T. Carpenter Jr., MD, John M. Kane, MD, et al.,
American Journal of Psychiatry 162, no. 3 (Mar. 2005): 441–49.
28. Alan S. Bellak, "Scientific and Consumer Models of Recovery in Schizophrenia: Concor-
dance, Contrasts, and Implications," *Schizophrenia Bulletin* 32, no. 3 (Feb. 2006): 432–42.

CHAPTER 18: RECOVERY AND WELLNESS
1. Patricia Deegan, "Recovery as a Self-Directed Process," 2001, https://d20wqiibvy9b23.cloud
front.net/resources/resources/000/000/615/original/Deegan_Recovery_as_a_Self_Directed
_Process.pdf?1468370243.
2. Patricia E. Deegan, "The Independent Living Movement and People with Psychiatric Disabilities: Taking Back Control over Our Own Lives," *Psychiatric Rehabilitation Journal* 15, no. 3
(Jan. 1992): 3–19.
3. "Anderson Cooper Tries a Schizophrenia Simulator," CNN, June 9, 2014, available at
https://www.youtube.com/watch?v=yL9UJVtgPZY.
4. Patricia E. Deegan, "Recovery: The Lived Experience of Rehabilitation," *Psychiatric Rehabilitation Journal* 3, no. 1 (1988): 23–31.
5. Robert E. Drake and Patricia E. Deegan, "Shared Decision Making Is an Ethical Imperative," *Psychiatric Services* 60, no. 8 (Aug. 2009): 1007.
6. *Shared Decision-Making in Mental Health Care: Practice, Research, and Future Directions*,
HHS Publication No. SMA-09-4371 (Rockville, MD: Center for Mental Health Services, Substance
Abuse and Mental Health Services Administration, 2010).
7. "Oregon State Hospital's Dark History Illuminated in a New Memorial for Forgotten Remains," *Oregonian*, July 7, 2014.
8. *From Numbers to Names*, documentary, dir. Pat Deegan, 2010, https://www.common
groundprogram.com/blog/from-numbers-to-names.
9. Patricia E. Deegan, "Recovering Our Sense of Value After Being Labeled: Mentally Ill,"
Journal of Psychosocial Nursing and Mental Health Services 31, no. 4 (Apr. 1993): 7–11.
10. "A Wellness Approach," *Psychiatric Rehabilitation Journal* 29, no. 4 (Spring 2006): 311–13.
11. Dana Foglesong et al., "National Practice Guidelines for Peer Support Specialists and Supervisors," *Psychiatric Services* (2021), https://ps.psychiatryonline.org/doi/pdf/10.1176/appi.ps
.202000901.
12. Sherry J. Tucker, Wendy Tiegreen, J. Toole, J. Banathy, D. Mulloy, and M. Swarbrick,
"Supervisor Guide: Peer Support Whole Health and Wellness Coach," Decatur, Georgia Mental
Health Consumer Network (2013), in author's possession; email communication with author from
Ike Powell, Sept. 8, 2021.
13. Email from Aaron Foster, director of consulting and education, RI International, Sept. 3,
2021; email from Ike Powell, Sept. 8, 2021.
14. Judith A. Cook et al., "Initial Outcomes of a Mental Illness Self-Management Program
Based on Wellness Recovery Action Planning," *Psychiatric Services* 60, no. 2 (Feb. 2009):
246–49.
15. Judith Cook et al., "Results of a Randomized Controlled Trial of Mental Illness Self-
Management Using Wellness Recovery Action Planning," *Schizophrenia Bulletin* 38, no. 4 (June 18,
2012): 881–91.

16. Nev Jones et al., "Outcomes of an Illness Self-Management Group Using Wellness Recovery Action Planning," *Psychiatric Rehabilitation Journal* 36, no. 3 (2013): 209–14.

17. "Peer Support, Wellness, and Respite Centers," Georgia Mental Health Consumer Network, https://www.gmhcn.org/peer-support-wellness-respite (accessed Dec. 21, 2021).

18. Laysha Ostrow, "A Case Study of Peer-Run Crisis Respite Organizing Process in Massachusetts" (Spring 2010), available from the website of the National Empowerment Center, https://power2u.org/wp-content/uploads/2020/07/Ostrow_Groundhogs-case-study.pdf.

19. David Covington, "The Retreat Model," July 2018, http://www.Davidwcovington.com.

20. "Peer 2.0: Valuing Recovery," n.d., http://www.Davidwcovington.com.

21. Email communication from Lisa St. George, Aug. 26, 2021.

22. Memo, Committee on Energy and Commerce, May 20, 2013, https://docs.house.gov/meetings/IF/IF02/20130522/100900/HHRG-113-IF02-20130522-SD002.pdf.

23. Greta Brawner and Tim Murphy, Mar. 5, 2013, C-SPAN, https://www.c-span.org/video/?311329-3/representative-tim-murphy-federal-mental-health-programs.

24. Insel made these remarks at a two-day meeting sponsored by the Forum on Global Violence Prevention, published as *Violence and Mental Health: Opportunities for Prevention and Early Detection: Proceedings of a Workshop, February 26–27, 2014* (Washington, DC: National Academies Press, 2018), chap. 2, https://doi.org/10.17226/24916.

25. Leah Harris, "Tim Murphy Raises Right Issues, Offers Wrong Solutions," *Pittsburgh Post-Gazette*, Sept. 10, 2014.

26. Testimony of Sally Satel, MD, US House Committee on Energy and Commerce Subcommittee on Oversight and Investigations Hearings on the Substance Abuse and Mental Health Services Administration Examining "SAMHSA's Role in Delivering Services to the Severely Mentally Ill," 113rd Congress, 1st session, May 22, 2013.

27. US Congress, House Subcommittee of the House Energy and Commerce Committee, "Examining HR 2646: The Helping Families in Mental Health Crisis Act," 114th Congress, 2nd session, June 16, 2015.

28. Oryx Cohen, "Mental Health Bill Caters to Big Pharma and Would Expand Coercive Treatments," *Truthout*, Nov. 6, 2015, https://truthout.org/articles/mental-health-bill-caters-to-big-pharma-and-would-expand-coercive-treatments.

29. Anne Harrington, *Mind Fixers: Psychiatry's Troubled Search for the Biology of Mental Illness* (New York: Norton, 2019), 274.

30. Molly Cate, "Psychiatric Solutions Forms Sunstone Unit," *Nashville Business Journal*, Dec. 31, 2000, https://www.bizjournals.com/nashville/stories/2001/01/01/story2.html.

31. Christina Jewett and Robin Fields, "Psychiatric Care's Peril and Profits," *Los Angeles Times*, Nov. 23, 2008.

32. These contracts are listed online at USASpending.gov.

33. *Business Week*, Sept. 24, 2007.

34. Rosalind Adams, "What the Fuck Just Happened?," *BuzzFeed News*, Dec. 7, 2016, https://www.buzzfeednews.com/article/rosalindadams/intakea.

35. Advisory Board, "The 45 Health Care Companies on This Year's Fortune 500," June 3, 2021, https://www.advisory.com/daily-briefing/2021/06/03/fortune-500.

36. Dominic A. Sisti, Andrea G. Segal, and Ezekiel J. Emanuel, "Improving Long-Term Psychiatric Care: Bring Back the Asylum," *Journal of the American Medical Association* 313, no. 3 (Jan. 20, 2015): 243–44.

37. Renée Binder, MD, "From the President: Return to Asylums? NEVER!" *Psychiatric News* 50, no. 6 (Aug. 13, 2015).

38. Pub Med, the database of the National Library of Medicine, recorded nearly 3,500 articles about recovery in scientific journals between 2000 and 2014; https://pubmed.ncbi.nlm.nih.gov/?term=Recovery+in+mental+illness+%2F+psychiatry&filter=years.2000-2014.

39. Benedict Carey, "Programs Expand Schizophrenic Patients' Role in Their Own Care," *New York Times*, Dec. 28, 2015.

40. Elinore F. McCance-Katz, MD, PhD, "The Federal Government Ignores the Treatment Needs of Americans with Serious Mental Illness," *Psychiatric Times* 33, no. 4 (Apr. 21, 2016).

41. Brianna Ehley, "Trump's Nominee for Mental Health Chief Wants to Shake Up the Agency," *Politico*, Apr. 28, 2017.

42. Elinore F. McCance-Katz, "The Substance Abuse and Mental Health Services Administration (SAMHSA): New Directions," *Psychiatric Services* 69, no. 10 (Oct. 2018): 1046–48.

43. David W. Oaks, "Trump Appoints Leader Who Campaigned for Involuntary Outpatient Drugging," MindFreedom International, https://mindfreedom.org/front-page/trumps-new -forced-psychiatric-drugging-czar-ellie-mccance-katz-doesnt-believe-you-should-have-the -right-to-own-your-own-body/.

44. Elinore F. McCance-Katz, *SAMHSA Looking Forward: Priorities and Plans*, Apr. 19, 2018, https://static1.squarespace.com/static/58739f64e6f2e14a3527a002/t/5aff261c70a6adafa2b15a7b /1526670877035/NYAPRS+4–18+DA.pdf.

45. NYAPRS reprinted the Oct. 4, 2018, *Politico* announcement in Dan Diamond, "PT: Del Vecchio Leaves CMHS Post," https://www.nyaprs.org/e-news-bulletins/2018/10/10/pt-del -vecchio-leaves-cmhs-post.

46. Kate Mulligan, "Recovery Model Seeks More than Symptom Relief," *Psychiatric News* 41, no. 18 (Sept. 16, 2005); Aaron Levin, "Moving to Recovery Model Called 'Marathon, Not a Sprint,'" *Psychiatric News*, Jan. 15, 2010.

47. Rich Daly, "Recovery Model Needs More Adherents, Says Psychiatrist," *Psychiatric News*, Nov. 20, 2009, https://doi.org/10.1176/pn.44.22.psychnews_44_22_017.

48. Robert H. Felix, "The National Mental Health Program," *American Journal of Public Health* 54, no. 11 (Nov. 1964): 1804–9; "A Model for Comprehensive Mental Health Centers," *American Journal of Public Health* 54, no. 10 (Dec. 1964): 1964–69.

49. CMI Report, Dec. 2017 (https://store.samhsa.gov/).

50. Institute of Medicine, *Priority Areas for National Action: Transforming Health Care Quality* (Washington, DC: National Academy Press, 2003).

EPILOGUE

1. Sara Hendren, *What Can a Body Do?* (New York: Riverhead Books, 2020), 199–206, 190.

2. Group for the Advancement of Psychiatry, Roadmap to the Ideal Crisis System: Essential Elements, Measurable Standards and Best Practices for Behavioral Health Crisis Response (Washington, DC: National Council for Behavioral Health, 2021).

3. Alisa Roth, *Insane: America's Criminal Treatment of Mental Illness* (New York: Basic Books, 2018), 250–54.

4. "Fatal Force," *Washington Post*, Oct. 31, 2021, https://www.washingtonpost.com/graphics /investigations/police-shootings-database.

5. Group for the Advancement of Psychiatry, *Roadmap to the Ideal Crisis System*, 3.

6. Ellis Amdur, "Police, Hospitals and Mentally Ill Subjects: A Better Way Forward," *Police1*, July 9, 2021, https://www.police1.com/crisis-intervention-training/articles/police-hospitals-and -mentally-ill-subjects-a-better-way-forward-1X4YBpofrYoAYQnd.

7. Sandhya Raman, "Mental Health Advocates Seek Crisis Hotline Expansion," *Roll Call*, Aug. 4, 2021, https://www.rollcall.com/2021/08/04/mental-health-advocates-seek-crisis-hotline -expansion-resources.

8. Lisa Jobe-Shields and Katharine Hawkes, "988, Shared Accountability, and Equity in Behavioral Health Crisis Services," Crisis Talk, Jan. 4, 2022, https://talk.crisisnow.com/988-shared -accountability-and-equity-in-behavioral-health-crisis-services; SAMHSA, "988 Appropriations Report, December 2021," https://www.samhsa.gov/sites/default/files/988-appropriations-report.pdf.

9. Centers for Disease Control and Prevention, "Evaluating Behavioral Health Surveillance Systems," *Implementation Evaluation* 15 (May 10, 2018), https://www.cdc.gov/pcd/issues/2018/17 _0459.htm.

10. Valerie A. Canady, "Bill Would Provide Medicare Reimbursement for Peer Services," *Mental Health Weekly* 31, no. 18 (May 10, 2021): 3–4.

11. Zusha Elinson, "When Mental-Health Experts, Not Police, Are the First Responders," *Wall Street Journal*, Nov.r 24, 2018.

12. J. D. Capelouto, "Atlanta on Track to See 450 Arrests Averted This Year through Diversion Program," *Atlanta Journal-Constitution*, July 13, 2021.

13. Grace Hauck, "Denver Successfully Sent Mental Health Professionals, Not Police, to Hundreds of Calls," *USA Today*, Feb. 6, 2021.

14. US Senate Committee on Finance, press release, July 13, 2021, https://www.finance.senate.gov/chairmans-news/wyden-cheers-open-applications-for-mental-health-crisis-intervention-services-.

15. Roth, *Insane*, 3, 98–99, 108, 199.

16. Author interview with Judge Steven Leifman (Jan. 2019).

17. John Iglehart, "Decriminalizing Mental Illness," *New England Journal of Medicine* 374, no. 18 (May 5, 2016): 1701–3; Daniel Change, "Criminal Mental Health Program in Miami-Dade Seen as a Model for Nation," *Miami Herald*, May 22, 2016.

18. Eleventh Judicial Court of Florida, Jail Diversion Services, https://www.jud11.flcourts.org/Self-Help-Center/Mental-Health/Jail-Diversion (accessed Jan. 30, 2022).

19. Quoted in Roth, *Insane*, 186.

20. Rachel Looker, "Miami-Dade County Builds Center for Mental Health and Recovery," National Association of Counties, Nov. 7, 2019, https://www.naco.org/articles/miami-dade-county-builds-center-mental-health-and-recovery.

21. J. Steven Lamberti, MD, and Robert L. Weisman, MD, "Essential Elements of Forensic Assertive Community Treatment," *Harvard Review of Psychiatry* 29, no. 4 (July–Aug. 2021): 278–97.

INDEX